WHAT TO **EAT** WHEN YOU'RE **EATING OUT**

2nd Edition

What to Eat in America's Most Popular Chain Restaurants

by Hope S. Warshaw, MMSc, RD

Director, Book Publishing, Robert Anthony; *Managing Editor, Book Publishing,* Abe Ogden; *Editor,* Rebekah Renshaw; *Production Manager,* Melissa Sprott; *Composition,* ADA; *Cover Design,* Vis-à-Vis Creative Concepts; *Printer,* United Graphics Inc.

Printed in the United States of America
3 5 7 9 10 8 6 4 2

Small Steps Press is an imprint of the American Diabetes Association. For infomation about Small Steps Press or the American Diabetes Association, in English or Spanish, call 1-800-342-2383. To order other Small Steps Press books, call 1-800-232-6733.

Consult a health care professional before trying any of the suggestions in this publication. Small Steps Press and ADA assume no responsibility for any injury that may result from the suggestions or information in this publication.

∞ The paper in this publication meets the requirements of the ANSI Standard Z39.48-1992 (permanence of paper).

Small Steps Press titles may be purchased for business or promotional use or for special sales. To purchase more than 50 copies of this book at a discount, or for custom editions of this book with your logo, contact Small Steps Press at the address below, at booksales@diabetes.org, or by calling 703-299-2046.

Small Steps Press
1701 North Beauregard Street
Alexandria, Virginia 22311

Library of Congress Cataloging-in-Publication Data

Warshaw, Hope S., 1954-
What to eat when you're eating out / Hope S. Warshaw. -- 2nd ed.
p. cm.
Includes bibliographical references and index.
ISBN 978-1-58040-316-0 (alk. paper)
1. Nutrition. 2. Restaurants--United States. I. Title.
RA784.W366 2009
613.2--dc22

2009005420

To people who strive to eating healthy as a
means to living a healthy lifestyle.
May the knowledge and information
you gather from this book help you achieve
your health and nutrition goals more
easily and effectively. And may your efforts
help you stay healthy for many years to come.

— HSW

Contents

Alphabetical Index of Restaurants ix

Preface xi

Acknowledgments xv

Today's Healthy Eating Goals 1
Restaurant Pitfalls and Strategies for Self-Defense 9
Restaurants Can Help or Hinder Your Healthy Eating Efforts 16
Put Your Best Guess Forward 23
Resources for Nutrition Information of Foods 27
How This Book Works for You 30

Breakfast Eats, Drinks, Snacks, and More 43
- Auntie Anne's 48
- Caribou Coffee 55
- Dunkin' Donuts 64
- Einstein Bros Bagels 84
- Jamba Juice 99
- Krispy Kreme 106
- Orange Julius 112
- Starbucks 11
- Tim Hortons ..... [mouse icon]

[mouse icon] = Exclusive Web Content

Burgers, Fries, and More 139
Burger King 143
Carl's Jr. 158
Dairy Queen/Brazier 167
Hardee's 177
Jack in the Box 191
McDonald's 208
Sonic, America's Drive-In 226
Wendy's 246
Whataburger ....

Chicken—Fried, Roasted, or Grilled 257
Chick-fil-A 260
Church's Chicken 268
El Pollo Loco ....
KFC 274
Popeyes Louisiana Kitchen 285

Seafood Catches 293
Captain D's 295
Long John Silver's 307

Family Fare 313
Bob Evans Restaurants 317
Boston Market 350
Denny's 361
Romano's Macaroni Grill 383
Zaxby's ....

= Exclusive Web Content

Soups, Sandwiches, Salads, and Subs **403**
Arby's **406**
Au Bon Pain **423**
Blimpie Subs and Salads **464**
Jersey Mike's Subs ....
Jimmy John's Gourmet Sandwiches ....
Panera Bread **484**
Schlotzsky's **510**
Steak 'n' Shake **528**
Subway **564**
Wienerschnitzel ....

Chinese and Asian Fare **629**
Panda Express **633**
P.F. Chang's China Bistro **638**
Pei Wei Asian Diner **661**

Pizza, Pasta, and All Else Italian **629**
CiCi's Pizza **633**
Domino's Pizza **638**
Fazoli's **661**
Godfather's Pizza ....
Little Caesars **672**
Papa John's Pizza **677**
Papa Murphy's Take 'N' Bake **695**
Pizza Hut **710**

Tacos, Burritos, and All Else Mexican **727**
Chipotle **731**
Del Taco ....

= Exclusive Web Content

Moe's Southwest Grill 735
Taco Bell 742
Taco John's 756

Frozen Sweets and Treats 769
Baskin Robbins 772
Carvel .... 🖱
Cold Stone Creamery 802
Freshëns .... 🖱
TCBY 814

🖱 = Exclusive Web Content

Exclusive Web Content

Be sure to visit the following restaurants online at http://www.diabetes.org/healthyrestaurant

Carvel	**Godfather's**	**Whataburger**
Del Taco	**Jersey Mike's**	**Wienerschnitzel**
El Pollo Loco	**Jimmy John's**	**Zaxby's**
Frëshens	**Tim Hortons**	

Alphabetical Index of Restaurants

Arby's 406
Au Bon Pain 423
Auntie Anne's 48
Baskin Robbins 772
Blimpie Subs and Salads 464
Bob Evans Restaurants 317
Boston Market 350
Burger King 143
Captain D's 295
Caribou Coffee 55
Carl's Jr. 158
Carvel ....
Chick-fil-A 260
Chipotle 731
Church's Chicken 268
CiCi's Pizza 633
Cold Stone Creamery 802
Dairy Queen/Brazier 167
Del Taco ....
Denny's 361
Domino's Pizza 638
Dunkin' Donuts 64
Einstein Bros Bagels 84
El Pollo Loco ....
Fazoli's 661
Freshëns ....
Godfather's Pizza ....

= Exclusive Web Content

Hardee's 177
Jack in the Box 191
Jamba Juice 99
Jersey Mike's Subs .... 🖱
Jimmy John's Gourmet Sandwiches .... 🖱
KFC 274
Krispy Kreme 106
Little Caesars 672
Long John Silver's 307
McDonald's 208
Moe's Southwest Grill 735
Orange Julius 112
P.F. Chang's China Bistro 591
Panda Express 585
Panera Bread 484
Papa John's Pizza 677
Papa Murphy's Take 'N' Bake 695
Pei Wei Asian Diner 615
Pizza Hut 710
Popeyes Louisiana Kitchen 285
Romano's Macaroni Grill 383
Schlotzsky's 510
Sonic, America's Drive-In 226
Starbucks 118
Steak 'n' Shake 528
Subway 564
Taco Bell 742
Taco John's 756
TCBY 814
Tim Hortons .... 🖱
Wendy's 246
Whataburger .... 🖱
Wienerschnitzel .... 🖱
Zaxby's .... 🖱

🖱 = Exclusive Web Content

Preface

In today's fast-paced and convenience-focused world, Americans frequently choose restaurant meals, eaten in or out of restaurants, to get the job of eating done. Restaurant foods contribute about one-third of our calories. According to the most recent statistics from the National Restaurant Association, we're, on average, eating 6 meals out per week and spending half our food dollars away from home.

Current trends indicate that we will be eating more restaurant meals and spending more of our food dollars on restaurant foods in the future. *What to Eat When You're Eating Out* gives you the nutrition information you need to make healthy food choices whenever you eat away from home.

Today, more nutrition information is available than ever before for "walk up and order" national chain restaurants. These are the restaurants in which you walk up to the counter or drive up to the window and place your order. *What to Eat When You're Eating Out* includes nutrition information for nearly 5,000 menu items from 60 restaurants.

Sparse nutrition information is available for the "sit down and order" national chain restaurants. They may boast about providing nutritional information for a few healthier items, but they remain hush-hush when it comes to full nutrition disclosure for the bulk of their menu offerings.

There continues to be virtually no nutrition information from independent chains, single unit restaurants, or most ethnic restaurants beyond the national walk up and order Mexican, Chinese, and Italian chains. This is understandable, because it is expensive to obtain and provide nutrition information. Even local and federal legislation that is being written and enacted only pertains to restaurant chains with 20 or more restaurants serving the same foods.

What hasn't changed much—even though there's a lot of talk about the epidemics of obesity in children and adults, heart disease, pre-diabetes, and type 2 diabetes—is the huge portions served in restaurants. Plenty of portions are enough for two or more, and you're consistently prompted to overeat with meal deals, two-for-one specials, mounds of French fries, and all-you-can-eat buffet restaurants.

This means you'll need all the portion-control pointers you'll find in the pages ahead. Portion control is one of your best defenses to limit overeating.

You'll also welcome the many tips to "guesstimate" restaurant portions in the "Put Your Best Guess Forward" section (page 23) and throughout this book. Good "guesstimating" skills are essential to your success.

I hope you find *What to Eat When You're Eating Out* helpful in your quest to eat healthy, get to or stay at a healthy weight, prevent or manage medical conditions, and enjoy good health for many years to come.

I encourage you to ask for nutrition information from restaurants that don't provide it. If enough of us keep asking, eventually they'll give us the facts. I also urge you to support federal and state legislative efforts to require national chain restaurants to tell us the nutrition content of the foods they serve. These initiatives have the potential to help all of us make healthier food choices.

To your health,

Hope S. Warshaw, MMSc, RD

Acknowledgments

This book would have been impossible to create without the willingness of many large national and regional restaurant chains to be forthcoming with the nutrition numbers for their foods by making them available on the Internet. On behalf of people who will use and benefit from the nutrition information in the pages ahead, I am indebted to these restaurant chains. They set an example of public responsibility for the rest of the chain restaurant industry.

No book is completed by just the author alone. In this case, many manuscript pages and a large nutrient database became a book with many people's help. I am grateful to Paula Payne, RD, who assisted with the development of the nutrient database and other aspects of the book. Thanks also to all those at Small Steps Press who supported this effort: Rebekah Renshaw, Development Editor; Melissa Sprott, Production Manager; Abe Ogden, Managing Editor; and Rob Anthony, Director, Book Publishing.

A final thanks goes to my professional colleagues who consistently lend their ears and ideas. They continue to be a source of inspiration and encouragement.

Today's Healthy Eating Goals

The Dietary Guidelines for Americans and the MyPyramid provide healthy eating guidelines that are straightforward and relatively easy to understand.

The difficulty, as you well know, is not in understanding the recommendations. It is the challenge of applying these healthy eating goals when you are faced with choosing foods and eating meals in our fast-paced and convenience-oriented world.

With an easy-to-digest understanding of today's healthy eating goals, plenty of tips and tactics from this guide, and a myriad of restaurant nutrition facts, you'll be a pro in no time at putting together healthier restaurant meals.

Healthy Eating Goals in a Nutshell

The Dietary Guidelines for Americans focus on six general themes for healthy eating. Learn more at: www.healthierus.gov/dietaryguidelines. These themes were echoed in the USDA's revised food pyramid. Check out the new food pyramid at: www.mypyramid.gov.

Think about each of these healthy eating themes and how you can make small changes in your food choices to take steps toward achieving these goals.

1. **Eat a variety of foods within the basic food groups.** Eat a variety of vegetables, fruits, whole grains, low-fat dairy foods (milk and yogurt), lean meats, and

healthy oils. Different foods in the same food groups provide an array of different nutrients. Yes, the phrase "variety is the spice of life" is very true when it comes to food choices.

2. **Make your calories count.** With our automated gadgets, cars, elevators, and more; Americans use fewer and fewer calories each day. This means you've got to get maximum nutrition out of the calories you eat. Make a habit out of choosing foods packed with essential vitamins and minerals. Keep foods that are heavy on added fats and sugars, and light on nutrition, such as desserts, to a bare minimum.
3. **Stay within your calorie needs to control your weight.** To maintain a healthy weight, eat just the number of calories you need each day. If you splurge one day, lighten up the next. If you find your weight creeping up the scale, watch your portions at home and when you choose to eat restaurant meals. Eat only smaller amounts of foods that provide concentrated sources of calories—those with added fats and sugars—regular soda and sugary drinks, fried foods and sweets. Research shows it is much easier to stay at a healthy weight than it is to try to lose weight and keep it off.
4. **Limit processed foods.** Eating fewer processed foods can help you eat less added sugars and solid fats (saturated and trans fats), along with fewer calories. It can also help you eat more foods from the basic food groups—vegetables, fruit, and dairy, for example—which often pack in more nutrients for the same or fewer calories.
5. **Eat less sodium.** Achieve this goal by eating fewer processed foods and restaurant meals. Research shows that Americans get most of their sodium—and

too much of it—from processed foods. Restaurant foods are processed or partially processed. Another contributor of sodium is salt. Lower your sodium count further by using less salt when you prepare foods at home or at restaurants.

6. **Be physically active.** Getting to, or staying at, a healthy weight and keeping yourself in shape, needs to be achieved through a balance between food choices and adequate physical activity. Physical activity is also good for your heart, bones, and mental outlook. Today's recommendations suggest you get at least 30 minutes of activity most days. Many people, especially people who have lost weight and are working to keep it off, need up to 60 to 90 minutes most days to accomplish and maintain their health goals. The easiest form of physical activity for many people is walking.

Those are the six key goals for healthy eating. Next, you need the details about what foods to eat and in what amounts to achieve these healthy eating goals.

The following are the key messages with a few practical tips:

- Eat more (six or more servings) grains, beans, and starchy vegetables each day. Make at least three (or half) of the servings you eat each day whole grains. A few tips:
  - Choose whole-grain hot and dry cereals and whole-wheat breads. Look for the words "whole" or "whole-grain" in the ingredients.
  - Select whole-wheat pasta and brown rice.
  - Include beans, peas, lentils, and corn in soups, side dishes, or entrees.

- Choose popcorn, whole-wheat pretzels, or whole-wheat crackers instead of fried snack foods.

■ Eat more fruits and vary your choices. Strive for 2 cups of fruit a day. Fruit is one of the most difficult foods to get in restaurants so try to eat fruit at home and/or bring a couple of pieces along with you to work, school, or wherever your daily life takes you. A few tips:

- Use fresh, frozen, canned, or dried fruit.
- Limit juices unless they are calcium fortified (and only drink these in small amounts).
- Have fruit at the ready—grapes, berries, bananas, and apples.
- Take a serving or two of fresh or dried fruit with you each day.

■ Eat more vegetables and vary your choices. Strive for 2 1/2 cups of vegetables a day. It's difficult to tank up on vegetables in restaurants, so eat plenty when you eat meals at home, and go out of your way to fit them into your restaurant meals.
A few tips:

- Eat a wide variety of vegetables. Rotate between dark green vegetables (broccoli, spinach, collards, chard, and kale) and orange vegetables (carrots, winter squash, and yams).
- Keep a stock of frozen or canned (no-salt) vegetables (not in sauces).
- Keep baby carrots, grape tomatoes, and celery sticks for easy-to-grab vegetables.

■ Include at least two to three servings of fat-free or low-fat dairy foods each day—milk, yogurt, and cheese—within your calorie allotment. (Children, pregnant and breastfeeding women, and some adults have higher requirements for dairy foods.) Low-fat dairy foods provide calcium and other important nutrients for your health. Milk has become easier to find at restaurants.

A few tips:

- 8 oz of milk or yogurt or 1 1/2 oz of cheese equals one dairy serving.
- Opt for fat-free milk rather than regular soda or a fruit drink.
- Enjoy yogurt as a snack, part of a healthy breakfast, or to top fresh fruit.

■ Eat a moderate amount of meat and other protein foods. Two 3-ounce servings each day are enough for most people. Not only does eating less meat help you eat less protein, it also makes it easier for you to eat less total fat, saturated fat, trans fat, and dietary cholesterol.

A few tips:

- Choose lean cuts of meat—round, sirloin, flank steak, or extra lean ground beef, and enjoy them prepared in low fat ways: grilled, steamed, broiled, or baked.
- Don't eat poultry skin.
- Choose lean turkey, ham, or roast beef for sandwiches, rather than high-fat bologna or salami.
- Eat more fish and order it grilled, baked, or poached.
- Use nutrition-packed legumes (beans and peas) in soups, side dishes, entrees, and on salads.

■ Go light on fats and oils. Limit fats and oils high in saturated fat and trans fat, such as butter, cheese, solid shortenings, and coconut and palm oils. Limit partially hydrogenated fats, which contain trans fats. Trans fats find their way into restaurant food mainly in the frying oil. Limiting fried foods is a good way to limit trans fats, as well as many calories, when you eat in restaurants.

A few tips:

- Buy and use liquid oil, such as canola, soy, olive, or corn oil. Use one of these as much as possible to sauté or cook rather than butter, margarine, or shortening.
- Keep the amount of saturated and trans fat low. Use few processed crackers, cookies, and fried foods. Choose fat-free dairy foods, reduced-fat cheeses, and lean meats.

■ Enjoy small amounts of sugary foods and sweets once in a while. If you have some pounds to shed or your blood glucose or blood fats are not in a healthy range, eat sweets more sparingly. If you're on the slim side, you can splurge on sweets a bit more often if you want to.

A few tips:

- Choose a few favorite desserts. Decide how often to eat them and in what portions. Consider only enjoying desserts when you eat out.
- Split a dessert in a restaurant or take half home. Portions are generally too big.
- Take advantage of smaller portions available in fast-food restaurants or frozen dessert spots—kiddie, small, or regular are the words to look for.

■ Drink no more than one alcoholic drink a day if you are a woman and two drinks a day if you are a man. One drink is defined as 1 1/2 oz of hard liquor (a shot), 12 oz of beer, or 5 oz of wine.

A few tips:

- Consider limiting your alcoholic beverages when you eat in restaurants as a way to minimize the amount of alcohol you consume.
- Sip an alcoholic drink slowly to make it last.
- If you order an alcoholic drink at a meal, also order a non-alcoholic and non-caloric drink to have by your side. Use the non-alcoholic drink to quench your thirst.

How Much Should You Eat?

In order to make the long-term changes in your eating habits that will keep you healthy, you need to continue to eat at least some of the foods you have enjoyed for years, albeit in smaller quantities. The quantities of food you eat and when you eat need to match your lifestyle and schedule. Another critical element is to determine what foods and times for meals and snacks work best to help you keep your weight and other health parameters in control.

The number of calories you need each day should be based on your needs. No set number of calories or amounts of foods or nutrients is right for everyone. Your needs depend on many factors: your height, your age, your current weight and whether you want to lose weight or are at a healthy weight, whether you have a hard or easy time losing weight, your daily activity level, the type of physical activity you do, and more. To develop an individualized eating plan and/or set healthy eating goals to make lifestyle changes, work with a registered dietitian (RD). A dietitian can help you learn how to work almost any food into a healthy eating plan and support your efforts to change your eating habits over time.

A valuable online resource to estimate your calorie needs and learn more about the number of servings you need from the different food groups is www.mypyramid.gov.

Restaurant Pitfalls and Strategies for Self-Defense

Eating out healthfully is no small task. It's downright challenging! You need willpower and perseverance. It's tough enough to eat healthfully in your own house, but even more challenges confront you when you are not able to control the portions or the condiments. You can't march into a restaurant's kitchen and hold the cook's hand while they ladle on more butter, slather on more mayonnaise, or shake more salt onto your once healthy foods.

Healthy restaurant eating is a challenge because of numerous pitfalls—from huge portions to the use of large quantities of fats, oils, sugar, and salt. Don't despair. You can learn to *choose* to eat healthfully in 99% of restaurants. To help make it easier on you, it's important to learn the pitfalls of restaurant eating. You'll find these discussed below. Next, you'll want to become well versed on healthy eating strategies. As you thumb though the tips and tactics in the pages ahead, you'll note that these strategies emerge repeatedly.

Pitfalls of Restaurant Eating

- **You think of restaurant ventures as special occasions.** Yes, once upon a time, people only ate in restaurants to celebrate a birthday, Mother's Day, or an anniversary.

Not today. According to the latest statistics from the National Restaurant Association, the average American eats six meals away from home each week. And you may easily top that number. When you eat that many meals away from home, your waistline can quickly spread if you treat each meal as a special occasion. So, do you give up restaurant foods? There's no need to take that drastic step. Plus, depending on your schedule, cutting out eating out may not be possible for you. Today, restaurant meals for most people are just part of a fast-paced life and no longer just special occasions.

- **You're not the cook.** Your methods to control both portions and how your food is prepared are to ask questions about the food on the menu, to make special requests to get an item delivered the way you want it, and to practice portion control when you order and when you eat. Yes, assertiveness will be required!
- **Fats are here, there, and everywhere.** Remember, fat makes food taste good and stay moist. Restaurants love it. Fat is in high-fat ingredients, such as butter, sour cream, or cream; in high-fat foods, such as cheese, bacon, or potato chips; and in high-fat cooking methods, such as deep-fat frying, breading and frying, and sautéing. It's also at the table in the form of fried Chinese noodles, tortilla chips, or butter or oil for breads. You need to master the craft of being a fat sleuth. You'll get plenty of tips ahead.
- **Sodium can skyrocket.** Along with fat, salt makes food taste good. Salt or high sodium preservatives are also used in many pre-prepared restaurant foods to keep them safe. Sodium can be particularly high in fast-food restaurants and others that use pre-packaged foods. It's nearly impossible for you

to cut the sodium count of pre-packaged foods. The sodium can also be high in restaurants that prepare food from scratch, simply because they maximize taste by lathering the food in salt. Some ethnic foods, particularly Asian cuisines, can be high in sodium because of seasonings and sauces, like soy and teriyaki sauce. If you're watching your sodium intake, you will need to learn the preparation methods that boost sodium and know where and how you can make reasonable special requests.

- **Portions are oversized.** Restaurants simply serve too much food. Unfortunately, we've evolved to a value = volume proposition in restaurants. Portions of food, particularly those produced and provided inexpensively, such as chips, fries, and drinks, are often enough for two. If there's one place to focus your attention and slowly change your behaviors, it's to develop and implement strategies that help you not overeat. Hopefully you have a few willing dining partners in your midst.
- **Meat is front and center.** A primary focus of the American diner is summed up in the catchphrase "Where's the beef?" Whether it is fish, chicken, or beef, the "meat" or main source of protein often takes center stage, particularly in restaurant meals. For example, a portion of red meat in table service restaurants is often 8 oz or more cooked. (It's easier to order just-right portions of meats in fast-food restaurants by sticking with those small portions.) A chicken breast is often a whole chicken breast. A goal to eat healthier is to think about moving meat from front and center to the side where the portion takes up only one-quarter of your plate. Fill about half of the rest of your plate with vegetables and the other

quarter with whole-grain starches. Yes, a goal to strive for, but not easy to do with restaurant meals!

Americans Eat Out: How Much and How Often?

According to the National Restaurant Association, in 1950 the average American spent only a quarter of his or her food dollar eating away from home. Today, an average American spends about half of every food dollar on food eaten away from home. Americans eat about one-third of their calories away from home, and eat six meals out of the house each week. Lunch is the meal eaten out most often, with dinner a close second. Breakfast is eaten out least often (keep in mind it is also the meal skipped most often, though it is known that eating breakfast has been shown to help people maintain weight losses). Men eat out more than women. Fast-food restaurants, or walk up and order restaurants (as this book defines them)—from hamburger joints to pizza and sub shops—represent about a quarter of all restaurants. As for ethnic food, Americans' favorites are Mexican, Chinese, and Italian.

Let's face it, restaurant meals are just part of dealing with our fast-paced world. And remember, whether you eat in the restaurant or take food out to the soccer field, your office, or the kitchen table, you face the same decisions. In fact, you have to make similar choices in today's supermarkets, because they have begun to look a bit like restaurants, with ready-to-eat parts of meals, complete meals, sandwiches, salads, and salad bars. One advantage to the supermarket is that the nutrition facts constantly stare you in the face. Not so in restaurants. At best, you have to have consulted the pages ahead and made decisions before you cross the threshold of the restaurant.

Ten Strategies to Eat Out Healthfully

Develop a can-do attitude. Too many people think in negative equations: Eating out equals pigging out; a restaurant meal is a special occasion; or eating out means blowing your "diet." These attitudes defeat your efforts to eat healthfully before you even start to try. Get ready to develop a can-do attitude about restaurant meals. Slowly begin to change how you order and the types of restaurants in which you choose to eat.

Decide when to eat out—or not. Take a look at how often you eat out. If your count verges on the excessive—at least once a day—then ask yourself why you eat out so frequently and how you can reduce your restaurant meals. If you reduce the restaurant meals you eat, you'll more easily eat healthier. Also, if you eat out more frequently, you need to keep splurges to a minimum. If you eat out only once a month, you might take a few more liberties—perhaps with an alcoholic drink or a dessert you split.

Zero in on the site. Seek out restaurants that offer at least a smattering of healthier options. If not, you'll set yourself up for failure. Believe it or not, there is an advantage to eating in chain restaurants. You know the menu all too well. This can help you plan ahead, no matter which one of the chain's locations you pop into.

Set your game plan in place prior to arrival. On your way to the restaurant—whether it's a quick fast-food lunch or a leisurely weekend dinner—envision a healthy and enjoyable outcome. Plan your strategy, or at least what you might have if you aren't familiar with the restaurant. Don't become a victim of hasty choices or be swayed by the sights and smells that come your way.

Become a fat sleuth. Learn to focus on fats and the calories within. Fat is the densest form of calories, and it often gets lost in the sauce, on the salad, on the bread, or in the chips. Watch out for high-fat ingredients—butter, cream, and sour cream. Be alert for high-fat foods, such as cheese, avocado, or sausage. Steer clear of high-fat preparation methods like frying of any kind. Look out for high-fat dishes—Mexican chimichangas, broccoli with cheese sauce, or stuffed potato skins, for starters.

Let your healthy eating goals or food plan be your guide. Choose foods with your healthy eating goals or plan in mind. For example, if you're trying to eat more vegetables, focus on how you can accomplish this. Try to fulfill each food group with menu items or substitute foods to make your meal complete.

Practice portion control from the start. The best way not to eat too much is to order less. Order with your stomach in mind, not your eyes. You need to outsmart the menu to get the right amount of food for you. Because practicing portion control is central to healthy restaurant eating, you'll get plenty of tips and tricks in the pages ahead.

Be creative with the menu. You outsmart the menu by being creative. You also control portions by being creative. Remember, no sign at the entrance says, "All who enter must order an entree." Take advantage of appetizers, soups, and salads; split menu items, including the entree, with your dining partner; order one or two fewer dishes than the number of people at the table and eat family or Asian style; or mix and match two entrees to achieve nutritional balance. For example, in a steak house, one person orders the steak, baked potato, and salad bar and the other orders just the potato and salad bar, and then they split the steak. In an Italian restaurant, one person orders pasta with a tomato-based sauce and the other orders a chicken or veal dish with a vegetable.

Get foods made to order. Don't be afraid to ask for what you want, even in a fast-food restaurant. Restaurants today need your business and want you back. Make sure your requests are practical—leave an item such as potato chips off the plate; substitute mustard for mayonnaise on a sandwich; make a sandwich on whole-wheat bread rather than on a croissant; or serve the salad dressing on the side. Restaurants can abide by these requests; however, don't expect to have your special requests greeted with a smile at noon in a fast-food restaurant or when you try to remake a menu item. Be reasonable and pleasant.

Know when enough is enough. Many people grew up being members of the "clean-plate club." Now you need to reserve a membership in the "leave-a-few-bites-on-your-plate club." To keep from overeating, don't order too much, order creatively, and push your plate away when you meet your calorie needs. Remember, take-home containers are at-the-ready in most restaurants.

Restaurants Can Help or Hinder Your Healthy Eating Efforts

The pendulum swings back and forth on how helpful restaurants are when it comes to efforts to provide healthier choices. During the 1980s and early 1990s, when the voices of people concerned about what they ate and about their health were loud, restaurants developed healthier options. Lower-calorie and lower-fat menu items were introduced. Restaurateurs willingly made lower-fat milk and reduced-calorie salad dressings available. Some restaurants even marked their menus with little hearts or other notations to indicate which menu items met specific health criteria.

The pendulum in restaurants then swung back in the late 1990s and early 2000s. McDonald's dropped the McLean hamburger and meal-sized salads. Belly-busting portions became commonplace again. Taco Bell's Border Lights line bombed because it was introduced toward the end of this round of the health craze. We were back in the era of triple-decker burgers, meal deals, and more all-you-can-eat buffets.

But then the pendulum swung again due to another round of interest in low-carb diets and, more important, a focus on childhood and adult obesity. Restaurant chains have responded in small ways. A few examples: McDonald's has stopped supersizing; several large hamburger chains are offering healthier side options including fruits and vegetables; Subway has taken on healthier eating in a big way, offering 6-inch subs and a handful of sandwiches with a minimal number of grams of fat; and, in many restaurants, it's easier to split and share items as well as get a range of items prepared your way.

Other interconnected movements are afoot in restaurant cuisine. One is the slow food movement, which promotes less processed and more made-from-scratch foods. Another is the push for restaurants to use more locally grown fruits and vegetables and meats raised and processed more humanely and without hormones. Additionally, organic items are finding their way onto menus.

Unfortunately, a majority of Americans still cast most health and nutrition cares to the wind when they set foot in any restaurant. It's easy to see where that is leading us. Today, nearly two-thirds of American adults are overweight, nearly 24 million people have diabetes, and about 57 million more have pre-diabetes.

This "no cares" nutrition attitude makes it harder for people who are health conscious. But don't feel pessimistic. Lower-fat milk, reduced-calorie salad dressings, and lower-fat frozen desserts are still widely available. There's also a greater ease in making special requests—ordering half portions and splitting items or meals down the middle with your dining partner. With skills and a bit of fortitude, you can eat healthfully at most restaurants. Granted, you still have to pick and choose among the menu offerings.

Chains That Give the Nutrition Lowdown

The restaurants included in this second edition provide complete nutrition information. The "walk up and order" type restaurants—pizza, chicken, Mexican and Chinese food, subs and sandwiches, donuts and bagels, and frozen desserts—provide the most complete nutrition information.

The types of restaurants that, for the most part, either do not have or do not provide nutrition information are chain sit-down restaurants. Several of these restaurants are all too happy to give you nutrition information about their healthier items; however, they either don't have the information, or are unwilling to disclose the nutrition information for the complete menu.

Why don't some restaurants provide nutrition information? There are a few reasons. First, it's expensive to obtain nutritional analyses on all menu items. Second, restaurants that do not provide information tend to change their menus frequently. As soon as they print nutrition information, it would need to be revised. Third, they want you to stay blindfolded to the nutrition lowdown on their foods. An important point here is that you need to keep asking for nutrition information at restaurants that don't give it.

How to Get the Latest Nutrition Lowdown

This book has over 60 restaurants. There are more chain restaurants that provide nutrition information. Here are a few hints on how to get the nutrition information for other restaurants.

- If you have access to the Internet, use it. Usually the nutrition information is tucked into the menu information.
- If you don't have Internet access, ask for nutrition information at the store location you frequent. You

might get lucky and have a nutrition pamphlet put right into your hands. Make sure you check the date on the nutrition pamphlet to be sure it is current.

- If the restaurant does not have the information, ask where you can call or write for it. You might need to call or write the corporate headquarters and have them send you a pamphlet.
- If you have a question about the nutrition content or ingredients used in a few items, contact the company either through the Internet or by phone.

A Bit of Help from Your Government

The Nutrition Facts panel on most canned and packaged foods in the supermarket hardly seems new. It's now been around since about 1994. The Nutrition Labeling and Education Act (NLEA) changed the nutrition label, increased the number of foods with information, and required restaurants to comply with several aspects of this law. Restaurants must provide nutrition information to customers when nutrition and health claims are made on signs and placards. If any restaurant makes a health claim about a food, that it is "low-fat," for instance, the nutrition information has to comply with the meaning of that nutrition claim according to the NLEA. This helps you know that when you see the word "healthy" to describe a can of beans or a fast-food sandwich, it has the same meaning. Restaurants from small one-unit sandwich shops to McDonald's have to abide by these regulations. Table 1 (see page 22) provides terms you might see on restaurant menu items and their definitions.

The law permits restaurants to make:

- Specific claims about a menu item's nutritional content.
- One of the approved health claims about the relationship between a nutrient or food and a disease or health condition. The criteria to make the health claim must be met. (There are about 15 FDA-approved health claims. These are different than nutrition claims.)

If the restaurant makes a nutrition or health claim, it must provide you with the nutrition information to back it up. The claim can be substantiated by a nutrition database, nutrition information in the cookbook from which the recipe was made, or another source that provides nutrition information. Further, restaurants do not have to give you the information in the nutrition label format you are familiar with from the supermarket. They can provide it in any format they choose.

There is a move in a handful of cities and states to require chain restaurants with more than 20 outlets to provide some basic nutrition information, such as calories, saturated fat, trans fat, carbohydrate, and sodium at the point of purchase, such as right next to the price of the item on menus or menu boards (not just on their Internet sites, on posters, or in brochures available in the restaurants).

This is great news because it's the key information you need to make wise choices. Legislation began to snowball in 2008 with New York City and Seattle putting legislation into action. In September 2008, California's governor signed a bill into law that requires restaurant chains to provide brochures with nutrition information in their restaurants (this will start in July

2009 and take full effect in 2011). Federal, state, and city legislators in other areas are forging ahead to put this legislation into effect across the nation. Check out what's going on federally by searching the Internet for "restaurant nutrition labeling laws." Consider weighing in with your support of the legislation to your federal representatives.

TABLE 1 Meaning of Nutrition Claims on Menus, Signs, and Placards*

Nutrition Claim	Meaning
Cholesterol-Free	Less than 2 mg of cholesterol per serving and 2 g or less of saturated fat per serving
Low Cholesterol	20 mg or less of cholesterol per serving and 2 g or less of saturated fat per serving
Fat Free	Less than 0.5 g of fat per serving
Low Fat	3 g or less of fat per serving
Light/Lite	Cannot be used by restaurants as a nutrient content claim, but can be used to describe a menu item, such as "lighter fare" or "light size"
Sodium Free	Less than 5 mg of sodium per serving
Low Sodium	140 mg or less of sodium per serving
Sugar Free	Less than 0.5 g of sugar per serving
Low Sugar	May not be used as a nutrient claim
Healthy	The food item is low in fat, low in saturated fat, has limited amounts of cholesterol and sodium, and provides significant amounts of one or more key nutrients—vitamins A and C, iron, calcium, protein, or fiber.
Heart Healthy (These claims will indicate that a diet low in saturated fat and cholesterol may reduce the risk of heart disease.)	The item is low in fat, saturated fat, and cholesterol, and provides significant amounts (not added) of one or more key nutrients—vitamins A and C, iron, calcium, protein, or fiber. OR The item is low in fat, saturated fat, and cholesterol, and provides significant amounts of one or more key nutrients—vitamins A and C, iron, calcium, protein—and is a significant source of soluble fiber.

*The definitions of these claims are the same as those used for food labels in the supermarket. Learn more about nutrient claims and health claims at the U.S. Food and Drug Association website (www.fda.gov).

Put Your Best Guess Forward

- Have measuring equipment at home and use it. Have a set of measuring spoons and measuring cups, as well as a food scale. There's a gamut of food scales available, from the inexpensive under $10 type, to expensive food scales that utilize an internal database to provide their nutrient counts based on the weight of the food. For more information on the more expensive scales, visit www.diabetesnet.com. If you are unfamiliar with portions, weigh and measure foods at home regularly to familiarize yourself with the portions you should eat. Then on occasion, weigh and measure foods, especially the starches, fruits, and meats. Weighing and measuring foods at home regularly helps you keep portions in control and can help you estimate them in restaurants. Estimating with the precise portion size helps you estimate the nutrient content correctly.
- Use these "handy" hand guides to estimate portions:
  - Tip of the thumb (to first knuckle)—1 teaspoon
  - Whole thumb—1 tablespoon
  - Palm of your hand—3 ounces (this is the portion size of cooked meat that most people need at a meal). Other 3-ounce portion guides: the size of a deck of regular size playing cards or the size of a household bar of soap.
  - Tight fist—1/2 cup
  - Loose fist or open handful—1 cup

Note: These guidelines hold true for most women's hands, but some men's hands are much larger. Check the size of your hands out for yourself with real weighing and measuring equipment.

- Use the scales in the produce aisle of the supermarket to educate yourself about the servings of food you may be served in a restaurant, such as white or sweet potatoes, an ear of corn, a banana, or half a grapefruit. Weigh individual pieces of these foods. Check out how many ounces a potato or an ear of corn is that you may be served in a restaurant. Note that you are weighing these foods raw, but their weight doesn't change that much if they are served cooked.
- If there are no data for a particular restaurant you frequent, use the information available from other similar restaurants. If you want to get a feel for the nutrient content of a food like French fries, baked potato, stuffing, pizza, or bagels, look at the serving size and nutrition information for those foods in restaurants that are included. You might want to take a few examples and then do an average. For example: if you regularly eat at a local pizza shop rather than a national chain and they have no nutrition information, take the nutrition information from this book for two slices of medium-sized regular crust cheese pizza from three restaurants. Then do an average. You will come pretty close to the nutrition content of the two slices of cheese pizza you eat.
- You can also use the nutrition information from the nutrition facts of foods in the supermarket to estimate what you might eat in a restaurant. You might find some similar foods in the frozen or pack-

aged convenience foods area. Again, take a couple of examples and then average.

- If you regularly eat particular ethnic foods for which you find no nutrition information, you might want to get a few cookbooks out of the library (or use your own) that contain recipes for the foods you enjoy. Use a nutrient database or book with nutrition information (see pages 27–29) to determine the estimated nutrient content for each ingredient. Do this for a couple of similar recipes. Get an average to help you estimate the nutrient content of what you are eating in the restaurant. This might work well for ethnic foods such as Indian, Mexican, or Chinese.

Most people regularly eat just 50 to 100 foods, including restaurant foods. People tend to frequent the same restaurants and order similar items. For this reason, it makes sense to spend a few hours estimating the nutrient content of your favorite restaurant items for which nutrition information is not available. Once you have this figured out, put it in a notebook, develop a computer file that you print out and keep with you, or put it into a personal data device that you always have with you.

Keep in mind that most restaurants serve portions that are larger than most average-sized people need to eat. So, even if you choose healthy foods that combine to make a healthy meal, you will likely also need to limit the amount you eat. Portion control is clearly not an easy task. Learn some techniques by reading the "Strategies for Self-Defense" on pages 9–15.

A word to the wise: avoid all-you-can-eat restaurants and other settings that promote overeating, such as hotel breakfast buffets or salad or food bars. This is best if you don't have much willpower or it bothers you to think that the restaurant is making money on you because you will not walk out feeling like a stuffed turkey. However, if you feel these settings work well because they help you control portions, use them to your advantage.

If you frequently eat particular items in a large chain restaurant that isn't in this book, contact the restaurant. Several restaurants note that while they don't provide nutrition information for all their items they would provide information for several items.

Even when you have consulted the nutrition facts for your menu items, practice defensive counting. Recognize that the nutrition information provided by restaurants is obtained from several samples of the foods prepared according to corporate specifications or based on the various ingredients. For this reason, on any given day, the portions of foods and ingredients you are served may be slightly more or less. Even in the fast-food hamburger chains, the same burger can include more or less ketchup, tomatoes, mayonnaise, or other ingredients. So, before you dig in, reassess your counts and ask yourself if the nutrition numbers provided by the chain add up based on your nutrition knowledge. If not, revise your counts.

Resources for Nutrition Information of Foods

BOOKS

The Ultimate Calorie, Carbohydrate, and Fat Gram Counter, by Lea Ann Holzmeister, RD, CDE. Small Steps Press, 2006. This book provides the carbohydrate count, as well as other nutrition information, for thousands of foods including fruits, vegetables,and other produce; meats, poultry, and seafood; desserts; many foods you know by their brand name; frozen entrees; and more.

The Doctor's Pocket Calorie, Fat, and Carb Counter, by Allan Borushek. Allan Borushek and Associates (revised annually). This book lists calorie, fat, and carbohydrate information for thousands of basic and brand-name foods. (See www.calorieking.com to order the book or to download food and restaurant databases.)

Calories and Carbohydrates, by Barbara Kraus. Signet, 16th edition, 2005. Carbohydrate and calorie counts for more than 8,500 items are included in this food dictionary. It covers brand name and basic foods of every variety.

The Corinne T. Netzer Carbohydrate Counter, by Corinne T. Netzer. Dell, 7th edition, 2001. This book features carbohydrate counts for thousands of foods, including fresh and frozen produce, dairy products, breads, grains, pastas, sweets, fast foods, and more.

INTERNET

www.diabetes/org/myfoodadvisor.html. This nutrient database, introduced in mid-2008, is provided for your use at no charge by the American Diabetes Association. It contains about 5,000 commonly eaten foods and for most of them provides the key nutrients: calories, carbohydrate, saturated fat, sodium, and fiber, as well as several other nutrients and the percent daily value for some vitamins and minerals. There are many ways to use this searchable database to learn more about the nutrient content of foods and improve your food choices, such as searching for healthier alternatives, compiling the nutrient counts for your favorite recipes, or searching through the ADA's recipe box.

www.ars.usda.gov. This is the U.S. federal government's nutrient database. It contains extensive nutrition information for about 7,000 basic and commercial foods. It is searchable and downloadable.

www.calorieking.com

www.healthydiningfinder.com. This is a joint venture between the Healthy Dining organization and the National Restaurant Association.

www.myfooddiary.com

www.nutritiondata.com

www.dietfacts.com

How This Restaurant Guide Works for You

You might open this book and be thrilled to see many of the restaurants you frequent. Then again, you might wonder why certain restaurants that you've never laid eyes on are included, or why your favorite hamburger or pizza stop is nowhere to be found.

Each July, a restaurant trade association magazine, *Restaurants and Institutions,* publishes a list of the top 400 restaurant chains based on several categories of criteria. The chain restaurants in this book were selected based on the number of locations they operate and whether the restaurant's business was growing or not.

If one of your favorite restaurants is not included, it is for one of the following reasons:

- The restaurant might not have been willing or able to provide sufficient menu and/or nutrition information to warrant their inclusion. This is especially true for sit-down restaurants.
- The restaurant chain may not be large enough across the country, although it appears to you that in your area there are many locations.

Where to Find the Restaurant in this Book

Clearly, you know to look in "Burgers and More" to find McDonald's or Wendy's, or in "Pizza, Pasta, and All Else Italian" to find Domino's or Pizza Hut; however, because Boston Market's menu today includes more than just chicken, you might not guess that it is in the section "Family Fare." The "best fit" approach was used. Nine times out of ten you'll guess correctly; however, if you don't find a restaurant in the chapter where you think it should be, then check the alphabetical listing of restaurants on page ix–x in the beginning of the book.

Close but Not Exact

You should be aware that the nutrition information from restaurants is close but not exact. Many restaurants state that their nutrition information is based on the specified ingredients and preparation; however, the same restaurant has locations all over the country and often the world, and different regions purchase their ingredients and foods from different food wholesalers. For example, a Wendy's in California might purchase lettuce, tomatoes, and hamburger buns from one food supplier, whereas a Wendy's in Connecticut will buy foods from another company. The same is true internationally. When international chains make varied nutrition information available for their restaurants, the information used in this book used the U.S. figures. The nutrition analysis of these items is close, but not identical. However, it is close enough to help you to make food decisions and eat healthy.

Restaurant foods are also prepared by different people. Even in the same restaurant, on different days you might get more or less cheese on your pizza, more pickles or ketchup on your hamburger, or a slightly smaller or larger steak, even though you order the 6-oz filet. Wherever humans are involved, portions aren't exact.

Beverages and Condiments

There are two categories of items that are not listed separately in the information provided for each restaurant. The first is beverages. Regularly sweetened drinks, such as carbonated beverages (soda), lemonade, noncarbonated fruit drinks, as well as noncaloric beverages, milk, and 100% juice and the like, are not listed repetitively within the information for each restaurant. The nutrition information for the most commonly served regular and diet beverages is found in Table 2 on page 34–35.

The second category of items not repeated for each restaurant is common condiments, such as ketchup, mustard, mayonnaise, and honey. Find this nutrition information in Table 3 on page 36–37. Information for items such as salad dressing, barbecue sauces, and other special sauces are provided within the specific restaurant.

The Nutrition Numbers Ahead

The nutrition information for these restaurants are in the pages ahead in the following order.

- Calories
- Fat (in grams)
    - Percentage of calories from fat. Look at this in relation to grams of fat. Keep in mind that the per-

centage of calories from fat might be high, but the grams of fat might be low, or vice versa.

- Saturated fat (in grams). Saturated fat is the type of fat that raises blood cholesterol levels. Try to keep your saturated fat intake to 10% or less of your total calories.
- Trans fat (in grams). Trans fat is a type of fat that is saturated and unhealthy for your heart and blood vessels. It is mainly found in processed foods, but is also present in foods of animal origin, such as dairy foods, meats, poultry, and seafood. You are encouraged to eat as little trans fat as possible. (Trans fat is a new addition for the 2nd edition.) Due to the attention on trans fats and the inclusion of it on packaged food's nutrition facts since 2006, restaurants have felt the pressure to include it.

- Cholesterol (in milligrams)
- Sodium (in milligrams)
- Carbohydrate (in grams)
    - Dietary fiber (in grams). Dietary fiber is a subcomponent of carbohydrate. Most people don't eat enough dietary fiber (less than 15 grams a day). You are encouraged to eat 20–35 grams of dietary fiber each day.
- Protein (in grams)
- Food servings/exchanges. The terms "servings" and "exchanges" are considered the same in this book (this is not true when it comes to the nutrition facts on food labels). Servings/exchanges have been calculated using the booklet *Choose Your Foods: Exchange Lists for Diabetes,* published by the ADA and the American Dietetic Association in 2008. A "best-fit" approach was used to calculate servings or exchanges.

TABLE 2 Nutrition Information for Beverages

Beverage	Amount	Cal.	Fat (g)	Sat. Fat (g)	Chol. (mg)	Sod. (mg)	Carb. (g)	Pro. (g)	Choices/Exchanges
Beer (regular)	12 oz	150	0	0	0	11	13	1	1 alc. equiv. + 1 carb*
Beer (light)	12 oz	103	0	0	0	18	5	1	1 alc. equiv. + 1/2 carb*
Wine, white	6 oz	120	0	0	0	7	1	0	1 alcohol equivalent
Wine, red	6 oz	125	0	0	0	6	4	1	1 alcohol equivalent
Coffee, black (regular and decaffeinated)	12 oz	4	0	0	0	7	0	0	free
Tea (hot, nothing added)	12 oz	4	0	0	0	7	1	0	free
Cola (regular)	20 oz	227	0	0	0	25	59	0	3 carb
Cola (diet)	20 oz	12	0	0	0	47	2	1	free
Soda, non-cola (regular)	20 oz	246	0	0	0	55	63	0	3 carb
Soda, non-cola (diet)	20 oz	0	0	0	0	95	0	0	free
Iced Tea (unsweetened)	12 oz	4	0	0	0	6	1	0	free

Liquor (any type)	1 1/2 oz	96	0	0	0	0	0	0	1 alcohol equivalent
Lemonade (regular)	12 oz	148	0	0	0	15	39	0	3 carb
Lemonade (sugar-free)	12 oz	11	0	0	0	14	2	0	free
Milk (whole)	8 oz	146	8	5	24	98	11	8	1 whole milk
Milk (reduced-fat/2%)	8 oz	122	5	3	20	100	11	8	1 low-fat milk
✓Milk (low-fat/1%)	8 oz	102	2	2	12	107	12	8	1 fat-free milk, 1/2 fat
✓Milk (fat-free)	8 oz	83	0	0	5	103	12	8	1 fat-free milk
Milk, chocolate (low-fat)	8 oz	160	3	2	8	152	26	8	1 fat-free milk, 1 carb
✓Apple juice	8 oz	175	0	0	0	11	43	0	3 fruit
✓Orange juice	8 oz	164	0	0	0	4	38	3	2 1/2 fruit

Source for nutrition information: U.S. Department of Agriculture, National Nutrient Database, http://www.ars.usda.gov. Consider the nutrition information as an estimate and not specific to the actual product you eat. If possible, use specific information when it is available.

*According to the calculation provided in *Choose Your Foods: Exchange Lists for Diabetes*, American Diabetes Association and American Dietetic Association, 2008. Talk to your diabetes educator or health care provider about how to work alcoholic beverages into your meal plan.

✓Healthiest Bets

TABLE 3 Nutrition Information for Condiments

Condiment	Amount	Cal.	Fat (g)	Sat. Fat (g)	Chol. (mg)	Sod. (mg)	Carb. (g)	Pro. (g)	Choices/Exchanges
Bacon, thinly sliced	1 slice	43	3	1	9	185	0	3	1 fat
Butter, stick	1 t	34	4	2	10	27	0	0	1 fat
Cheese, American	1-oz slice	105	9	6	26	416	0	6	1 high-fat meat
Cheese, Swiss	1-oz slice	95	7	5	24	388	1	7	1 high-fat meat
Cheese, mozzarella	1 oz shredded	85	6	4	22	178	1	6	1 medium-fat meat
Cream Cheese (regular)	1 T	51	5	3	16	43	0	1	1 fat
Cream Cheese (light)	1 T	35	3	2	8	44	1	2	1/2 fat
Half & Half, regular	2 T	39	3	2	11	12	1	1	1/2 fat
Honey	1 t	21	0	0	0	0	6	0	1/2 carb
Honey Mustard	1 t	7	0	0	0	16	1	0	free

Ketchup	1 T	15	0	0	0	167	4	0	free
Margarine (regular stick)	1 t	31	4	1	0	30	0	0	1 fat
Margarine (regular tub)	1 t	33	4	1	0	31	0	0	1 fat
Mayonnaise (regular)	1 T	57	5	1	4	105	4	0	1 fat
Mayonnaise (light)	1 T	49	5	1	5	101	1	0	1 fat
Mustard (regular)	1 t	3	0	0	0	57	0	0	free
Non-Dairy Creamer	1/2 oz/1 T	30	2	2	0	0	3	0	free
Olive Oil	1 t	40	5	1	0	0	0	0	1 fat
Pancake Syrup (regular)	1 T	47	0	0	0	16	12	0	1 carb
Pancake Syrup (light)	1 T	25	0	0	0	27	7	0	1/2 carb
Relish, sweet pickle-type	1 T	20	0	0	0	122	5	0	free
Salsa, tomato-based	1 T	4	0	0	0	96	1	0	free
Sour Cream (regular)	1 T	26	3	2	5	6	1	0	1/2 fat

(*Continued*)

There is not one right way to fit restaurant foods into your eating plan. Figuring out what food group the grams of carbohydrate come from is the biggest challenge to figuring servings or exchanges. This is how it was approached: When it appears that the grams of carbohydrate come from a starch—be it potato, bread, or starchy vegetable—the servings or exchanges are called starches. If the carbohydrate comes from vegetable, fruit, or milk, the servings or exchanges are designated as such.

A food group in *Choose Your Foods: Exchange Lists for Diabetes* is Sweets, Desserts, and Other Carbohydrate. This group contains sweets, frozen desserts, spaghetti sauce, jam, and maple syrup, to name a few. The calories and carbohydrate in many of these foods come from simple sugars. Therefore, in calculating the servings or exchanges for this book, we've called foods that fit into the "other carbohydrate" group "carb." Exchanges for fast-food shakes and frozen and regular desserts, for example, are calculated as carbs.

When it comes to meat dishes, the servings or exchanges were calculated based on the group that the meat fits into regardless of how it's prepared. For example, fish fillet sandwiches and chicken fingers are considered to fall into the lean meat group even though they have a lot of fat by the time they are served. On the other hand, sausage in any form is classified as a high-fat meat because that's the food group sausage fits into.

Putting It All Together

Perhaps one of the hardest parts of meal planning is figuring out how to put together healthy, well-balanced meals. This is a particular challenge in restaurants. To show you how to design healthier restaurant meals, we've put together two sample meals for most of the restaurants. In doing this, we've tried to show you variety and how you can mix and match foods to achieve your nutrition goals. We applied the following criteria to put together the meals. Please note that the criteria might be less strict than what you would consider for a healthy meal at home. That's because restaurant meals tend to be higher in calories, fat, and sodium.

In some restaurants, putting together healthier meals is easier, while in others it was virtually impossible to meet these criteria, especially for fat and sodium. Consider what the nutrition profile of meals in these restaurants would be if you weren't choosing with care. Also, keep in mind that you can make special requests to have higher fat or sodium ingredients left out, so that the items you eat are healthier.

An effort was made to minimize the amount of saturated and trans fat in all meals. This can be a challenge in restaurant meals. If you eat a restaurant meal that is high in fat and its components, balance this out with healthier meals other times of the day.

THE LIGHT 'N' LEAN CHOICE

- 400–700 calories (based on about 1,200–1,600 calories per day)
- 30–40 percent of calories from fat
- 100–200 milligrams of cholesterol (total per day should be 300 milligrams or less)
- 1,000–1,800 milligrams of sodium (total per day should be no more than 2,300 milligrams)

THE HEALTHY 'N' HEARTY CHOICE

- 600–1,000 calories (based on about 1,800–2,400 calories per day)
- 30–40 percent of calories from fat
- 100–200 milligrams of cholesterol (total per day should be 300 milligrams or less)
- 1,000–1,800 milligrams of sodium (total per day should be no more than 2,300 milligrams)

*An effort was consistently made to minimize the amount of saturated and trans fat in all meals. This can be a challenge in restaurant meals. If you eat a restaurant meal that is high in fat and its components, balance this out with healthier meals other times of the day.

Healthiest Bets

With nutrition information in hand, we've made it easy for you to zero in on healthier restaurant offerings. We've marked these "Healthiest Bets" with a ✓. Remember, foods that are not marked as Healthiest Bets are not necessarily foods you should never eat. Healthiest Bets just steer you toward healthier choices.

When you're putting together healthy meals, don't look at only the Healthiest Bets. You can feel free to mix and match healthier and less healthy foods to make up overall healthy meals. Also keep in mind that if you split or share some less healthy bets, such as shakes, desserts, or fried items, they then fit into Healthiest Bets. That's why you'll see some Healthiest Bets and some less healthy items mixed and matched in the two sample meals for most restaurants. What's most important is that you eat a healthy balance of foods and meals over the course of the day and from week to week. So if you want a juicy hamburger and French fries for lunch one day a month, go ahead and enjoy.

The Healthiest Bets were chosen on the basis of the following criteria:

- Breakfast entrees: Less than 400 calories per serving, 45 grams of carbohydrate, less than 15 grams of fat (3 fat exchanges [about 30% fat]), and 1,000 milligrams of sodium.
- Lunch or dinner entrees, including entree salads: Less than 600–750 calories, 60 grams of carbohydrate, less than 20 grams of fat (4 fat exchanges [about 30% fat]), and 1,000 milligrams of sodium.
- Pizza, sandwiches (including breakfast sandwiches), hamburgers, etc.: Less than 500 calories per reasonable serving (for example, 2 slices of pizza), 60 grams of carbohydrate, 20 grams of fat (4 fat exchanges [about 30% fat]), and 1,000 milligrams of sodium.
- Side items: For items such as fruit, vegetables (raw and cooked), grains, legumes, starches, and meats, no more than 20 grams of carbohydrate, 5 grams of fat (1 fat exchange). For fried items, such as French fries, hash browns, chicken pieces, fried chicken, onion rings, and potato chips, less than 10 grams of fat (2 fat exchanges); less than 500 milligrams of sodium per serving.
- Soups: Less than 30 grams of carbohydrate, 10 grams of fat (2 fat exchanges), and 1,000 milligrams of sodium per serving.
- Salad dressings, cream cheeses, spreads, and condiments: Less than 50 calories, 10 grams of carbohydrate, 5 grams of fat (1 fat exchange), and 250 milligrams of sodium per tablespoon.

- Breads (such as rolls, biscuits, bagels, bread, croissants, scones, donuts, muffins, pretzels, and scones): Less than 400 calories, 45 grams of carbohydrate, 10 grams of fat (2 fat exchanges), and 800 milligrams of sodium per serving.
- Frozen desserts: Less than 300 calories, 30 grams of carbohydrate, and 10 grams of fat (2 fat exchanges) per serving.
- Beverages (such as milk, juice, milk shakes, and special coffees): Less than 300 calories, 30 grams of carbohydrate, and 5 grams of fat (1 fat exchange). Less than 400 milligrams of sodium. (Coffee and diet beverages, though minimal in calories, were not checked as Healthiest Bets.)

Bon Appetit!

Breakfast Eats, Drinks, Snacks, and More

RESTAURANTS

Auntie Anne's
Caribou Coffee
Dunkin' Donuts
Einstein Bros Bagels
Jamba Juice
Krispy Kreme
Orange Julius
Starbucks

EXCLUSIVE WEB CONTENT

Tim Hortons (http://www.diabetes.org/healthyrestaurant)

Note: Restaurants in this chapter generally devote their menus to bagels, donuts, pastries, coffees (regular and fancy), tea (regular and fancy), and other hot and cold drinks. A couple restaurants serve mainly fruit shakes or pretzels. Some also serve soups, sandwiches, and more. Look in "Burgers, Fries, and More" for fast-food breakfast fare. Look in "Family Fare" for restaurants that serve breakfast and brunch as well as lunch and dinner. Look in "Soups, Sandwiches, and Subs" for Au Bon Pain and Panera Bread, which also serve breakfast items.

The healthy meal choices for the restaurants in this section have slightly fewer calories and other nutrients than the criteria noted on page 54. That's because meals you eat in these restaurants are most likely breakfasts, light meals, or snacks.

Healthy Tips

- ★ Stick with coffee without a lot of added cream, whole milk, or sugar. These add fat and empty calories. Use a sugar substitute. You will often have three choices in restaurants—Splenda, Equal, and Sweet 'N' Low.
- ★ Try half of a soft-baked pretzel as an accompaniment to a salad or as a snack.
- ★ Opt for one of the light bagel spreads, but keep in mind that they are not free of calories or fat. Spread them thinly.
- ★ Cake donuts have slightly less fat than yeast donuts.
- ★ Do eat breakfast. Skipping breakfast keeps your engine in low gear and may help you rationalize overeating at meals during the rest of the day. Plus, if you take diabetes medications that can cause low blood glucose, skipping breakfast puts you at risk of hypoglycemia. Need another reason to eat breakfast? Research shows that people who eat breakfast have an easier time maintaining weight loss over the long term.
- ★ In breakfast sandwiches, choose ham, egg, and/or cheese and pass on the bacon or sausage.
- ★ Read the fine print when you see the words "low-fat," "fat-free," or "sugar-free." These phrases don't mean that there are no calories or no carbohydrate in the food. In fact, some of these foods can contain more

carbohydrate and/or more calories than the regular food.

★ If jam or jelly is an option, take it. Jams and jellies have no fat and just a small amount of carbs. Spread them thinly all the same.

NUTRITION PROS

- Bagels are a popular breakfast item. Without a spread, bagels contain nearly no fat (except if they contain cheese). That's good. However, bagels have been on a growth curve—they've gotten bigger and bigger. Today's bagels can be equal to about four slices (or more) of bread. You might consider eating only one-half or two-thirds of a bagel to control your carbohydrate count. Apply spreads thinly and wisely.
- Light cream cheese spreads are available in most bagel shops. Although not completely free of calories or fat, they still have less than the regular versions.
- Soft-baked pretzels—as long as they aren't loaded with lots of fat or sugar—are a healthy snack or side item. Just half might provide plenty of carbs, so share it.
- Whole-wheat pretzels and bagels are a great source of dietary fiber.
- Dunkin' Donuts and Krispy Kreme aren't just for donuts anymore. They also serve bagels, low-fat muffins, and coffees.
- Muffin mania has died down, but you'll still find them at many breakfast spots. Low-fat muffins are usually available. A regular muffin is often a better choice than some donuts or loaded bagels. But watch

the size. They can be huge. Consider splitting one in half and definitely choose a high-fiber type.

- English muffins and yeast rolls are healthy choices as long as you use only a small amount of butter or margarine. Choose whole grain, if possible.
- One of the quickest and healthiest breakfast foods—dry or cooked cereal with fat-free milk—is rarely served. When it's an option, grab it.

NUTRITION CONS

- Bagels can quickly become high in fat and calories if large ones are topped with a quarter inch of high-fat cream cheese or spread.
- Bagels in most bagel shops average at least 3–4 oz and 250–340 calories. That's equal to at least three or four slices of bread. And on the streets of New York? These bagels equal five or six slices of bread.
- Pretzels may sound healthy, but their calorie and fat content rise when they are rolled in glazes or butter or dipped in cheese sauce, cream cheese, or caramel.
- Croissants are high in fat by their very nature—that's how they become puffy and flaky. You add insult to injury when you stuff a croissant with bacon, sausage, cheese, tuna salad, or chicken salad. Skip 'em.
- Donuts are high in fat (but surprisingly, not as unhealthy as you might think because the servings are small). Save them for a rare splurge.
- Biscuits are loaded with fat. When sausage, bacon, eggs, and/or cheese are added, they give you your daily allotment of fat (and possibly saturated and trans fat) in one fell swoop.
- Fancy coffees and teas—both hot and iced, from mochas to chai teas—are not just coffee and tea. If they

contain whole milk, half and half, or whipped cream, then they are blended with sugar and fat. In their larger sizes, these drinks can supply 300–400 calories.

Get It Your Way

- ★ Order bagel spreads on the side so that you can control how much is put on.
- ★ Order butter or margarine on the side.
- ★ Opt for fat-free milk in specialty coffees and teas.
- ★ Order a sandwich on a bagel or roll, not on a high-fat croissant or biscuit.

Exclusive Web Content

Be sure to visit the following restaurants online at http://www.diabetes.org/healthyrestaurant

Carvel	**Godfather's**	**Whataburger**
Del Taco	**Jersey Mike's**	**Wienerschnitzel**
El Pollo Loco	**Jimmy John's**	**Zaxby's**
Frëshens	**Tim Hortons**	

(*Continued*)

Auntie Anne's (www.auntieannes.com)

Light 'n Lean Choice

Jalapeno Pretzel, without butter

Calories	270	Cholesterol (mg)	0
Fat (g)	1	Sodium (mg)	280
% calories from fat	3	Carbohydrate (g)	58
Saturated fat (g)	0	Fiber (g)	2
Trans fat (g)	0	Protein (g)	8

Exchanges: 3 1/2 starch

Healthy 'n Hearty Choice

Sour Cream & Onion Pretzel, without butter

Calories	310	Cholesterol (mg)	0
Fat (g)	1	Sodium (mg)	920
% calories from fat	9	Carbohydrate (g)	66
Saturated fat (g)	0	Fiber (g)	2
Trans fat (g)	0	Protein (g)	9

Exchanges: 4 starch

Auntie Anne's

	Amount	Cal.	Fat (g)	% Cal. Fat	Sat. Fat (g)	Trans Fat (g)	Chol. (mg)	Sod. (mg)	Carb. (g)	Fiber (g)	Pro. (g)	Choices/Exchanges
DIPPING SAUCES												
✔Caramel	1.5 oz	135	3	2	2	0	5	110	27	0	1	2 carb, 1/2 fat
✔Cheese Sauce	1.25 oz	100	8	7	4	0	10	510	4	0	3	2 fat
✔Hot Salsa Cheese Dip	1.25 oz	100	8	7	4	0	10	550	4	0	2	1 veg, 2 fat
✔Light Cream Cheese	1.25 oz	70	6	8	4	0	25	140	1	0	3	1 1/2 fat
✔Marinara Sauce	1.25 oz	10	0	0	0	0	0	180	4	0	0	Free
✔Sweet Mustard Sauce	1.25 oz	60	2	3	1	0	40	120	8	0	1	1/2 carb
✔Sweet Pretzel Sauce	1.4 oz	40	0	0	0	0	0	0	10	0	0	1/2 carb
DUTCH ICE												
Blue Raspberry	14 oz	165	0	0	0	0	0	20	38	0	0	2 1/2 carb

✔ = Healthiest Bets

(Continued)

DUTCH ICE *(Continued)*	Amount	Cal.	Fat (g)	% Cal. Fat	Sat. Fat (g)	Trans Fat (g)	Chol. (mg)	Sod. (mg)	Carb. (g)	Fiber (g)	Pro. (g)	Choices/Exchanges
Grape	14 oz	180	0	0	0	0	0	20	43	0	0	3 carb
Kiwi-Banana	14 oz	190	0	0	0	0	0	30	44	0	0	3 carb
Lemonade	14 oz	315	0	0	0	0	0	0	77	0	0	5 carb
Mocha	14 oz	400	10	2	9	0	0	100	74	0	0	5 carb, 1 fat
Orange Cream	14 oz	280	0	0	0	0	0	35	64	0	0	4 1/2 carb
Pina Colada	14 oz	220	0	0	0	0	0	150	53	0	0	3 1/2 carb
Strawberry	14 oz	220	0	0	0	0	0	40	50	0	0	3 1/2 carb
Strawberry Lemonade	14 oz	330	0	0	0	0	0	0	81	0	0	5 1/2 carb
Watermelon	14 oz	200	0	0	0	0	0	35	50	0	0	3 1/2 carb
Wild Cherry	14 oz	210	0	0	0	0	0	25	48	0	0	3 carb
DUTCH LATTE												
Caramel	14 oz	350	15	4	11	0	55	170	49	0	4	3 1/2 carb, 2 1/2 fat

Coffee	14 oz	290	14	4	9	0	50	135	38	0	4	2 1/2 carb, 3 fat
Mocha	14 oz	360	17	4	11	0	55	135	47	0	5	3 carb, 3 fat
DUTCH SHAKE												
Chocolate	14 oz	580	27	4	18	0	105	380	75	0	10	5 carb, 5 fat
Coffee	14 oz	590	27	4	18	0	105	304	77	0	10	5 carb, 5 fat
Strawberry	14 oz	610	27	4	18	0	105	304	78	0	10	5 carb, 5 fat
Vanilla	14 oz	510	27	5	17	0	105	300	58	0	10	4 carb, 5 fat
DUTCH SMOOTHIE												
Blue Raspberry	14 oz	230	8	3	5	0	30	100	34	0	3	2 1/2 carb, 1 1/2 fat
Grape	14 oz	230	8	3	5	0	30	100	36	0	3	2 1/2 carb, 1 1/2 fat
Kiwi-Banana	14 oz	240	8	3	5	0	30	100	38	0	3	2 1/2 carb, 1 fat
Lemonade	14 oz	300	8	2	5	0	30	80	53	0	3	3 1/2 carb, 1 fat
Mocha	14 oz	330	13	4	9	0	30	130	50	0	3	3 1/2 carb, 2 fat

✓ = Healthiest Bets

(Continued)

DUTCH SMOOTHIE ***(Continued)***	Amount	Cal.	Fat (g)	% Cal. Fat	Sat. Fat (g)	Trans Fat (g)	Chol. (mg)	Sod. (mg)	Carb. (g)	Fiber (g)	Pro. (g)	Choices/Exchanges
Orange Cream	14 oz	280	8	3	5	0	30	100	46	0	3	3 carb, 1 1/2 fat
Pina Colada	14 oz	260	8	3	5	0	30	90	44	0	3	3 carb, 1 fat
Strawberry	14 oz	250	8	3	5	0	30	100	40	0	3	2 1/2 carb, 1 fat
Wild Cherry	14 oz	250	8	3	5	0	30	90	41	0	3	2 1/2 carb, 1 fat
LEMONADE												
Lemonade	22 oz	180	0	0	0	0	0	0	43	0	0	3 carb
Strawberry Lemonade	22 oz	190	0	0		0	0	0	48	0	0	3 carb
PRETZELS WITH BUTTER												
Almond Pretzel	1	400	8	2	5	0	20	400	72	2	9	5 starch, 1 fat
Cinnamon Sugar Pretzel	1	450	9	2	5	0	25	430	83	3	8	5 1/2 starch, 1 fat
Garlic Pretzel	1	350	5	1	3	0	10	850	68	2	9	4 1/2 starch
Glazin Raisin Pretzel	1	510	4	1	2	0	10	480	107	4	11	7 starch

Jalapeno Pretzel	1	310	5	1	3	0	10	940	59	2	8	4 starch, 1/2 fat
Original Pretzel	1	370	4	1	2	0	10	930	72	3	10	5 starch, 1/2 fat
Pretzel Dog	1	290	16	5	7	1	40	600	25	1	10	1 1/2 starch, 3 fat
Sesame Pretzel	1	410	12	3	4	0	15	860	64	7	12	4 1/2 starch, 2 fat
Sour Cream & Onion Pretzel	1	340	5	1	3	0	10	930	66	2	9	4 1/2 starch, 1/2 fat
Stix	6 sticks	370	4	1	2	0	10	930	72	3	10	5 starch
Whole Wheat Pretzel	1	370	5	1	2	0	10	1120	72	7	11	5 starch, 1/2 fat
PRETZELS WITHOUT BUTTER												
Almond Pretzel	1	350	2	1	0.5	0	0	390	72	2	9	5 starch
Cinnamon Sugar Pretzel	1	350	2	1	0	0	0	410	74	2	9	5 starch
Garlic Pretzel	1	320	1	0	0	0	0	830	66	2	9	4 1/2 starch
Glazin Raisin Pretzel	1	470	1	0	0	0	0	460	104	3	11	6 1/2 starch
Jalapeno Pretzel	1	270	1	0	0	0	0	780	58	2	8	3 1/2 starch

✓ = Healthiest Bets

(Continued)

PRETZELS WITHOUT BUTTER *(Continued)*	Amount	Cal.	Fat (g)	% Cal. Fat	Sat. Fat (g)	Trans Fat (g)	Chol. (mg)	Sod. (mg)	Carb. (g)	Fiber (g)	Pro. (g)	Choices/Exchanges
Original Pretzel	1	340	1	0	0	0	0	900	72	3	10	4 1/2 starch
Sesame Pretzel	1	350	6	2	1	0	0	840	63	3	11	4 starch, 1/2 fat
Sour Cream & Onion Pretzel	1	310	1	0	0	0	0	920	66	2	9	4 starch
Stix	6 sticks	340	1	0	0	0	0	900	72	3	10	5 starch
Whole Wheat Pretzel	1	350	2	1	0	0	0	1100	72	7	11	5 starch

✓ = Healthiest Bets

Caribou Coffee (www.cariboucoffee.com)

Light 'n Lean Choice

Northern Lite Vanilla Latte, skim milk, no whipped cream *(small)*
Turkey & Roasted Red Pepper on Grilled Flatbread

Calories	470	Cholesterol (mg)	70
Fat (g)	12	Sodium (mg)	1,495
% calories from fat	23	Carbohydrate (g)	52
Saturated fat (g)	6	Fiber (g)	3
Trans fat (g)	0	Protein (g)	37

Exchanges: 2 1/2 starch, 3 lean meat, 1 milk, 1/2 fat

Healthy 'n Hearty Choice

Northern Lite Chocolate Cooler, no whipped cream *(small)*
Turkey & Smoked Mozzarella

Calories	650	Cholesterol (mg)	65
Fat (g)	18	Sodium (mg)	1,795
% calories from fat	25	Carbohydrate (g)	104
Saturated fat (g)	11	Fiber (g)	4
Trans fat (g)	0	Protein (g)	34

Exchanges: 3 1/2 starch, 2 1/2 carb, 3 lean meat, 1 milk, 2 fat

Caribou Coffee

	Amount	Cal.	Fat (g)	% Cal. Fat	Sat. Fat (g)	Trans Fat (g)	Chol. (mg)	Sod. (mg)	Carb. (g)	Fiber (g)	Pro. (g)	Choices/Exchanges
CLASSICS W/ 2% MILK, W/O WHIP												
Hot Cocoa	sm	270	6	2	4	0	25	180	43	0	12	2 carb, 1 milk, 1 fat
Kids Cocoa	sm	300	7	2	5	0	25	210	48	0	12	2 carb, 1 milk, 1 1/2 fat
Reindeer Drinks	sm	230	6	2	4	0	25	135	34	0	11	1 carb, 1 milk, 1 fat
White Hot Cocoa	sm	320	10	3	8	0	25	125	47	0	10	2 carb, 1 milk, 2 fat
COLD W/ 2% MILK, W/O WHIP												
✔Blended Chai Tea Latte	sm	170	3.5	2	2	0	15	80	28	0	6	1 carb, 1 milk, 1/2 fat

✔Iced Americana	sm	10	0	0	0	0	0	25	2	0	0	Free
✔Iced Chai Tea Latte	sm	170	3.5	2	2	0	15	80	28	0	6	1 carb, 1 milk, 1/2 fat
✔Iced Latte	sm	120	5	4	3	0	20	110	11	0	8	1 milk, 1 fat
Iced Mocha	sm	190	3	1	1.5	0	10	70	35	1	5	1 carb, 1 milk, 1/2 fat
COOLERS W/O WHIP												
Caramel	sm	240	1.5	1	1.5	0	0	70	55	0	2	2 1/2 carb, 1 milk, 1/2 fat
Chocolate	sm	250	3.5	1	2.5	0	0	70	51	2	3	2 carb, 1 milk, 1/2 fat
✔Coffee	sm	110	2	2	2	0	0	35	23	0	1	1/2 carb, 1 milk, 1/2 fat
✔Espresso	sm	90	1.5	2	1.5	0	0	40	18	0	1	1 milk, 1/2 fat
Vanilla	sm	280	4.5	1	4.5	0	0	80	56	0	3	2 1/2 carb, 1 milk, 1 fat
ESPRESSO W/ 2% MILK, W/O WHIP												
✔Americana	sm	5	0	0	0	0	0	10	1	0	0	Free

✔ = Healthiest Bets; na = not available

(*Continued*)

ESPRESSO W/ 2% MILK, W/O WHIP *(Continued)*	Amount	Cal.	Fat (g)	% Cal. Fat	Sat. Fat (g)	Trans Fat (g)	Chol. (mg)	Sod. (mg)	Carb. (g)	Fiber (g)	Pro. (g)	Choices/Exchanges
Breve	sm	310	26	8	16	0	80	105	11	0	7	1 milk, 5 fat
✔Cappuccino	sm	90	3.5	4	2	0	15	80	8	0	6	1 milk, 1/2 fat
✔Espresso	sm	5	0	0	0	0	0	10	1	0	0	Free
✔Latte	sm	140	6	4	3.5	0	20	125	13	0	9	1 milk, 1 fat
✔Macchiato	sm	5	0	0	0	0	0	15	1	0	1	Free
Mocha	sm	250	6	2	4	0	20	150	41	0	9	2 carb, 1 milk, 1 fat
White Chocolate Mocha	sm	310	10	3	8	0	20	100	46	0	8	2 carb, 1 milk, 2 fat
FRUIT												
✔Fresh Fruit Medley	1	120	0.5	0	0	0	0	30	29	2	2	2 fruit
NORTHERN LITE COOLERS W/O WHIP												
Caramel	sm	210	3	1	3	0	0	80	53	6	3	2 carb, 1 milk, 1/2 fat
Chocolate	sm	210	5	2	4.5	0	0	125	54	9	4	2 1/2 carb, 1 milk, 1 fat

Coffee	sm	130	4	3	3.5	0	0	100	36	8	3	1 carb, 1 milk, 1 fat
✔Espresso	sm	100	3	3	3	0	0	85	27	6	3	1 carb, 1 milk, 1/2 fat
Vanilla	sm	220	6	2	6	0	0	110	53	8	4	2 carb, 1 milk, 1 fat
NORTHERN LITE LATTES W/ SKIM MILK, W/O WHIP												
✔Caramel	sm	80	0	0	0	0	5	125	12	0	8	1 milk
✔Hazelnut	sm	80	0	0	0	0	5	125	12	0	8	1 milk
✔Raspberry	sm	80	0	0	0	0	5	125	12	0	8	1 milk
✔Turtle	sm	80	0	0	0	0	5	125	12	0	8	1 milk
✔Vanilla	sm	80	0	0	0	0	5	125	12	0	8	1 milk
SALADS												
Blue Ribbon Popcorn Chicken	1	530	35	6	8	0	130	640	10	2	43	1 starch, 3 veg, 6 lean meat, 3 fat

✔ = Healthiest Bets; na = not available

(*Continued*)

SALADS *(Continued)*	Amount	Cal.	Fat (g)	% Cal. Fat	Sat. Fat (g)	Trans Fat (g)	Chol. (mg)	Sod. (mg)	Carb. (g)	Fiber (g)	Pro. (g)	Choices/Exchanges
Italian Antipasto	1	584	42	6	9	0	37	1026	37	3	18	1 starch, 3 veg, 2 lean meat, 7 fat
Turkey & Cherry Pasta	1	457	27	5	4	0	53	486	35	3	18	1 starch, 3 veg, 2 lean meat, 4 fat
SANDWICHES												
Chicken Salad	1	637	35	5	6	0	98	695	49	4	29	3 1/2 starch, 3 lean meat, 5 fat
✔Chicken Salad on Marble Rye	1	450	21	4	3.5	0	75	610	33	4	31	2 starch, 3 lean meat, 2 fat
Cold Cut Combo	1	510	20	4	8	0	75	2000	50	2	24	3 1/2 starch, 2 medium-fat meat, 2 fat
Turkey & Roasted Red Pepper on Grilled Flatbread	1	390	12	3	6	0	65	1370	40	3	29	2 1/2 starch, 3 lean meat, 1/2 fat
Turkey & Smoked Mozzarella	1	440	13	3	6	0	65	1670	50	3	30	3 1/2 starch,

												3 lean meat, 1 fat
✔Turkey Breast	1	431	16	3	7	0	29	917	42	2	28	3 starch, 3 lean meat, 1 fat
SMOOTHIES												
Passion Fruit Green Tea	sm	200	0	0	0	0	0	35	48	0	1	2 carb, 1 fruit
Pom-A-Mango	sm	250	0	0	0	0	0	35	60	1	1	3 carb, 1 fruit
Strawberry Banana	sm	260	0	0	0	0	0	25	65	2	2	3 1/2 carb, 1 fruit
Wild Berry	sm	230	0	0	0	0	0	30	57	2	2	2 1/2 carb, 1 fruit
SNOWDRIFTS W/ 2% MILK, W/O WHIP												
Cookies & Cream	sm	470	13	2	10	0	15	290	79	1	9	3 carb, 2 milk, 2 fat
Mint	sm	350	10	3	8	0	15	110	58	0	8	2 carb, 2 milk, 1 1/2 fat
WILD W/O WHIP												
Campfire Mocha w/ Skim Milk	med	480	8	2	5	0	20	200	90	0	12	5 carb, 1 milk, 1 fat

✔ = Healthiest Bets; na = not available

(*Continued*)

WILD W/O WHIP *(Continued)*	Amount	Cal.	Fat (g)	% Cal. Fat	Sat. Fat (g)	Trans Fat (g)	Chol. (mg)	Sod. (mg)	Carb. (g)	Fiber (g)	Pro. (g)	Choices/Exchanges
Caramel High Rise w/ Skim Milk	med	320	7	2	4.5	0	30	210	53	0	12	2 1/2 carb, 1 milk, 1 1/2 fat
✔Chai Tea Latte, 2% Milk	sm	210	6	3	4	0	25	125	30	0	10	1 carb, 1 milk, 1 fat
Hot Apple Blast	med	340	0.5	0	0	0	0	75	84	1	1	5 1/2 carb
Lite White Berry w/ Skim Milk	med	390	6	1	5	0	5	140	74	0	10	4 carb, 1 milk, 1 fat
Mint Condition w/ 2% Milk	med	480	9	2	7	0	20	210	86	0	13	4 1/2 carb, 1 milk, 1 1/2 fat
Turtle Mocha w/ 2% Milk	med	500	7	1	4	0	20	250	96	0	13	5 carb, 1 milk, 1 1/2 fat
WRAPS												
Chicken Caesar	1	560	26	4	9	0	105	960	32	3	47	2 starch, 6 lean meat, 1 1/2 fat
Chipotle Turkey	1	450	12	2	2	0	53	3037	57	8	30	4 starch, 3 lean meat, 1 fat

Curry Chicken	1	590	32	5	7	0	50	850	57	2	22	4 starch, 2 lean meat, 5 fat
YOGURTS												
Low Fat Yogurt Parfait	1	239	4	2	2	0	6	169	44	2	7	2 carb, 1 milk, 1 fat

✔ = Healthiest Bets; na = not available

Dunkin' Donuts (www.dunkindonuts.com)

Light 'n Lean Choice

Egg Cheese English Muffin
Orange Juice

Calories	365	Cholesterol (mg)	190
Fat (g)	13	Sodium (mg)	1,081
% calories from fat	32	Carbohydrate (g)	47
Saturated fat (g)	5	Fiber (g)	0
Trans fat (g)	0	Protein (g)	15

Exchanges: 2 starch, 1 high-fat meat, 1 fruit, 1 fat

Healthy 'n Hearty Choice

Glazed Cake Donuts *(2)*
Latte *(10 oz)*

Calories	580	Cholesterol (mg)	25
Fat (g)	26	Sodium (mg)	735
% calories from fat	40	Carbohydrate (g)	70
Saturated fat (g)	14	Fiber (g)	2
Trans fat (g)	0	Protein (g)	14

Exchanges: 4 carb, 1 milk, 1/2 fat

Dunkin' Donuts

	Amount	Cal.	Fat (g)	% Cal. Fat	Sat. Fat (g)	Trans Fat (g)	Chol. (mg)	Sod. (mg)	Carb. (g)	Fiber (g)	Pro. (g)	Choices/Exchanges
BAGELS												
Blueberry	1	330	3	1	1	0	0	600	66	2	10	4 1/2 starch, 1/2 fat
Cinnamon Raisin	1	330	3	1	1	0	0	430	65	3	10	4 starch, 1/2 fat
Everything	1	370	6	1	1	0	0	650	67	3	14	4 1/2 starch, 1 fat
Multigrain	1	380	6	1	1	0	0	650	68	5	14	4 1/2 starch, 1 fat
Onion	1	320	4	1	1	0	0	610	61	3	12	4 starch, 1/2 fat
Plain	1	320	3	1	1	0	0	650	62	2	12	4 starch, 1/2 fat
Poppy seed	1	370	7	2	1	0	0	650	65	3	14	4 starch, 1 fat
Salt	1	320	3	1	1	0	0	4520	62	2	12	4 starch, 1/2 fat
Sesame	1	380	8	2	1	0	0	650	64	3	14	4 starch, 1 fat

✓ = Healthiest Bets

(*Continued*)

BAGELS *(Continued)*	Amount	Cal.	Fat (g)	% Cal. Fat	Sat. Fat (g)	Trans Fat (g)	Chol. (mg)	Sod. (mg)	Carb. (g)	Fiber (g)	Pro. (g)	Choices/Exchanges
Wheat	1	330	4	1	1	0	0	610	62	4	12	4 starch, 1/2 fat
BREAKFAST SANDWICHES												
Bacon Egg Cheese Bagel	1	540	18	3	7	0	200	1400	69	2	18	4 1/2 starch, 1 medium-fat meat, 2 1/2 fat
Bacon Egg Cheese Croissant	1	440	25	5	12	0	150	910	33	1	19	2 starch, 2 high-fat meat, 2 fat
Bacon Egg Cheese English Muffin	1	360	16	4	6	0	200	1300	36	0	17	2 starch, 2 high-fat meat
Bacon Lover's Supreme	1	640	43	6	19	1	280	1120	36	2	26	2 starch, 3 high-fat meat, 4 fat
Egg Cheese Bagel	1	470	15	3	6	0	190	1120	65	2	20	4 starch, 1 high-fat meat, 1 1/2 fat
Egg Cheese Biscuit	1	540	29	5	17	0	125	1390	53	2	16	3 1/2 starch, 1 high-fat meat, 4 fat

Egg Cheese Croissant	1	430	26	5	11	0	190	780	33	1	14	2 starch, 1 high-fat meat
Egg Cheese English Muffin	1	310	13	4	5	0	190	1080	35	1	14	2 starch, 1 high-fat meat, 1 fat
Ham Egg Cheese Bagel	1	510	16	3	6	0	200	1390	65	2	26	4 starch, 2 medium-fat meat, 1 fat
Ham Egg Cheese Croissant	1	460	27	5	12	0	205	1040	33	1	20	2 starch, 2 medium-fat meat, 3 1/2 fat
Ham Egg Cheese English Muffin	1	310	10	3	5	0	160	1270	34	1	21	2 starch, 2 medium-fat meat
Hash Browns	9 pcs	180	9	5	1	0	0	730	22	3	2	1 1/2 starch, 2 fat
Sausage Egg Cheese Bagel	1	660	35	5	13	.5	225	1450	63	3	28	4 starch, 2 high-fat meat, 3 1/2 fat
Sausage Egg Cheese Biscuit	1	800	32	4	24	0	235	1960	54	2	24	3 1/2 starch, 2 high-fat meat, 3 fat
Sausage Egg Cheese Croissant	1	630	45	6	17	1	230	1250	34	1	24	2 starch, 2 high-fat meat, 6 fat

✓ = Healthiest Bets

(*Continued*)

BREAKFAST SANDWICHES *(Continued)*	Amount	Cal.	Fat (g)	% Cal. Fat	Sat. Fat (g)	Trans Fat (g)	Chol. (mg)	Sod. (mg)	Carb. (g)	Fiber (g)	Pro. (g)	Choices/Exchanges
Sausage Egg Cheese English Muffin	1	530	32	5	12	.5	235	1610	37	1	23	2 1/2 starch, 3 high-fat meat, 1 fat
Supreme Omelet Sandwich on a Croissant	1	530	33	6	14	0	255	1070	35	2	21	2 starch, 2 medium-fat meat, 5 fat
COOKIES												
Chocolate Chunk	4.5 oz	540	23	4	13	0	50	550	80	3	7	5 carb, 4 1/2 fat
Oatmeal Raisin Pecan	4.5 oz	480	14	3	7	0	40	310	83	5	8	5 carb, 3 fat
Peanut Butter Cup	4.5 oz	590	29	4	13	0	50	530	73	3	11	5 carb, 6 fat
COOLATTA												
Cherry Lime SoBe	16 oz	250	0	0	0	0	0	65	62	2	0	4 carb
Coffee w/ 2% milk	16 oz	190	2	1	1.5	0	10	80	41	0	4	2 1/2 carb
Coffee w/ cream	16 oz	350	22	6	14	0	75	65	40	0	3	2 1/2 carb, 4 fat

Coffee w/ milk	16 oz	210	4	2	2.5	0	15	80	42	0	4	3 carb, 1 fat
Coffee w/ skim milk	16 oz	170	0	0	0	0	0	80	41	0	4	3 carb
Lemonade	16 oz	240	0	0	0	0	0	35	59	0	0	4 carb
Strawberry Fruit	16 oz	290	0	0	0	0	0	30	72	1	0	4 1/2 carb
Tropicana Orange	16 oz	370	0	0	0	0	0	50	92	3	1	6 carb
Vanilla Bean	16 oz	500	17	3	17	0	0	95	85	2	1	5 carb, 3 fat
CRAVINGS SANDWICHES												
Chicken Bruschetta	1	580	25	4	8	0	85	1450	48	4	42	3 starch, 5 lean meat, 2 fat
Chipotle Chicken	1	620	26	4	9	0	110	1730	49	4	49	3 starch, 6 lean meat, 1 1/2 fat
Pastrami Supreme	1	760	42	5	17	0	130	1990	47	5	48	3 starch, 6 medium-fat meat, 2 1/2 fat
Turkey Pesto	1	530	23	4	8	0	65	1630	48	4	33	3 starch, 3 lean meat, 3 fat

✓ = Healthiest Bets

(*Continued*)

	Amount	Cal.	Fat (g)	% Cal. Fat	Sat. Fat (g)	Trans Fat (g)	Chol. (mg)	Sod. (mg)	Carb. (g)	Fiber (g)	Pro. (g)	Choices/Exchanges
CREAM CHEESE												
✓Chive	4 T	170	17	9	11	0	45	230	4	2	4	3 fat
✓Garden Vegetable	4 T	170	15	8	11	0	45	340	4	0	2	3 1/2 fat
✓Lite	4 T	120	9	7	6	0	30	280	5	0	4	2 fat
✓Lite Garden Vegetable	4 T	100	8	7	5	0	25	270	5	0	3	1 1/2 fat
✓Plain	4 T	190	17	8	13	0	55	190	4	0	4	3 1/2 fat
Reduced Carb w/ Cheese	1	380	12	3	5	0	20	780	45	14	25	3 starch, 2 1/2 fat
✓Salmon	4 T	170	17	9	11	0	45	180	2	0	4	3 1/2 fat
✓Strawberry	4 T	190	17	8	9	0	45	150	9	0	4	3 1/2 fat
DANISH												
Apple	1	330	20	5	9	0	30	260	32	1	4	2 carb, 4 fat
Cheese	1	340	22	6	10	0	35	270	30	1	4	2 carb, 4 1/2 fat

Strawberry Cheese	1	320	20	6	9	0	30	260	31	1	4	2 carb, 4 fat
DELI CLASSICS SANDWICHES												
Ham and Swiss	1	360	11	3	5	0	45	1120	44	4	23	3 starch, 2 lean meat, 1 fat
Roast Beef and Swiss	1	530	25	4	8	0	80	1290	45	4	31	3 starch, 3 lean meat, 3 fat
Tuna	1	550	26	4	5	0	35	830	49	4	29	3 starch, 3 lean meat, 3 fat
Turkey and Cheese	1	510	22	4	6	0	65	1380	45	4	35	3 starch, 4 lean meat, 2 fat
Vegetarian	1	420	21	5	3	0	5	480	51	8	9	3 starch, 1 veg, 4 fat
DONUTS												
✔Gingerbread	1	280	4	1	1	0	45	400	56	1	5	3 1/2 carb, 1 fat
Wheat Glazed Cake	1	310	19	6	8	0	0	380	32	2	4	2 carb, 4 fat
Apple Crumb	1	320	13	4	6	0	0	360	45	2	4	3 carb, 2 1/2 fat
Apple N' Spice	1	260	11	4	5	0	0	350	35	2	4	2 carb, 2 fat
Bavarian Kreme	1	250	6	2	6	0	20	460	52	1	4	3 1/2 carb, 1 fat

✔ = Healthiest Bets

(*Continued*)

DONUTS ***(Continued)***	**Amount**	**Cal.**	**Fat (g)**	**% Cal. Fat**	**Sat. Fat (g)**	**Trans Fat (g)**	**Chol. (mg)**	**Sod. (mg)**	**Carb. (g)**	**Fiber (g)**	**Pro. (g)**	**Choices/Exchanges**
✔Black Raspberry	1	270	10	3	5	0	0	350	40	1	4	2 1/2 carb, 2 fat
Blueberry Cake	1	290	16	5	6	0	10	400	35	1	3	2 carb, 3 fat
Blueberry Crumb	1	330	13	4	6	0	0	360	48	2	4	3 carb, 2 1/2 fat
Boston Kreme	1	270	12	4	5	0	0	370	38	1	4	2 1/2 carb, 3 fat
Chocolate Coconut	1	370	21	5	11	0	0	380	42	3	3	3 carb, 4 fat
Chocolate Frosted	1	330	19	5	9	0	15	260	36	2	4	2 1/2 carb, 4 fat
Chocolate Glazed	1	340	19	5	9	0	0	360	39	2	3	2 1/2 carb, 4 fat
Chocolate Kreme Filled	1	300	14	4	6	0	0	360	39	2	4	2 1/2 carb, 3 fat
Cinnamon	1	310	18	5	9	0	15	260	34	2	3	2 carb, 3 1/2 fat
Double Chocolate	1	340	20	5	9	0	0	360	36	3	3	2 carb, 4 fat
✔French Cruller	1	150	8	5	5	0	20	105	17	1	2	1 carb, 2 1/2 fat
Glazed	1	330	18	5	9	0	15	260	38	2	3	2 1/2 carb, 3 1/2 fat
✔Glazed Cake	1	230	10	4	5	0	0	320	30	1	4	2 carb

✔Jelly Filled	1	270	10	3	5	0	0	350	39	1	4	2 1/2 carb, 2 fat
✔Maple Frosted	1	240	10	4	5	0	0	320	31	1	4	2 carb, 2 fat
Marble Frosted	1	230	11	4	5	0	0	320	30	1	4	2 carb, 2 fat
Mini M&M	1	270	12	4	5	0	0	360	39	1	4	2 1/2 carb, 2 1/2 fat
Old Fashioned Cake	1	280	18	6	9	0	15	260	26	2	3	1 1/2 carb, 3 1/2 fat
Powdered	1	310	18	5	9	0	15	260	34	2	3	3 carb, 3 1/2 fat
Pumpkin Glazed	1	280	6	2	6	0	20	460	52	1	4	3 1/2 carb, 1 fat
✔Strawberry Frosted	1	240	10	4	5	0	0	330	32	1	4	2 carb, 2 fat
✔Sugar Raised	1	210	10	4	5	0	0	320	27	1	4	2 carb, 2 fat
Vanilla Kreme Filled	1	320	16	5	7	0	0	360	39	1	4	2 1/2 carb, 3 fat
FANCIES												
Apple Fritter	1	290	13	4	6	0	0	360	35	2	4	2 carb, 2 1/2 fat
Bow Tie Donut	1	300	17	5	8	0	0	340	34	1	4	2 carb, 3 fat

✔ = Healthiest Bets

(*Continued*)

FANCIES *(Continued)*	Amount	Cal.	Fat (g)	% Cal. Fat	Sat. Fat (g)	Trans Fat (g)	Chol. (mg)	Sod. (mg)	Carb. (g)	Fiber (g)	Pro. (g)	Choices/Exchanges
Chocolate Frosted Coffee Roll	1	340	20	5	9	0	0	340	36	1	4	2 carb, 4 fat
Chocolate Iced Bismarck	1	340	15	4	6	0	0	290	50	1	3	3 1/2 carb, 3 fat
Coffee Roll	1	340	20	5	9	0	0	340	33	1	4	2 carb, 4 fat
Éclair	1	300	15	5	6	0	0	260	39	1	3	2 1/2 carb, 3 fat
Glazed Fritter	1	250	13	5	6	0	0	330	31	1	4	2 carb, 2 1/2 fat
Maple Frosted Coffee Roll	1	340	20	5	9	0	0	340	36	1	4	2 carb, 4 fat
Vanilla Frosted Coffee Roll	1	340	20	5	9	0	0	340	36	1	4	2 carb, 4 fat
FAVORITES SANDWICHES												
Avocado and Turkey	1	500	22	4	3	0	40	1330	49	8	38	3 starch, 4 lean meat, 2 fat
Chicken Cordon Bleu	1	550	19	3	7	0	95	1370	51	4	45	3 starch, 5 lean meat, 1 fat
Steak and Cheese	1	510	23	4	6	0	75	1830	45	4	30	3 starch, 3 medium-fat meat, 1 1/2 fat

Toasted Italian	1	630	34	5	12	0	90	2330	49	5	35	3 starch, 5 medium-fat meat, 2 fat
FLAT BREAD SANDWICHES												
Ham and Swiss	1	350	12	3	5	0	35	1040	41	2	20	3 starch, 2 lean meat, 1 fat
Three Cheese	1	460	24	5	12	0	55	1000	42	2	20	3 starch, 2 high-fat meat, 1/2 fat
Turkey, Cheddar and Bacon	1	360	13	3	5	0	35	1060	41	2	20	3 starch, 2 lean meat, 1 fat
HOT CHOCOLATE												
Dunkaccino	10 oz	230	11	4	9	0	10	5	35	0	2	2 carb, 2 fat
Hot Chocolate	10 oz	230	7	3	7	0	0	290	39	2	2	2 1/2 carb, 2 fat
Milky Way Hot Chocolate	10 oz	200	7	3	6	0	0	410	37	1	1	2 1/2 carb
Vanilla Chai	10 oz	230	8	3	6	0	5	50	40	0	1	3 carb
White Hot Chocolate	10 oz	230	9	4	7	0	0	290	37	0	2	2 1/2 carb

✓ = Healthiest Bets

(*Continued*)

	Amount	Cal.	Fat (g)	% Cal. Fat	Sat. Fat (g)	Trans Fat (g)	Chol. (mg)	Sod. (mg)	Carb. (g)	Fiber (g)	Pro. (g)	Choices/Exchanges
HOT ESPRESSO DRINKS												
✔Cappuccino	10 oz	80	5	6	2.5	0	20	70	7	0	4	1 milk
✔Cappuccino w/ Soy Milk	10 oz	70	3	4	0	0	0	80	6	1	4	1 milk
✔Cappuccino w/ Soy Milk & Sugar	10 oz	120	3	2	0	0	0	80	20	1	4	1/2 carb, 1 milk
✔Cappuccino w/ Sugar	10 oz	130	5	3	2.5	0	15	65	21	0	4	1/2 carb, 1 milk, 1 fat
Caramel Cream Latte	10 oz	260	9	3	6	0	20	125	40	0	8	2 carb, 1 milk, 2 fat
Caramel Swirl Latte	10 oz	230	6	2	3.5	0	25	140	36	0	8	2 carb, 1 milk
Caramel Swirl Latte w/ Soy Milk	10 oz	210	4	2	0	0	0	160	34	1	8	1 1/2 carb, 1 milk
✔Espresso	2 oz	0	0	0	0	0	0	5	1	0	0	Free
✔Espresso w/ Sugar	2 oz	30	0	0	0	0	0	5	7	0	0	1/2 carb
Gingerbread Latte	10 oz	330	9	2	5	0	30	160	54	0	9	3 carb, 1 milk, 2 fat

✔Hot Latte Lite	10 oz	70	0	0	0	0	50	80	10	0	6	1 milk
✔Latte	10 oz	120	6	5	3.5	0	25	95	10	0	6	1 milk, 1/2 fat
✔Latte w/ Soy Milk	10 oz	90	4	4	0	0	0	110	8	1	6	1 milk
✔Latte w/ Soy Milk & Sugar	10 oz	150	4	2	0	0	0	110	22	1	6	1/2 carb, 1 milk
Latte w/ Sugar	10 oz	160	6	3	3.5	0	25	95	22	0	6	1/2 carb, 1 milk, 1 fat
Mocha Almond Latte	10 oz	290	10	3	7	0	20	115	46	1	8	2 carb, 1 milk, 2 fat
Mocha Swirl Latte	10 oz	230	7	3	4	0	25	110	37	1	6	2 carb, 1/2 milk, 1 fat
Mocha Swirl Latte w/ Soy Milk	10 oz	210	5	2	1	0	0	130	35	2	7	2 carb, 1/2 milk, 1 fat
Pumpkin Spice Latte	10 oz	220	6	2	3.5	0	20	130	34	0	8	1 1/2 carb, 1 milk
Turbo Hot Latte	10 oz	130	6	4	3.5	0	20	55	20	0	1	1/2 carb, 1 milk
✔Vanilla Latte Lite	10 oz	80	0	0	0	0	5	80	10	0	6	1 milk

✔ = Healthiest Bets

(*Continued*)

	Amount	Cal.	Fat (g)	% Cal. Fat	Sat. Fat (g)	Trans Fat (g)	Chol. (mg)	Sod. (mg)	Carb. (g)	Fiber (g)	Pro. (g)	Choices/Exchanges
ICED ESPRESSO DRINKS												
Iced Caramel Cream Latte	16 oz	260	9	3	6	0	20	125	40	0	8	2 carb, 1 milk
Iced Caramel Swirl Latte	16 oz	240	7	3	4	0	25	150	37	0	8	1 1/2 carb, 1 milk, 1 fat
Iced Caramel Swirl Latte w/ fat-free milk	16 oz	180	0	0	0	0	0	150	36	0	8	1 1/2 carb, 1 milk
✔Iced Latte	16 oz	120	7	5	4	0	25	105	11	0	6	1 milk
✔Iced Latte Lite	16 oz	80	0	0	0	0	0	110	13	0	7	1 milk
✔Iced Latte w/ fat-free milk	16 oz	70	0	0	0	0	0	110	11	0	7	1 milk
✔Iced Latte w/ fat-free milk and sugar	16 oz	120	0	0	0	0	0	110	23	0	7	1/2 carb, 1 milk
✔Iced Latte w/ Sugar	16 oz	170	7	4	4	0	25	110	23	0	6	1 carb, 1 milk
Iced Mocha Almond Latte	16 oz	290	10	3	7	0	20	115	46	1	8	2 carb, 1 milk

Iced Mocha Swirl Latte	16 oz	240	8	3	4.5	0	25	125	38	1	7	1 1/2 carb, 1 milk
Iced Mocha Swirl Latte w/ fat-free milk	16 oz	180	1	1	1	0	0	115	37	1	7	1 1/2 carb, 1 milk
Turbo Ice	16 oz	120	7	5	3.5	0	20	25	14	0	1	1 carb, 1 1/2 fat
MUFFINS & MISC.												
Banana Walnut Muffin	1	540	25	4	3.5	0	65	520	69	3	10	4 1/2 carb, 4 fat
Biscuit	1	440	22	5	13	0	0	980	51	2	7	3 1/2 starch, 4 1/2 fat
Blueberry Muffin	1	470	17	3	3	0	60	500	73	2	8	5 carb, 2 fat
Chocolate Chip Muffin	1	630	26	4	8	0	70	560	89	2	10	5 1/2 carb, 4 fat
Cinnamon Cake	4	270	15	5	3.5	4	25	210	31	1	3	2 carb, 2 1/2 fat
Coffee Cake Muffin	1	580	19	3	3	0	65	520	78	1	9	5 carb, 4 fat
Corn Muffin	1	510	18	3	3.5	0	75	860	77	1	8	5 carb, 3 fat
Cranberry Orange Muffin	1	440	17	3	3	0	65	480	66	3	8	4 1/2 carb, 3 fat

✔ = Healthiest Bets

(*Continued*)

MUFFINS & MISC. *(Continued)*	Amount	Cal.	Fat (g)	% Cal. Fat	Sat. Fat (g)	Trans Fat (g)	Chol. (mg)	Sod. (mg)	Carb. (g)	Fiber (g)	Pro. (g)	Choices/Exchanges
Croissant	1	27	14	47	6	0	0	300	30	1	6	2 starch, 3 fat
✔English Muffin	1	160	1.5	1	0	0	0	340	31	2	1	2 starch
Honey Bran Raisin Muffin	1	480	15	3	2.5	0	60	480	79	5	8	5 carb, 2 fat
Reduced Fat Blueberry Muffin	1	400	5	1	2	0	60	480	78	3	8	5 carb, 1 fat
MUNCHKINS												
Cinnamon Cake	4	260	15	5	7	0	10	210	29	2	3	2 carb, 3 fat
Glazed	4	300	15	5	7	0	10	210	38	2	3	2 1/2 carb, 1 1/2 fat
Glazed Cake	4	300	15	5	7	0	10	210	38	1	3	2 1/2 carb, 1 1/2 fat
Glazed Chocolate Cake	4	300	15	5	7	0	10	290	38	1	3	2 1/2 carb, 1 1/2 fat
✔Jelly Filled	5	240	8	3	3.5	0	0	280	37	1	3	2 1/2 carb, 1 1/2 fat
Plain Cake	4	230	15	6	7	0	10	210	21	1	3	1 1/2 carb, 3 fat

Powdered Cake	4	260	15	5	7	0	10	210	29	2	3	2 carb, 3 fat
✔Sugar Raised	5	190	8	4	3.5	0	0	270	26	1	3	1 1/2 carb, 1 fat
PERSONAL PIZZA												
✔Cheese	1	400	19	4	10	0	25	820	46	2	18	3 starch, 1 high-fat meat, 3 fat
✔Pepperoni	1	410	19	4	9	0	35	960	45	2	19	3 starch, 1 high-fat meat, 2 fat
SALADS												
Caesar Salad	1	390	33	8	7	0	35	980	14	3	10	3 veg, 6 fat
Chicken Caesar	1	520	36	6	8	0	85	152	16	3	34	1/2 starch, 2 veg, 4 lean meat, 5 fat
Garden Salad	1	240	12	5	5	0	30	430	24	5	12	4 veg, 2 1/2 fat
Mediterranean Salad	1	220	11	5	4	0	15	760	23	5	10	4 veg, 2 fat

✔ = Healthiest Bets

(Continued)

SALADS *(Continued)*	Amount	Cal.	Fat (g)	% Cal. Fat	Sat. Fat (g)	Trans Fat (g)	Chol. (mg)	Sod. (mg)	Carb. (g)	Fiber (g)	Pro. (g)	Choices/Exchanges
Oriental Salad	1	580	35	5	5	1	45	1510	39	4	30	1 starch, 4 veg, 3 medium-fat meat, 4 fat
SMOOTHIE												
Mango Passion Fruit	24 oz	550	4	1	2.5	0	10	180	118	3	10	7 1/2 carb
Strawberry Banana	24 oz	550	4	1	2.5	0	10	180	118	3	10	7 1/2 carb
Wildberry	24 oz	550	4	1	2.5	0	10	180	118	2	10	7 1/2 carb
SOUPS												
Broccoli and Cheese	1 cup	180	13	7	8	0	40	1310	10	1	7	1 starch, 1 medium-fat meat, 1 1/2 fat
✔Chicken Noodle	1 cup	140	4	3	1	0	45	840	20	1	8	1 starch, 1 lean meat
Clam Chowder	1 cup	230	11	4	4	0	30	990	20	1	10	1 starch, 1 milk, 2 fat
Lasagna Soup	1 cup	250	13	5	5	0	35	810	21	2	11	1 1/2 starch, 1 lean meat, 2 fat

✔Timberline Chili w/ Beans	1 cup	230	8	3	3	0	35	890	26	8	15	1 starch, 2 veg, 1 lean meat
STICKS												
Cinnamon Cake	1	340	20	5	10	0	15	290	37	2	4	2 1/2 carb, 4 fat
Glazed Cake	1	360	20	5	10	0	15	280	41	2	4	3 carb, 4 fat
Glazed Chocolate	1	370	21	5	10	0	0	390	41	2	3	3 carb, 4 fat
Jelly	1	420	20	4	10	0	15	310	53	2	4	3 1/2 carb, 4 fat
Plain Cake	1	310	20	6	10	0	15	250	29	2	4	2 carb, 4 fat
Powdered Cake	1	340	20	5	10	0	15	280	37	2	4	2 1/2 carb, 4 fat

✔ = Healthiest Bets

Einstein Bros Bagels (www.einsteinbros.com)

Light 'n Lean Choice

Pumpernickel Bagel
Whipped Garden Vegetable Cream Cheese, Reduced-Fat *(2 Tbsp)*
Nonfat Milk Cappuccino *(12 oz)*

Calories	390	Cholesterol (mg)	20
Fat (g)	7	Sodium (mg)	905
% calories from fat	16	Carbohydrate (g)	70
Saturated fat (g)	3.5	Fiber (g)	3
Trans fat (g)	0	Protein (g)	17

Exchanges: 4 starch, 1 milk, 1 fat

Healthy 'n Hearty Choice

Deli Tuna Sandwich
Fruit Salad *(5 oz)*

Calories	500	Cholesterol (mg)	35
Fat (g)	15	Sodium (mg)	935
% calories from fat	27	Carbohydrate (g)	66
Saturated fat (g)	2.5	Fiber (g)	5
Trans fat (g)	0	Protein (g)	30

Exchanges: 3 1/2 starch, 1 fruit, 3 lean meat, 1 fat

Einstein Bros Bagels

	Amount	Cal.	Fat (g)	% Cal. Fat	Sat. Fat (g)	Trans Fat (g)	Chol. (mg)	Sod. (mg)	Carb. (g)	Fiber (g)	Pro. (g)	Choices/Exchanges
BAGEL PRETZELS												
Asiago Cheese	1	300	5	2	2	0	5	740	57	2	12	4 starch, 1 fat
Cinnamon Sugar	1	330	3	1	0.5	0	0	660	71	3	9	4 1/2 starch, 1/2 fat
✔Plain	1	270	3	1	0.5	0	0	660	57	2	9	4 starch, 1/2 fat
Salt	1	270	3	1	0.5	0	0	1770	57	2	9	4 starch, 1/2 fat
BAGELS												
Asiago Cheese	1	320	5	1	3	0	15	660	58	2	15	4 starch, 1 fat
Blueberry	1	290	2	1	0	0	0	480	64	3	9	4 starch
Chocolate Chip	1	290	3	1	1	0	0	460	60	3	10	4 starch, 1/2 fat

✔ = Healthiest Bets

(*Continued*)

BAGELS ***(Continued)***	**Amount**	**Cal.**	**Fat (g)**	**% Cal. Fat**	**Sat. Fat (g)**	**Trans Fat (g)**	**Chol. (mg)**	**Sod. (mg)**	**Carb. (g)**	**Fiber (g)**	**Pro. (g)**	**Choices/Exchanges**
Cinnamon Raisin Swirl	1	290	1	0	0	0	0	450	64	3	10	4 starch
Cinnamon Sugar	1	310	3	1	0.5	0	0	510	66	3	9	4 starch, 1/2 fat
Cranberry	1	290	1	0	0	0	0	450	64	3	9	4 starch
Egg	1	300	6	2	1.5	0	150	480	52	2	12	3 1/2 starch, 1 fat
Everything	1	290	2	1	0	0	0	650	60	2	10	4 starch
Fruit and Nut Power Bagel	1	380	6	1	1	0	0	330	72	5	13	4 1/2 starch, 1 fat
Garlic Dip'd	1	290	3	1	0	0	0	490	60	2	10	4 starch, 1/2 fat
Good Grains	1	290	3	1	0	0	0	480	63	4	10	4 starch, 1/2 fat
Honey Whole Wheat	1	270	1	0	0	0	0	480	61	3	9	4 starch
Onion Dip'd	1	290	1	0	0	0	0	490	63	2	9	4 starch
Plain	1	270	1	0	0	0	0	490	59	2	9	4 starch
Poppy Dip'd	1	290	3	1	0	0	0	490	60	2	10	4 starch, 1/2 fat
Potato	1	260	1	0	0	0	0	540	58	2	9	3 1/2 starch

Pumpernickel	1	270	2	1	0	0	0	710	58	3	10	4 starch
Sesame Dip'd	1	310	3	1	0	0	0	530	62	2	11	4 starch, 1/2 fat
Sun dried Tomato	1	270	2	1	0	0	0	570	58	3	10	4 starch
BREAKFAST SANDWICHES												
Bacon & Spinach Panini	1 srvg	870	50	5	15	0	465	1700	69	7	40	4 1/2 starch, 3 high-fat meat, 5 fat
Egg Way w/ Bacon	1 srvg	620	26	4	12	0	435	1120	63	2	36	4 starch, 4 medium-fat meat, 1 fat
Egg Way w/ Black Forest Ham	1 srvg	590	23	4	10	0	440	1390	62	2	40	4 starch, 4 medium-fat meat, 1/2 fat
Egg Way w/ Sausage	1 srvg	620	25	4	11	0	450	1050	63	2	39	4 starch, 4 medium-fat meat, 1 fat
Egg Way, Spinach Mushroom & Swiss Omelets	1 srvg	550	22	4	9	0	410	880	65	3	30	4 starch, 2 medium-fat meat, 2 fat

✓ = Healthiest Bets

(*Continued*)

BREAKFAST SANDWICHES *(Continued)*	Amount	Cal.	Fat (g)	% Cal. Fat	Sat. Fat (g)	Trans Fat (g)	Chol. (mg)	Sod. (mg)	Carb. (g)	Fiber (g)	Pro. (g)	Choices/Exchanges
Original Egg Way	1 srvg	550	21	3	10	0	420	870	62	3	31	4 starch, 3 medium-fat meat
Sausage Ranchero Panini	1 srvg	700	30	4	13	0	465	1410	66	5	44	4 1/2 starch, 4 high-fat meat
Vegetable Breakfast Panini	1 srvg	740	36	4	17	0	445	1330	70	4	38	4 starch, 1 veg, 3 medium-fat meat, 4 fat
BREAKFAST WRAPS												
Sante Fe	1 srvg	760	35	4	13	0	450	1440	76	8	35	5 starch, 3 high-fat meat, 2 fat
Spicy Elmo	1 srvg	740	42	5	18	0	465	1100	56	6	36	4 starch, 3 high-fat meat, 4 fat
CREAM CHEESE												
✔Plain	2 T	70	7	9	4.5	0	20	65	1	0	1	1 1/2 fat

✔Whipped Garden Vegetable Reduced Fat	2 T	60	5	8	3.5	0	15	100	3	0	1	1 fat
✔Whipped Garlic Herb Reduced Fat	2 T	60	5	8	3.5	0	15	100	3	0	1	1 fat
✔Whipped Honey Almond Reduced Fat	2 T	70	5	6	3	0	15	45	6	0	1	1 fat
✔Whipped Jalapeno Salsa Reduced Fat	2 T	60	5	8	3.5	0	15	105	3	0	1	1 fat
✔Whipped Onion and Chive	2 T	70	6	8	4	0	20	60	3	0	1	1 fat
✔Whipped Plain Reduced Fat	2 T	60	5	8	3.5	0	15	100	2	0	1	1 fat
✔Whipped Smoked Salmon	2 T	60	6	9	3.5	0	20	120	2	0	1	1 fat
✔Whipped Strawberry Reduced Fat	2 T	70	5	6	3.5	0	15	50	5	0	1	1 fat

✔ = Healthiest Bets

(Continued)

	Amount	Cal.	Fat (g)	% Cal. Fat	Sat. Fat (g)	Trans Fat (g)	Chol. (mg)	Sod. (mg)	Carb. (g)	Fiber (g)	Pro. (g)	Choices/Exchanges
DELI MELTS												
Ham Deli Melt	1	540	18	3	10	0	80	1810	62	3	38	4 starch, 4 lean meat, 1/2 fat
Pastrami Deli Melt	1	560	19	3	10	0.5	95	1800	64	3	40	4 starch, 4 medium-fat meat
Tuna Salad Deli Melt	1	610	25	4	11	0.5	80	1160	64	3	40	4 starch, 4 medium-fat meat, 1 fat
Turkey Deli Melt	1	530	17	3	9	0	85	1520	62	3	40	4 starch, 4 lean meat, 1 fat
Veggie Deli Melt	1	660	30	4	17	0	75	1400	76	5	25	4 starch, 2 veg, 2 high-fat meat, 3 fat
DELI SANDWICHES												
Deli Bacon	1 srvg	830	52	6	14	0.5	105	1930	52	4	39	3 1/2 starch, 4 high-fat meat, 4 fat
Deli Chicken Salad	1 srvg	970	79	7	12	1.5	70	850	51	4	16	3 1/2 starch, 1 lean meat, 15 fat

Deli Ham	1	590	32	5	9	0	100	1770	45	2	32	3 starch, 3 lean meat, 4 fat
Deli Pastrami	1	650	34	5	9	1	85	1960	53	5	36	3 1/2 starch, 4 high-fat meat
✔Deli Tuna Salad	1	440	15	3	2.5	0	35	920	50	4	29	3 1/2 starch, 3 lean meat, 1 fat
Deli Turkey and Swiss	1	700	42	5	9	1	85	1530	49	4	37	3 starch, 3 medium-fat meat, 6 fat
GOURMET BAGELS												
Dutch Apple	1	350	4	1	2	0	0	570	71	3	9	4 1/2 starch, 1 fat
Green Chili	1	370	9	2	5	0	25	740	60	2	16	4 starch, 2 fat
Six-Cheese	1	340	6	2	4	0	15	680	58	2	15	4 starch, 1 fat
Spinach Florentine	1	360	9	2	5	0	25	630	59	3	16	4 starch, 2 fat
ICED SPECIALTY COFFEE												
Iced Mocha	12 oz	210	6	3	4	0	15	120	33	0	7	1 carb, 1 milk, 1 fat

✔ = Healthiest Bets

(*Continued*)

ICED SPECIALTY COFFEE *(Continued)*	Amount	Cal.	Fat (g)	% Cal. Fat	Sat. Fat (g)	Trans Fat (g)	Chol. (mg)	Sod. (mg)	Carb. (g)	Fiber (g)	Pro. (g)	Choices/Exchanges
✔Iced Nonfat Latte	16 oz	90	0	0	0	0	5	130	12	0	8	1 milk
Low Fat Iced Mocha	16 oz	180	3	2	2	0	5	115	32	0	7	1 carb, 1 milk
Whole Milk Iced Latte	16 oz	190	9	4	5	0	25	150	17	0	9	1 milk, 2 fat
OTHER HOT BEVERAGES												
Chai Tea w/ 2% Milk	12 oz	220	2	1	1	0	5	65	47	0	3	4 carb
Chai Tea w/ Nonfat Milk	12 oz	210	0	0	0	0	0	65	47	0	3	4 carb
Chai Tea w/ Whole Milk	12 oz	230	3	1	1.5	0	10	55	47	0	3	3 1/2 carb, 1/2 fat
Hot Chocolate	12 oz	290	11	3	8	0	20	160	39	0	9	1 carb, 1 milk, 2 fat
Hot Chocolate w/ Whole Milk	12 oz	320	14	4	10	0	30	160	39	0	9	1/2 carb, 1 milk, 3 fat
PANINI SANDWICHES												
Italian Chicken	1	810	40	4	12	0	125	2490	67	5	47	4 1/2 starch, 4 medium-fat meat, 4 fat

Turkey Club	1	790	39	4	11	0	110	2340	68	7	47	4 1/2 starch, 4 medium-fat meat, 4 fat
SALAD DRESSING												
Caesar	2 T	150	16	10	2.5	0	10	350	1	0	1	3 fat
✔Chile Lime	2 T	60	4	6	0	0	0	650	5	0	1	1 fat
Raspberry Vinaigrette	2 T	160	14	8	2	0	0	0	8	0	0	3 fat
SALADS												
Bros Bistro Salad	10.5 oz	820	68	7	11	0	25	320	38	7	14	1/2 starch, 6 veg, 1 high-fat meat, 12 fat
Bros Bistro Salad w/ Chicken	14 oz	940	71	7	12	0	105	810	39	7	36	1/2 starch, 6 veg, 4 lean meat, 12 fat
Caesar Salad w/ Chicken	14 oz	700	54	7	11	0	120	1840	23	4	34	1/2 starch, 4 veg, 4 lean meat
Chipotle Salad	12 oz	600	39	6	9	0	20	1490	53	10	13	1 starch, 8 veg, 1 high-fat meat, 6 fat

✔ = Healthiest Bets

(*Continued*)

SALADS *(Continued)*	Amount	Cal.	Fat (g)	% Cal. Fat	Sat. Fat (g)	Trans Fat (g)	Chol. (mg)	Sod. (mg)	Carb. (g)	Fiber (g)	Pro. (g)	Choices/Exchanges
Chicken Chipotle Salad	15 oz	720	41	5	10	0	100	1980	54	10	35	1 starch, 8 veg, 4 lean meat, 5 1/2 fat
Half Bros. Bistro Salad	5.3 oz	410	34	7	5	0	15	160	19	3	7	4 veg, 1 high-fat meat, 3 fat
Half Bros. Bistro Salad w/ Chicken	7.3 oz	480	36	7	6	0	55	440	19	3	19	4 veg, 2 lean meat, 6 fat
Half Caesar Salad	4.5 oz	270	25	8	5	0	20	630	8	2	6	2 veg, 5 fat
Half Caesar Salad w/ Chicken	6.5 oz	340	27	7	6	0	65	920	9	2	18	2 veg, 2 lean meat, 4 fat
Half Chicken Chipotle Salad	7.9 oz	370	22	5	5	0	45	990	27	5	19	5 veg, 2 lean meat, 3 fat
✔Half Chipotle Salad	5.9 oz	300	19	6	4.5	0	10	750	26	6	7	5 veg, 1 high-fat meat, 3 fat

SIDE SALADS AND EXTRAS												
Candied Walnuts	1.5 oz	260	22	8	0	0	0	20	9	3	4	1/2 carb, 1 high-fat meat, 3 fat
Cole Slaw	5 oz	650	65	9	10	1	50	340	17	1	1	3 veg, 13 fat
✔Fruit Salad	5 oz	60	0	0	0	0	0	15	16	1	1	1 fruit
SIDES												
✔Bagel Croutons	1.2 oz	100	4	4	1	0	0	250	16	1	2	1 starch
✔Fruit and Yogurt Plate	1 srvg	180	1	1	0	0	5	140	36	4	9	1 1/2 fruit, 1 milk
✔Fruit Salad	11 oz	140	0	0	0	0	0	35	36	3	2	2 fruit
Kettle Classic Potato Chips	1 oz	100	10	9	2	0	0	130	11	1	1	1 starch, 2 fat
Traditional Potato Salad	1/2 cup	355	29	7	4	0	20	550	20	2	3	1 starch, 6 fat
SPECIALTY BREAD												
✔Braided Challah Roll	1	220	4	2	0.5	0	60	500	41	1	8	3 starch, 1 fat

✔ = Healthiest Bets

(*Continued*)

SPECIALTY BREAD *(Continued)*	Amount	Cal.	Fat (g)	% Cal. Fat	Sat. Fat (g)	Trans Fat (g)	Chol. (mg)	Sod. (mg)	Carb. (g)	Fiber (g)	Pro. (g)	Choices/Exchanges
Ciabatta bread	1	290	3	1	0	0	0	640	60	2	10	4 starch, 1/2 fat
✔Multi-Grain Bread	1 slice	130	3	2	0	0	0	220	23	2	5	1 1/2 starch, 1/2 fat
✔Americano	8 oz	1	0	0	0	0	0	0	0	0	0	Free
✔Espresso	2 oz	1	0	0	0	0	0	0	0	0	0	Free
SPECIALTY COFFEE												
Low Fat Regular Mocha	11 oz	240	10	4	6	0	40	135	29	0	7	1/2 carb, 1 milk, 2 fat
✔Nonfat Milk Cappuccino	12 oz	60	0	0	0	0	5	95	9	0	6	1 milk
Regular Mocha	12 oz	230	6	2	4.5	0	15	135	34	0	8	1/2 carb, 1 milk, 1 fat
Whole Milk Cappuccino	12 oz	150	8	5	4.5	0	25	110	12	0	7	1 milk, 1 1/2 fat
Whole Milk Regular Mocha	12 oz	270	9	3	5	0	25	150	38	0	8	1/2 carb, 1 milk, 2 fat

SPECIALTY SANDWICHES

Club Mex on Challah	1	600	30	5	9	0	120	1810	48	2	38	3 starch, 4 high-fat meat
Grilled Chicken, Bacon and Swiss	1	760	47	6	12	0.5	170	1260	45	2	41	3 starch, 3 high-fat meat, 4 fat
Rachel, overstuffed	1	1050	71	6	19	1.5	185	3310	53	2	55	3 1/2 starch, 6 high-fat meat, 4 fat
Rachel, regular	1	930	66	6	17	1.5	135	2200	51	2	37	3 1/2 starch, 4 high-fat meat, 6 fat
Reuben, overstuffed	1	800	44	5	15	1	165	3570	49	3	55	3 starch, 5 high-fat meat, 1 fat
Reuben, regular	1	670	40	5	13	1	115	2460	47	3	37	3 starch, 4 high-fat meat, 1 1/2 fat
Roasted Turkey and Swiss	1	700	42	5	9	1	85	1530	49	4	37	3 starch, 3 high-fat meat, 3 fat

✓ = Healthiest Bets

(*Continued*)

SPECIALTY SANDWICHES *(Continued)*	Amount	Cal.	Fat (g)	% Cal. Fat	Sat. Fat (g)	Trans Fat (g)	Chol. (mg)	Sod. (mg)	Carb. (g)	Fiber (g)	Pro. (g)	Choices/Exchanges
Tasty Turkey on Asiago Bagel	1	570	20	3	12	0	100	1560	68	3	38	4 1/2 starch, 3 medium-fat meat, 1 fat
Turkey Rachel, overstuffed	1	970	65	6	16	1	170	2610	50	1	59	3 1/2 starch, 6 high-fat meat, 4 fat
Turkey Rachel, regular	1	890	64	6	16	1	130	1860	50	1	39	3 1/2 starch, 4 high-fat meat, 6 fat
Turkey Rueben, overstuffed	1	720	39	5	12	1	150	2870	45	3	59	3 starch, 6 high-fat meat
Turkey Rueben, regular	1	630	37	5	12	1	110	2120	45	3	39	3 starch, 4 high-fat meat, 1 fat
Veg Out on Sesame Bagel	1	450	14	3	7	0	30	800	70	4	17	4 starch, 1 veg, 1 high-fat meat, 1 fat

✔ = Healthiest Bets

Jamba Juice (www.jambajuice.com)

Light 'n Lean Choice

Orange Mango Passion *(1/2, 8 oz)*

Calories	370	Cholesterol (mg)	20
Fat (g)	10	Sodium (mg)	225
% calories from fat	24	Carbohydrate (g)	64
Saturated fat (g)	0	Fiber (g)	8
Trans fat (g)	0	Protein (g)	7

Exchanges: 3 carb, 1 1/2 fruit, 2 fat

Healthy 'n Hearty Choice

Blueberry Oatcake *(1 slice)*
Orange Carrot Banana Juice *(16 oz)*

Calories	450	Cholesterol (mg)	20
Fat (g)	11	Sodium (mg)	310
% calories from fat	22	Carbohydrate (g)	82
Saturated fat (g)	2.5	Fiber (g)	8
Trans fat (g)	0	Protein (g)	9

Exchanges: 3 carb, 1 veg, 2 fruit, 2 fat

(*Continued*)

Jamba Juice

	Amount	Cal.	Fat (g)	% Cal. Fat	Sat. Fat (g)	Trans Fat (g)	Chol. (mg)	Sod. (mg)	Carb. (g)	Fiber (g)	Pro. (g)	Choices/Exchanges
ALL FRUIT												
Mega Mango	16 oz.	220	0.5	0	0	0	0	5	54	4	2	3 1/2 fruit
Peach Perfection	16 oz.	200	0	0	0	0	0	20	50	4	1	3 1/2 fruit
Pomegranate Paradise	16 oz.	220	0.5	0	0	0	0	20	57	4	1	3 1/2 fruit
Strawberry Whirl	16 oz.	200	0	0	0	0	0	15	50	4	1	3 1/2 fruit
BAKED GOODS												
Apple Cinnamon Pretzel	1	380	4	1	0	0	0	250	76	4	11	5 starch, 1 fat
Blueberry Oatcake	1 slice	280	10	3	2.5	0	20	220	42	7	6	3 carb, 2 fat
✓Omega-3 Chocolate Brownie Cookie	1	150	4	2	1	0	0	15	30	2	3	2 carb, 1 fat
✓Omega-3 Oatmeal Cookie	1	150	6	4	1.5	0	5	85	26	3	2	1 1/2 carb, 1 fat

Reduced-Fat Blueberry Lemon Loaf	1 slice	290	8	2	2	0	20	220	53	2	2	3 1/2 carb, 1 1/2 fat
Reduced-Fat Cranberry Orange Loaf	1 slice	310	9	3	2	0	20	200	52	4	6	3 1/2 carb, 2 fat
Sourdough Parmesan Pretzel	1	410	10	2	2	0	5	640	67	3	14	4 starch, 2 fat
✔Zucchini Walnut Loaf	1 slice	270	9	3	1.5	0	20	250	43	4	5	3 carb, 2 fat
BLENDED WITH A PURPOSE												
3G Energizer	16 oz.	310	1	0	0	0	5	20	73	4	2	3 carb, 2 fruit
Açaí Super-Antioxidant	16 oz.	270	4	1	2	0	5	50	55	4	4	1 carb, 2 fruit, 1 fat
Coldbuster	16 oz.	260	1.5	1	0	0	5	20	61	3	3	2 carb, 2 fruit
Fit n' Fruitful	16 oz.	240	3	1	0	0	0	15	54	4	2	1 carb, 2 fruit, 1/2 fat
Pomegranate Heart Defender	16 oz.	280	0.5	0	0	0	0	105	66	3	4	2 carb, 2 fruit
Protein Berry Workout w/ Soy Protein	16 oz.	280	1	0	0	0	0	160	56	4	14	1 carb, 2 fruit, 2 milk

✔ = Healthiest Bets; na = not available

(Continued)

BLENDED WITH A PURPOSE *(Continued)*	Amount	Cal.	Fat (g)	% Cal. Fat	Sat. Fat (g)	Trans Fat (g)	Chol. (mg)	Sod. (mg)	Carb. (g)	Fiber (g)	Pro. (g)	Choices/Exchanges
Protein Berry Workout w/ Whey	16 oz.	270	1	0	0	0	5	100	53	4	16	1 carb, 2 fruit, 2 milk
BOOSTS												
✔Green Caffeine Boost	1	5	0	0	na	na	0	na	2	2		Free
✔Omega-3 Super Boost	1	30	1.5	5	na	na	0	na	7	7	1	1/2 carb
✔Weight Burner Super Boost	1	30	3	9	0	0	0	na	na	na	na	Free
✔Whey Protein Super Boost	1	45	0	0	na	na	5	20	1	na	10	1 lean meat
CREAMY INDULGENCES												
Matcha Green Tea Blast	16 oz.	340	0	0	0	0	0	180	74	1	8	5 carb, 1 lean meat
Orange Dream Machine	16 oz.	340	1.5	0	0	0	5	160	73	0	8	2 carb, 2 fruit, 1 milk
Peanut Butter Moo'd	16 oz.	530	11	2	2	0	10	320	94	4	16	3 1/2 carb, 2 fruit, 1 milk, 1 lean meat, 2 fat

FRESH SQUEEZED JUICES												
✔Carrot Juice	16 oz.	90	0.5	1	0	0	0	230	22	0	4	4 veg
Orange Juice	16 oz.	220	1	0	0	0	0	0	52	0	3	4 veg
JAMBA CLASSICS												
Aloha Pineapple	16 oz.	300	1	0	0	0	5	20	69	3	6	2 1/2 carb, 2 fruit
Banana Berry	16 oz.	280	1	0	0	0	0	65	67	3	3	2 1/2 carb, 2 fruit
Caribbean Passion	16 oz.	270	1	0	0	0	5	35	62	3	2	2 carb, 2 fruit
Citrus Squeeze	16 oz.	280	1.5	0	0	0	5	20	66	3	3	2 carb, 2 fruit
Mango-a-go-go	16 oz.	300	1.5	0	0	0	5	35	71	2	2	3 carb, 2 fruit
Orange a Peel	16 oz.	260	1	0	0	0	0	95	60	3	8	2 carb, 2 fruit
Peach Pleasure	16 oz.	280	1	0	0	0	5	35	66	3	2	2 carb, 2 fruit
Razzmatazz	16 oz.	290	1.5	0	0	0	5	40	67	3	2	2 1/2 carb, 2 fruit
Strawberries Wild	16 oz.	260	0	0	0	0	0	100	61	2	3	2 carb, 2 fruit

✔ = Healthiest Bets; na = not available

(*Continued*)

JAMBA CLASSICS *(Continued)*	Amount	Cal.	Fat (g)	% Cal. Fat	Sat. Fat (g)	Trans Fat (g)	Chol. (mg)	Sod. (mg)	Carb. (g)	Fiber (g)	Pro. (g)	Choices/Exchanges
Strawberry Surf Rider	16 oz.	320	1	0	0	0	5	5	77	3	2	3 carb, 2 fruit
JAMBA LIGHT												
✔Berry Fulfilling	16 oz.	150	0.5	0	0	0	5	210	30	3	6	1 carb, 1 fruit
Mango Mantra	16 oz.	160	0.5	0	0	0	5	220	34	2	6	1 carb, 1 fruit
Strawberry Nirvana	16 oz.	150	0	0	0	0	5	210	32	3	6	1 carb, 1 fruit
JUICES												
Orange Carrot Banana	16 oz.	170	1	1	0	0	0	90	40	1	3	1 veg, 2 fruit
JUICIEST												
Orange Mango Passion	16 oz.	180	0.5	0	0	0	0	10	43	1	2	3 fruit
SHOTS												
✔Matcha Green Tea Shot - Orange Juice	Single - 4 oz.	60	0	0	0	0	0	0	13	0	1	1 fruit

✔Matcha Green Tea Shot - Soymilk	Single - 4 oz.	80	0	0	0	0	0	45	16	0	3	1 milk
✔Wheatgrass Shot	1 oz.	5	0	0	0	0	0	0	1	0	0	Free
SMOOTHIES W/ ORGANIC GRANOLA												
Berry Topper	16 oz.	490	10	2	2	0	5	130	80	10	13	5 carb, 1 fruit, 2 fat
Chunky Strawberry	16 oz.	570	17	3	2	0	5	160	91	9	17	5 carb, 1 fruit, 3 1/2 fat
Mango Peach Topper	16 oz.	500	10	2	2	0	5	130	95	9	13	5 carb, 1 fruit, 2 fat
YOGURT & FRUIT BLENDS												
Bright Eyed & Blueberry	16 oz.	220	0.5	0	0	0	5	70	43	2	11	1 fruit, 2 milk
Sunrise Strawberry	16 oz.	240	0.5	0	0	0	5	75	49	2	11	1 fruit, 2 milk

✔ = Healthiest Bets; na = not available

Krispy Kreme (www.krispykreme.com)

Light 'n Lean Choice

1 Glazed Cinnamon Doughnut
Low-Fat Milk (8 oz)

Calories	312	Cholesterol (mg)	17
Fat (g)	14	Sodium (mg)	207
% calories from fat	40	Carbohydrate (g)	36
Saturated fat (g)	6	Fiber (g)	0
Trans fat (g)	0	Protein (g)	10

Exchanges: 1 1/2 starch, 1 fat-free milk, 3 fat

Healthy 'n Hearty Choice

Cinnamon Bun
Orange Juice

Calories	370	Cholesterol (mg)	5
Fat (g)	16	Sodium (mg)	127
% calories from fat	39	Carbohydrate (g)	53
Saturated fat (g)	8	Fiber (g)	0
Trans fat (g)	0	Protein (g)	5

Exchanges: 2 carb, 2 fruit, 1 milk, 3 1/2 fat

Krispy Kreme

	Amount	Cal.	Fat (g)	% Cal. Fat	Sat. Fat (g)	Trans Fat (g)	Chol. (mg)	Sod. (mg)	Carb. (g)	Fiber (g)	Pro. (g)	Choices/Exchanges
CAKE DOUGHNUTS												
Chocolate Iced Cake	1	280	14	5	6	0	20	320	36	0	3	2 carb, 3 fat
Powdered Cake	1	290	14	4	6	0	20	320	37	0	3	2 1/2 carb, 3 fat
Traditional Cake	1	230	13	5	6	0	20	320	25	0	3	1 1/2 carb, 2 1/2 fat
CHILLERS												
Berries and Kreme	12 oz	620	28	4	24	0	30	220	92	0	3	6 carb, 5 1/2 fat
Berries and Kreme	20 oz	960	40	4	36	0	30	330	150	0	3	10 carb, 8 fat
Chocolate, Chocolate	12 oz	670	29	4	24	0	30	320	104	2	4	7 carb, 6 fat

✔ = Healthiest Bets

(*Continued*)

CHILLERS *(Continued)*	Amount	Cal.	Fat (g)	% Cal. Fat	Sat. Fat (g)	Trans Fat (g)	Chol. (mg)	Sod. (mg)	Carb. (g)	Fiber (g)	Pro. (g)	Choices/Exchanges
Chocolate, Chocolate	20 oz	1050	42	4	36	0	30	490	170	4	6	11 carb, 8 1/2 fat
Lemon Sherbet	12 oz	630	28	4	24	0	30	220	92	0	3	6 carb, 5 1/2 fat
Lemon Sherbet	20 oz	980	40	4	36	0	30	330	155	0	3	10 carb, 8 fat
Lotta Latte	12 oz	670	28	4	24	0	30	380	49	1	3	3 carb, 5 1/2 fat
Lotta Latte	20 oz	1050	40	3	36	0	30	580	79	2	5	5 carb, 8 fat
Mocha Dream	12 oz	670	28	4	24	0	30	320	105	1	3	7 carb, 5 1/2 fat
Mocha Dream	20 oz	1050	41	4	36	0	30	490	71	2	5	4 1/2 carb, 8 fat
Orange You Glad	20 oz	290	0	0	0	0	0	10	71	0	0	4 1/2 carb
Orange You Glad	12 oz	180	0	0	0	0	0	10	43	0	0	3 carb
Oranges and Kreme	12 oz	630	28	4	24	0	30	220	92	0	3	6 carb, 5 1/2 fat
Oranges and Kreme	20 oz	970	40	4	36	0	30	330	150	0	3	10 carb, 8 fat
Very Berry	20 oz	290	0	0	0	0	0	10	71	0	0	4 1/2 carb

Very Berry	12 oz	170	0	0	0	0	0	10	43	0	0	3 carb
CRULLERS												
Apple Fritter	1	380	20	5	10	0	5	220	47	2	4	3 carb, 4 fat
Chocolate Glazed Cruller	1	290	15	5	7	0	15	240	37	0	2	2 1/2 carb, 3 fat
Glazed Cruller	1	240	14	5	7	0	15	240	26	0	2	1 1/2 carb, 3 fat
DOUGHNUT HOLES												
Glazed Blueberry	4	220	12	5	5	0	20	280	27	0	3	1 1/2 carb, 2 1/2 fat
✔Glazed Cake	4	210	10	4	4.5	0	15	240	29	0	2	2 carb, 2 fat
✔Glazed Chocolate Cake	4	210	10	4	4.5	0	15	240	29	0	2	2 carb, 2 fat
✔Glazed Pumpkin Spice	4	210	10	4	4.5	0	15	240	29	0	2	2 carb, 2 fat
Original Glazed	4	200	11	5	5	0	5	90	25	0	2	1 1/2 carb, 2 fat

✔ = Healthiest Bets

(*Continued*)

	Amount	Cal.	Fat (g)	% Cal. Fat	Sat. Fat (g)	Trans Fat (g)	Chol. (mg)	Sod. (mg)	Carb. (g)	Fiber (g)	Pro. (g)	Choices/Exchanges
DOUGHNUTS												
Caramel Kreme Crunch	1	380	19	5	9	0	10	170	49	0	4	3 carb, 4 fat
Chocolate Iced w/ Sprinkles	1	270	12	4	6	0	5	100	38	0	3	2 1/2 carb, 2 fat
Cinnamon Bun	1	260	16	6	8	0	5	125	28	0	3	2 carb, 3 fat
Cinnamon Twist	1	240	15	6	7	0	5	130	23	0	3	1 1/2 carb, 3 fat
Dulce De Leche	1	300	18	5	9	0	5	160	31	0	3	2 carb, 3 1/2 fat
New York Cheesecake	1	340	20	5	10	0	15	200	34	0	4	2 carb, 4 fat
Original Glazed	1	200	12	5	6	0	5	95	22	0	2	1 1/2 carb, 2 fat
Sugar	1	200	12	5	6	0	5	95	21	0	2	1 1/2 carb, 2 1/2 fat
FILLED DOUGHNUTS												
Chocolate Iced Custard Filled	1	300	17	5	8	0	5	150	35	0	3	2 carb, 3 fat

Chocolate Iced Kreme Filled	1	350	20	5	11	0	5	140	39	0	3	2 1/2 carb, 4 fat
Cinnamon Apple Filled	1	290	16	5	8	0	5	150	32	0	3	2 carb, 3 fat
Glazed Kreme Filled	1	340	20	5	10	0	5	140	39	0	3	2 1/2 carb, 4 fat
Glazed Lemon Filled	1	290	16	5	8	0	5	135	35	0	3	2 carb, 3 fat
Glazed Raspberry Filled	1	300	16	5	8	0	5	125	36	0	3	2 carb, 3 fat
Powdered Strawberry Filled	1	290	16	5	8	0	5	135	33	0	3	2 carb, 3 fat
GLAZED DOUGHNUTS												
Chocolate Iced Glazed	1	250	12	4	6	0	5	100	33	0	3	2 carb, 2 1/2 fat
Glazed Chocolate Cake	1	300	15	5	7	0	20	250	42	2	3	3 carb, 3 fat
Glazed Cinnamon	1	210	12	5	6	0	5	100	24	0	2	1 1/2 carb, 2 1/2 fat
Glazed Pumpkin Spice	1	300	14	4	7	0	20	250	42	0	2	3 carb, 3 fat
Glazed Sour Cream	1	300	13	4	7	0	20	250	43	0	2	3 carb, 2 1/2 fat

✔ = Healthiest Bets

Orange Julius (www.orangejulius.com)

Light 'n Lean Choice

Strawberry Julius *(16 oz)*

Calories	220	Cholesterol (mg)	0
Fat (g)	<1	Sodium (mg)	10
% calories from fat	<10	Carbohydrate (g)	57
Saturated fat (g)	<1	Fiber (g)	1
Trans fat (g)	na	Protein (g)	1

Exchanges: 4 carb

Healthy 'n Hearty Choice

Cinnamon Bun
Orange Juice

Calories	350	Cholesterol (mg)	0
Fat (g)	8	Sodium (mg)	85
% calories from fat	21	Carbohydrate (g)	70
Saturated fat (g)	7	Fiber (g)	2
Trans fat (g)	na	Protein (g)	3

Exchanges: 4 1/2 carb

Orange Julius

	Amount	Cal.	Fat (g)	% Cal. Fat	Sat. Fat (g)	Trans Fat (g)	Chol. (mg)	Sod. (mg)	Carb. (g)	Fiber (g)	Pro. (g)	Choices/Exchanges
ADD ON												
Banana	1	110	1	1	0	na	0	0	27	2	1	2 fruit
Banana	1/2	60	0	0	0	na	0	0	13	1	1	1 fruit
NUTRIFIERS												
✔Energy	0.25 oz.	16	0	0	na				4		0	Free
✔Immunity	0.25 oz.	16	0	0	na				4		0	Free
✔Mind	0.25 oz.	16	0	0	na				4		0	Free
✔Mood	0.25 oz.	16	0	0	na				4		0	Free
✔Protein +	0.25 oz.	16	0	0	na				4		3	Free

✔ = Healthiest Bets; na = not available

(*Continued*)

NUTRIFIERS *(Continued)*	**Amount**	**Cal.**	**Fat (g)**	**% Cal. Fat**	**Sat. Fat (g)**	**Trans Fat (g)**	**Chol. (mg)**	**Sod. (mg)**	**Carb. (g)**	**Fiber (g)**	**Pro. (g)**	**Choices/Exchanges**
✔Vita Min	0.25 oz.	16	0	0	na				4		0	Free
ORIGINAL DRINKS												
Bananarilla	16 oz.	290	7	2	7	na	0	75	56	3	3	3 1/2 carb, 1 fat
Bananarilla	20 oz.	370	9	2	9	na	0	95	69	4	4	4 1/2 carb, 2 fat
Bananarilla	32 oz.	580	14	2	14	na	0	150	111	7	6	7 1/2 carb, 3 fat
Cool Cappuccino	16 oz.	390	10	2	7	na	10	210	69	1	12	4 1/2 carb, 2 fat
Cool Cappuccino	20 oz.	480	13	2	9	na	15	270	86	1	15	5 1/2 carb, 2 fat
Cool Cappuccino	32 oz.	770	20	2	14	na	20	430	138	2	24	9 carb, 4 fat
Orange Julius	16 oz.	220	1	0	<1	na	0	10	54	1	1	3 1/2 carb
Orange Julius	20 oz.	270	1	0	<1	na	0	10	68	1	1	4 1/2 carb
Orange Julius	32 oz.	440	1	0	1	na	0	15	108	1	2	7 carb
Piña Colada	16 oz.	330	7	2	7	na	0	50	70	3	2	4 1/2 carb, 1 fat

Piña Colada	20 oz.	410	9	2	9	na	0	65	87	4	3	6 carb, 2 fat
Piña Colada	32 oz.	660	14	2	14	na	0	100	139	6	4	9 1/2 carb, 3 fat
Raspberry	16 oz.	310	7	2	7	na	0	80	59	2	3	4 carb, 1 fat
Raspberry	20 oz.	400	10	2	9	na	0	105	78	2	4	5 carb, 2 fat
Raspberry	32 oz.	610	15	2	14	na	0	160	118	3	6	8 carb, 3 fat
Raspberry Julius	16 oz.	240	1	0	<1	na	0	25	61	1	1	4 carb
Raspberry Julius	20 oz.	300	1.5	0	1	na	0	35	76	1	2	5 carb
Raspberry Julius	32 oz.	480	2	0	1.5	na	0	50	121	2	3	8 carb
Strawberry Banana	16 oz.	400	7	2	7	na	0	70	77	1	3	5 carb, 1 fat
Strawberry Banana	20 oz.	500	9	2	9	na	0	90	97	2	4	6 1/2 carb, 2 fat
Strawberry Banana	32 oz.	800	14	2	14	na	0	140	155	2	6	10 1/2 carb, 3 fat
Strawberry Julius	16 oz.	220	0	0	<1	na	0	10	57	1	1	4 carb
Strawberry Julius	20 oz.	280	1	0	<1	na	0	10	72	1	1	5 carb
Strawberry Julius	32 oz.	450	1	0	<1	na	0	15	115	2	2	7 1/2 carb

✓ = Healthiest Bets; na = not available

(*Continued*)

ORIGINAL DRINKS *(Continued)*	Amount	Cal.	Fat (g)	% Cal. Fat	Sat. Fat (g)	Trans Fat (g)	Chol. (mg)	Sod. (mg)	Carb. (g)	Fiber (g)	Pro. (g)	Choices/Exchanges
Tripleberry	16 oz.	350	8	2	7	na	0	85	70	2	3	4 1/2 carb, 1 fat
Tripleberry	20 oz.	460	10	2	9	na	0	110	92	3	4	6 carb, 2 fat
Tripleberry	32 oz.	700	15	2	14	na	0	170	140	4	6	9 1/2 carb, 3 fat
Tropical	16 oz.	290	7	2	7	na	0	70	54	3	3	3 1/2 carb, 1 fat
Tropical	20 oz.	370	9	2	9	na	0	90	69	4	4	4 1/2 carb, 2 fat
Tropical	32 oz.	580	14	2	14	na	0	140	108	7	7	7 carb, 3 fat
PREMIUM FRUIT SMOOTHIES												
3-Berry Blast	20 oz.	610	1.5	0	0.5	na	0	250	144	3	9	9 1/2 carb
Berry Lemon Lively	20 oz.	450	1	0	0.5	na	0	250	101	1	9	6 1/2 carb
Blackberry Storm	20 oz.	630	8	1	7	na	0	310	129	2	10	8 1/2 carb, 1 fat
Blackberry Toner	20 oz.	440	1	0	0	na	0	250	96	1	9	6 1/2 carb
Blueberrathon	20 oz.	350	1.5	0	0	na	0	10	89	6	2	6 carb

Blueberry Burst	20 oz.	470	0.5	0	0	na	0	230	106	4	7	7 carb
Cocoa Latte Swirl	20 oz.	640	9	1	8	na	5	500	122	2	21	8 carb, 2 fat
Mango Passion	20 oz.	360	0	0	0	na	0	250	80	1	7	5 1/2 carb
Orange Swirl	20 oz.	490	10	2	9	na	10	135	96	2	4	6 1/2 carb, 2 fat
Peaches & Cream	20 oz.	500	0	0	0	na	0	250	116	4	8	7 1/2 carb
Raspberry Crème	20 oz.	540	7	1	7	na	0	300	107	2	11	7 carb
Raspberry Crush	20 oz.	330	2	1	0.5	na	0	35	83	3	3	5 1/2 carb
Strawberried Treasure	20 oz.	550	8	1	8	na	0	300	103	2	10	7 carb, 1 fat
Strawberry Sensation	20 oz.	430	0	0	0	na	0	230	98	2	7	6 1/2 carb
Strawberry Xtreme	20 oz.	410	0.5	0	0	na	0	250	87	1	8	6 carb
Tart 'N' Berry	20 oz.	450	1	0	0	na	0	250	102	5	9	7 carb
Tropical Tango	20 oz.	400	3	1	2	na	10	85	90	2	2	6 carb
Tropi-Colada	20 oz.	560	8	1	8	na	0	310	110	3	10	7 1/2 carb, 1 fat
Wild Blue Twist	20 oz.	490	0.5	0	0	na	0	230	115	4	7	7 1/2 carb

✔ = Healthiest Bets; na = not available

Starbucks (www.starbucks.com)

Light 'n Lean Choice

Raspberry Scone *(1/2)*
Caffe Latte, non-fat *(12 oz)*

Calories	345	Cholesterol (mg)	48
Fat (g)	11	Sodium (mg)	400
% calories from fat	29	Carbohydrate (g)	48
Saturated fat (g)	6	Fiber (g)	1
Trans fat (g)	0	Protein (g)	14

Exchanges: 2 carb, 1 fat-free milk, 2 fat

Healthy 'n Hearty Choice

Cranberry Orange Muffin
Coffee Frappuccino, with nonfat milk *(12 oz)*

Calories	520	Cholesterol (mg)	85
Fat (g)	12	Sodium (mg)	730
% calories from fat	21	Carbohydrate (g)	98
Saturated fat (g)	6.5	Fiber (g)	2
Trans fat (g)	0	Protein (g)	9

Exchanges: 5 1/2 carb, 1 milk, 2 1/2 fat

Starbucks

	Amount	Cal.	Fat (g)	% Cal. Fat	Sat. Fat (g)	Trans Fat (g)	Chol. (mg)	Sod. (mg)	Carb. (g)	Fiber (g)	Pro. (g)	Choices/Exchanges
BROWNIES, COOKIES, & BARS												
Black and White Cookie	1	240	12	5	1	0	40	160	32	1	2	2 carb, 2 1/2 fat
Blueberry Oat Bar w/ Organic Blueberries	1	390	15	3	5	0	0	300	59	3		4 carb, 5 medium-fat meat, 3 fat
Chewy Marshmallow Square	1	280	6	2	3	0	10	330	54	0	2	3 1/2 carb, 1 fat
Chocolate Chunk Cookie	1	370	18	4	11	0	60	150	50	2	4	3 1/2 carb, 3 1/2 fat
Chocolate Fudge Brownie	1	410	22	5	13	0	110	136	52	2	5	3 1/2 carb, 4 1/2 fat
Decorated Cookie	1	470	14	3	8	0	60	130	80	1	5	5 carb, 3 fat
Lemon Slice Cookie	1	460	22	4	10	0	25	250	60	1	5	4 carb, 4 fat
Oatmeal Raisin Cookie	1	350	12	3	7	0	50	95	56	3	5	3 1/2 carb, 2 1/2 fat

✓ = Healthiest Bets

(Continued)

BROWNIES, COOKIES, AND BARS *(Continued)*	Amount	Cal.	Fat (g)	% Cal. Fat	Sat. Fat (g)	Trans Fat (g)	Chol. (mg)	Sod. (mg)	Carb. (g)	Fiber (g)	Pro. (g)	Choices/Exchanges
Rainbow Cookie	1	480	20	4	13	1	70	210	71	1	6	4 1/2 carb, 4 fat
Toffee Almond Bar	1	400	19	4	8	0	50	340	53	1	4	3 1/2 carb, 4 fat
CLASSIC FAVORITES - NONFAT												
Apple Juice	12 oz	190	0	0	0	0	0	20	48	0	0	3 carb
Caramel Apple Spice - no whip	12 oz	240	0	0	0	0	0	20	57	0	0	4 carb
Caramel Apple Spice - whip	12 oz	300	7	2	4	0	25	25	59	0	0	4 carb
Chocolate Milk	12 oz	220	2	1	0	0	5	150	41	1	14	1 1/2 carb, 1 1/2 milk
Cinnamon Dolce Crème - no whip	12 oz	170	0	0	0	0	5	120	31	0	10	2 carb
Cinnamon Dolce Crème - whip	12 oz	230	6	2	4	0	30	25	33	0	10	2 carb, 1 fat
✔Honey Crème - no whip	12 oz	160	0	0	0	0	5	125	29	0	10	2 carb

Honey Crème - whip	12 oz	230	6	2	4	0	30	130	33	0	10	2 carb, 1 fat
Hot Chocolate - no whip	12 oz	190	2	1	0	0	5	110	37	1	11	1 1/2 carb, 1 milk
Hot Chocolate - whip	12 oz	250	8	3	4	0	30	115	39	1	11	2 carb, 1 milk, 1 1/2 fat
Pumpkin Spice Crème - no whip	12 oz	200	0	0	0	0	25	180	39	0	12	2 1/2 carb, 1 milk
Pumpkin Spice Crème - whip	12 oz	260	6	2	4	0	30	180	40	0	12	3 carb, 1 milk, 1 fat
Steamed Apple Juice	12 oz	170	0	0	0	0	0	15	43	0	0	3 carb
✔Vanilla Crème - no whip	12 oz	150	0	0	0	0	5	120	28	0	10	2 carb
Vanilla Crème - whip	12 oz	220	6	2	4	0	30	125	30	0	10	2 carb, 1 fat
White Hot Chocolate - no whip	12 oz	270	5	2	3.5	0	5	200	47	0	12	1 carb, 11 1/2 milk, 1 fat
White Hot Chocolate - whip	12 oz	330	10	3	7	0	20	100	49	0	12	1 carb, 1 1/2 milk, 2 fat

✔ = Healthiest Bets

(*Continued*)

	Amount	Cal.	Fat (g)	% Cal. Fat	Sat. Fat (g)	Trans Fat (g)	Chol. (mg)	Sod. (mg)	Carb. (g)	Fiber (g)	Pro. (g)	Choices/Exchanges
CROISSANTS, BAGELS & BREADS												
8 Grain Roll	1	270	1	0	0.5	0	0	400	56	5	8	3 1/2 starch
Butter Croissant	1	300	15	5	9	0	45	350	36	1	5	2 starch, 3 fat
Chocolate Croissant	1	470	26	5	13	0.5	60	440	65	2	7	4 starch, 5 fat
Plain Bagel	1	310	2	1	0.5	0	0	600	61	2	11	4 starch
DOUGHNUTS, SWEET ROLLS & DANISH												
Artisan Cinnamon Roll	1	400	22	5	10	0	20	310	48	1	4	3 carb, 4 1/2 fat
Cheese Danish	1	390	19	4	12	0.5	50	410	47	2	8	3 carb, 4 fat
Cinnamon Twist	1	420	20	4	12	0.5	50	400	51	2	8	3 1/2 carb, 4 fat
Top Pot Apple Fritter	1	490	22	4	10	0	0	290	65	1	4	4 carb, 4 1/2 fat
Top Pot Chocolate Old Fashioned Doughnut	1	480	25	5	7	0	20	350	60	2	5	4 carb, 5 fat

✔Top Pot Glazed Old Fashioned Mini Doughnut	1	150	7	4	1.5	0	5	120	19	0	1	1 carb, 1 1/2 fat
FRAPPUCCINO BLENDED COFFEE - NONFAT MILK												
Caffe Vanilla - no whip	12 oz	230	3	1	1.5	0	10	180	49	0	4	2 1/2 carb, 1 milk, 1/2 fat
Caffe Vanilla - whip	12 oz	320	10	3	6	0	40	190	52	0	4	2 1/2 carb, 1 milk, 2 fat
Caramel - no whip	12 oz	220	3	1	2	0	10	180	44	0	4	2 carb, 1 milk, 1/2 fat
Caramel - whip	12 oz	300	11	3	7	0	40	190	46	0	4	2 carb, 1 milk, 2 fat
Cinnamon Dolce - no whip	12 oz	210	3	1	1.5	0	10	180	43	0	4	2 carb, 1 milk, 1/2 fat
Cinnamon Dolce - whip	12 oz	290	10	3	6	0	40	190	45	0	4	2 carb, 1 milk, 2 fat
Espresso	12 oz	180	3	2	1.5	0	10	170	37	0	4	1 1/2 carb, 1 milk, 1/2 fat
Honey - no whip	12 oz	210	3	1	1.5	0	10	180	44	0	4	2 carb, 1 milk, 1/2 fat
Honey - whip	12 oz	300	10	3	6	0	40	180	47	0	4	2 carb, 1 milk, 2 fat
Java Chip - no whip	12 oz	260	6	2	4	0	10	480	50	1	5	2 1/2 carb, 1 milk, 1 fat

✔ = Healthiest Bets

(*Continued*)

FRAPPUCCINO BLENDED COFFEE - NONFAT MILK ***(Continued)***	**Amount**	**Cal.**	**Fat (g)**	**% Cal. Fat**	**Sat. Fat (g)**	**Trans Fat (g)**	**Chol. (mg)**	**Sod. (mg)**	**Carb. (g)**	**Fiber (g)**	**Pro. (g)**	**Choices/Exchanges**
Java Chip - whip	12 oz	340	14	4	9	0	40	180	52	1	6	2 1/2 carb, 1 milk, 3 fat
Mint Mocha Chip - no whip	12 oz	270	5	2	3.5	0	10	200	54	1	5	3 carb, 1 milk, 1 fat
Mint Mocha Chip - whip	12 oz	360	14	4	9	0	40	210	57	1	6	3 carb, 1 milk, 3 fat
Mocha - no whip	12 oz	200	3	1	1.5	0	10	170	41	0	4	1 carb, 1 milk, 1/2 fat
Mocha - whip	12 oz	280	11	4	6	0	40	180	43	0	5	1 1/2 carb, 1 milk, 2 fat
Pumpkin Spice - no whip	12 oz	230	3	1	1.5	0	10	210	47	0	5	1 1/2 carb, 1 milk, 1/2 fat
Pumpkin Spice - whip	12 oz	310	11	3	7	0	40	210	49	0	5	2 carb, 1 milk, 2 fat
White Chocolate Mocha - no whip	12 oz	240	4	2	2.5	0	10	200	47	1	5	2 carb, 1 milk, 1 fat
White Chocolate Mocha - whip	12 oz	320	12	3	7	0	40	210	49	0	5	2 1/2 carb, 2 1/2 milk

FRAPPUCCINO BLENDED CRÈME - NONFAT

Double Chocolaty Chip - no whip	12 oz	300	6	2	2.5	0	5	230	57	2	10	3 carb, 1 milk, 1 fat
Double Chocolaty Chip - whip	12 oz	380	14	3	8	0	35	240	59	2	11	3 carb, 1 milk, 3 fat
Honey - no whip	12 oz	250	2	1	0	0	5	240	50	1	8	2 1/2 carb, 1 milk
Honey - whip	12 oz	330	10	3	5	0	35	250	53	1	9	2 1/2 carb, 1 milk, 2 fat
Mint Chocolaty Chip - no whip	12 oz	310	5	1	2	0	5	240	61	2	9	3 carb, 1 milk, 1 fat
Mint Chocolaty Chip - whip	12 oz	400	14	3	8	0	35	250	64	2	10	3 carb, 1 milk, 3 fat
Pumpkin Spice - no whip	12 oz	280	2	1	0	0	5	270	55	0	10	3 carb, 1 milk
Pumpkin Spice - whip	12 oz	360	10	3	5	0	35	380	58	0	10	3 carb, 1 milk, 2 fat
Strawberries and Crème - no whip	12 oz	320	2	1	0	0	5	240	66	0	9	3 1/2 carb, 1 milk

✔ = Healthiest Bets

(*Continued*)

FRAPPUCCINO BLENDED CREME - NONFAT *(Continued)*	Amount	Cal.	Fat (g)	% Cal. Fat	Sat. Fat (g)	Trans Fat (g)	Chol. (mg)	Sod. (mg)	Carb. (g)	Fiber (g)	Pro. (g)	Choices/Exchanges
Strawberries and Crème - whip	12 oz	410	11	2	6	0	40	250	68	0	9	3 1/2 carb, 1 milk, 2 fat
Tazo Chai - no whip	12 oz	260	2	1	0	0	5	220	52	0	8	2 1/2 carb, 1 milk
Tazo Chai - whip	12 oz	340	10	3	5	0	24	120	55	0	9	3 carb, 1 milk, 2 fat
Tazo Green Tea - no whip	12 oz	290	2	1	0	0	5	230	60	1	9	3 carb, 1 milk
Tazo Green Tea - whip	12 oz	370	10	2	5	0	35	240	62	1	9	3 carb, 1 milk, 2 fat
Vanilla Bean - no whip	12 oz	260	2	1	0	0	5	230	53	0	9	2 1/2 carb, 1 milk
Vanilla Bean - whip	12 oz	340	10	3	5	0	35	240	55	0	9	3 carb, 1 milk, 2 fat
FRAPPUCCINO LIGHT BLENDED COFFEE - NONFAT												
✔Caffe Vanilla	12 oz	140	1	1	0	0	0	180	30	2	4	2 carb
✔Caramel	12 oz	130	1	1	0	0	5	180	25	2	4	1 1/2 carb
✔Cinnamon Dolce	12 oz	120	1	1	0	0	0	180	24	2	4	1 1/2 carb

Coffee	12 oz	180	3	2	1.5	0	10	170	37	0	4	2 1/2 carb
✔Espresso	12 oz	140	2	1	1	0	5	125	27	0	3	1 1/2 carb
✔Honey	12 oz	120	1	1	0	0	0	170	25	2	4	1 1/2 carb
✔Java Chip	12 oz	160	4	2	2	0	0	180	30	3	5	2 carb
Mint Mocha Chip	12 oz	170	3	2	1.5	0	0	180	32	3	5	2 carb
✔Mocha	12 oz	110	1	1	0	0	0	170	23	2	4	1 1/2 carb
✔Pumpkin Spice	12 oz	120	1	1	0	0	0	190	25	2	5	1 1/2 carb
✔White Chocolate Mocha	12 oz	140	2	1	1	0	0	190	27	2	5	2 carb
HOT ESPRESSO - 2% MILK												
Caffe Latte	12 oz	150	6	4	3.5	0	25	115	14	0	10	1 milk, 1 fat
Caffe Mocha - no whip	12 oz	200	6	3	3.5	0	20	100	31	1	10	1 carb, 1 milk, 1 fat
Caffe Mocha - whip	12 oz	270	12	4	7	0	40	105	33	1	10	1 carb, 1 milk, 2 fat
✔Cappuccino	12 oz	90	4	4	2	0	15	70	9	0	6	1 milk, 1 fat

✔ = Healthiest Bets

(*Continued*)

HOT ESPRESSO - 2% MILK *(Continued)*	Amount	Cal.	Fat (g)	% Cal. Fat	Sat. Fat (g)	Trans Fat (g)	Chol. (mg)	Sod. (mg)	Carb. (g)	Fiber (g)	Pro. (g)	Choices/Exchanges
Peppermint White Chocolate Mocha - whip	12 oz	410	15	3	10	0	40	90	60	0	11	3 carb, 1 milk, 3 fat
✔Syrup Flavored Latte	12 oz	190	5	2	3.5	0	20	110	27	0	9	1 carb, 1 milk, 1 fat
HOT ESPRESSO - NONFAT												
✔Caffe Americano	12 oz	10	0	0	0	0	0	5	2	0	1	Free
✔Caffe Latte	12 oz	100	0	0	0	0	5	120	15	0	10	1 milk
Caffe Mocha - no whip	12 oz	170	2	1	0	0	5	100	32	1	10	1 carb, 1 milk
Caffe Mocha - whip	12 oz	230	8	3	4	0	25	110	34	1	11	1 carb, 1 milk, 1 1/2 fat
✔Cappuccino	12 oz	60	0	0	0	0	5	70	9	0	6	1 milk
✔Caramel Macchiato	12 oz	140	1	1	0.5	0	5	105	25	0	8	1 carb, 1 milk
Cinnamon Dolce Latte - no whip	12 oz	160	0	0	0	0	5	110	31	0	9	1 carb, 1 milk

✔Cinnamon Dolce Latte - sugar free syrup	12 oz	90	0	0	0	0	5	125	14	0	9	1 milk
Cinnamon Dolce Latte - whip	12 oz	220	6	2	4	0	30	115	33	0	9	1 carb, 1 milk, 1 fat
Honey Latte - no whip	12 oz	160	0	0	0	0	5	115	31	0	9	1 carb, 1 milk
Honey Latte - whip	12 oz	220	6	2	4	0	30	120	33	0	9	1 carb, 1 milk, 1 fat
Peppermint White Chocolate Mocha - no whip	12 oz	320	5	1	3.5	0	5	180	59	0	11	3 carb, 1 milk
Peppermint White Chocolate Mocha - whip	12 oz	380	11	3	7	0	30	190	61	0	11	3 carb, 1 milk, 2 fat
Pumpkin Spice Latte - no whip	12 oz	200	0	0	0	0	5	170	38	0	11	1 1/2 carb, 1 milk
Pumpkin Spice Latte - whip	12 oz	260	6	2	4	0	30	170	40	0	11	1 1/2 carb, 1 milk, 1 fat
✔Skinny Caramel Latte - no whip	12 oz	90	0	0	0	0	5	125	14	0	9	1 milk

✔ = Healthiest Bets

(*Continued*)

HOT ESPRESSO - NONFAT *(Continued)*	Amount	Cal.	(g)	% Fat Fat	Sat. Cal. (g)	Trans Fat (g)	Fat (mg)	Chol. (mg)	Sod. (g)	Carb. (g)	Fiber (g)	Pro. Choices/Exchanges
✔Skinny Cinnamon Dolce Latte - no whip	12 oz	90	0	0	0	0	5	125	14	0	9	1 milk
✔Skinny Hazelnut Latte - no whip	12 oz	90	0	0	0	0	5	125	14	0	9	1 milk
✔Skinny Mocha - no whip	12 oz	90	0	0	0	0	5	125	14	0	9	1 milk
✔Skinny Vanilla - no whip	12 oz	90	0	0	0	0	5	125	14	0	9	1 milk
HOT ESPRESSO - SOY												
✔Caffe Latte	12 oz	130	4	3	0.5	0	0	100	18	1	7	1 milk, 1 fat
Caffe Mocha - no whip	12 oz	190	5	2	0.5	0	0	90	34	2	8	1 carb, 1 milk, 1 fat
Caffe Mocha - whip	12 oz	260	11	4	4.5	0	20	95	36	2	8	1 carb, 1 milk, 2 fat
✔Cappuccino	12 oz	80	3	3	0	0	0	60	11	1	4	1 milk, 1/2 fat

Peppermint White Chocolate Mocha - whip	12 oz	400	13	3	7	0	25	180	63	1	9	3 carb, 1 milk, 3 fat
Syrup Flavored Latte	12 oz	180	4	2	0.5	0	0	95	31	1	6	1 carb, 1 milk, 1 fat
HOT ESPRESSO - WHOLE MILK												
Caffe Latte	12 oz	180	9	5	5	0	30	115	14	0	10	1 milk, 2 fat
Caffe Mocha - no whip	12 oz	230	9	4	4.5	0	25	100	31	1	10	1 carb, 1 milk, 2 fat
Caffe Mocha - whip	12 oz	290	15	5	9	0	45	105	33	1	10	1 carb, 1 milk, 3 fat
Cappuccino	12 oz	110	6	5	3	0	15	70	9	0	6	1 milk, 1 fat
Peppermint White Chocolate Mocha - whip	12 oz	440	18	4	11	0	45	180	60	0	11	3 carb, 1 milk, 3 1/2 fat
Syrup Flavored Latte	12 oz	220	9	4	5	0	25	105	27	0	9	1 carb, 1 milk, 2 fat
ICED ESPRESSO - NONFAT												
✔Caffe Americano	12 oz	10	0	0	0	0	0	5	2	0	1	Free

✔ = Healthiest Bets

(*Continued*)

	Amount	Cal.	Fat (g)	% Cal. Fat	Sat. Fat (g)	Trans Fat (g)	Chol. (mg)	Sod. (mg)	Carb. (g)	Fiber (g)	Pro. (g)	Choices/Exchanges
✔Caffe Latte	12 oz	70	0	0	0	0	5	80	10	0	6	1 milk
✔Caffe Mocha - no whip	12 oz	130	2	1	0	0	4	65	27	1	7	1 carb, 1 milk
Caffe Mocha - whip	12 oz	210	10	4	5	0	30	70	29	1	7	1 carb, 1 milk, 2 fat
✔Caramel Macchiato - no whip	12 oz	140	1	1	1	0	5	100	25	0	7	1 carb, 1 milk
✔Double shot + Energy Beverage	12 oz	70	0	0	0	0	0	15	14	0	3	1 carb
✔Double shot Beverage	12 oz	60	0	0	0	0	0	15	14	0	2	1 carb
✔Honey Latte - no whip	12 oz	130	0	0	0	0	5	70	25	0	6	1 carb, 1 milk
Honey Latte - whip	12 oz	210	8	3	5	0	35	80	28	0	6	1 carb, 1 milk, 1 1/2 fat
Peppermint White Chocolate Mocha - no whip	12 oz	280	5	2	3.5	0	5	140	54	0	7	3 carb, 1 milk

Peppermint White Chocolate Mocha - whip	12 oz	360	13	3	8	0	35	150	56	0	8	3 carb, 1 milk, 2 fat
Pumpkin Spice Latte - no whip	12 oz	170	0	0	0	0	5	130	33	0	8	1 1/2 carb, 1 milk
Pumpkin Spice Latte - whip	12 oz	250	8	3	5	0	35	140	36	0	8	1 1/2 carb, 1 milk, 1 1/2 fat
✔Skinny Cinnamon Dolce Latte - no whip	12 oz	60	0	0	0	0	5	85	9	0	6	1 milk
✔Sugar-Free Syrup Flavored Latte	12 oz	60	0	0	0	0	5	85	9	0	6	1 milk
✔Syrup Flavored Latte	12 oz	120	0	0	0	0	0	90	24	0	6	1 carb, 1 milk
✔Vanilla Latte	12 oz	120	0	0	0	0	0	90	24	0	6	1 carb, 1 milk
White Chocolate Mocha - no whip	12 oz	230	5	2	3.5	0	5	150	42	0	8	2 carb, 1 milk

✔ = Healthiest Bets

(*Continued*)

ICED ESPRESSO - NONFAT *(Continued)*	Amount	Cal.	Fat (g)	% Cal. Fat	Sat. Fat (g)	Trans Fat (g)	Chol. (mg)	Sod. (mg)	Carb. (g)	Fiber (g)	Pro. (g)	Choices/Exchanges
White Chocolate Mocha - whip	12 oz	320	12	3	8	0	35	160	44	0	9	2 carb, 1 milk, 2 fat
LOAVES AND COFFEE CAKES												
Banana Nut Loaf	1 pc	470	23	4	3.5	0	40	220	59	3	5	4 carb, 4 1/2 fat
Classic Coffee Cake	1 pc	430	18	4	11	0	95	220	61	1	5	4 carb, 3 1/2 fat
Iced Lemon Pound Cake	1 pc	390	8	2	5	0	80	380	66	0	5	4 1/2 carb, 1 1/2 fat
No Sugar Added Banana Nut Coffee Cake	1 pc	480	28	5	4	0	45	210	63	3	7	4 carb, 5 1/2 fat
Pumpkin Loaf	1 pc	380	14	3	2	0	55	180	59	2	5	4 carb, 3 fat
Reduced Fat Banana Chocolate Chip Coffee Cake	1 pc	390	8	2	4.5	0	0	400	76	3	5	5 carb, 1 1/2 fat

Reduced Fat Blueberry Coffee Cake	1 pc	320	6	2	4.5	0	10	390	54	1	4	3 1/2 carb, 1 fat
MUFFINS AND SCONES												
Blueberry Muffin	1	430	16	3	10	0	70	270	64	2	7	4 carb, 3 fat
Blueberry Scone	1	500	23	4	13	0.5	75	640	68	2	7	4 1/2 carb, 4 1/2 fat
Bran Muffin	1	410	18	4	9	0	70	430	60	7	9	4 carb, 3 1/2 fat
Cranberry Orange Muffin	1	340	9	2	5	0	75	560	61	2	5	4 carb, 2 fat
Low Fat Blueberry Muffin	1	290	5	2	1	0	0	460	56	1	7	3 1/2 carb, 1 fat
Maple Oat Nut Scone	1	400	23	5	7	0	25	220	45	2	5	3 carb, 4 1/2 fat
✔Petite Vanilla Bean Scone	1	130	5	3	3	0	15	65	20	0	2	1 carb, 1 fat
Raspberry Scone	1	490	22	4	12	0.5	85	560	66	2	7	4 1/2 carb, 41/2 fat
TAZO TEA - NONFAT												
Iced Tazo Green Tea Latte	12 oz	160	0	0	0	0	5	85	32	1	7	2 carb

✔ = Healthiest Bets

(Continued)

TAZO TEA - NONFAT *(Continued)*	Amount	Cal.	Fat (g)	% Cal. Fat	Sat. Fat (g)	Trans Fat (g)	Chol. (mg)	Sod. (mg)	Carb. (g)	Fiber (g)	Pro. (g)	Choices/Exchanges
✓Tazo Black Shaken Iced Tea	12 oz	60	0	0	0	0	0	10	16	0	0	1 carb
✓Tazo Black Shaken Iced Tea Lemonade	12 oz	100	0	0	0	0	0	10	25	0	0	1 1/2 carb
Tazo Chai Iced Tea Latte	12 oz	150	0	0	0	0	5	70	33	0	5	2 carb
Tazo Chai Tea Latte	12 oz	150	0	0	0	0	5	75	33	0	6	2 carb
✓Tazo Green Shaken Iced Tea	12 oz	60	0	0	0	0	0	10	16	0	0	1 carb
✓Tazo Green Shaken Iced Tea Lemonade	12 oz	100	0	0	0	0	0	10	25	0	0	1 carb
✓Tazo Green Tea Latte	12 oz	150	0	0	0	0	5	65	30	1	6	2 carb
✓Tazo Passion Shaken Iced Tea	12 oz	60	0	0	0	0	0	10	16	0	0	1 carb

✔Tazo Passion Shaken Iced Tea Lemonade	12 oz	100	0	0	0	0	0	10	25	0	0	1 1/2 carb
✔Tazo Tea	12 oz	0	0	0	0	0	0	0	0	0	0	Free

✔ = Healthiest Bets

Exclusive Web Content

Be sure to visit the following restaurants online at http://www.diabetes.org/healthyrestaurant

Carvel	**Frëshens**	**Jimmy John's**	**Wienerschnitzel**
Del Taco	**Godfather's**	**Tim Hortons**	**Zaxby's**
El Pollo Loco	**Jersey Mike's**	**Whataburger**	

Exclusive Web Content

Be sure to visit the following restaurants online at http://www.diabetes.org/healthyrestaurant

Carvel
Del Taco
El Pollo Loco
Frëshens
Godfather's
Jersey Mike's
Jimmy John's
Tim Hortons
Whataburger
Wienerschnitzel
Zaxby's

Burgers, Fries, and More

RESTAURANTS

Burger King
Carl's Jr.
Dairy Queen/Brazier
Hardee's
Jack in the Box
McDonald's
Sonic, America's Drive-In
Wendy's

EXCLUSIVE WEB CONTENT

Whataburger (http://www.diabetes.org/healthyrestaurant)

NUTRITION PROS

- Small portions are easy to find at these restaurants as long as you know and use the right words, such as "regular," "small," "junior," and "single."
- There's no waiting for food. You order and then eat.
- No foods greet you at the table. What you order is what you eat. This means you don't have to keep your hands off of pre-meal extras like bread and butter.
- You can get a few grams of fiber from multigrain buns and baked potatoes. Of course, they often aren't available.
- It's easier than ever to partner a vegetable with a burger, usually as a salad or ready-to-eat carrots. Entrée salads are on nearly all menus. Be careful to limit the high-fat salad toppings, such as cheese, fried

chicken, fried noodles, and nuts. When it comes to salad dressing, choose wisely and drizzle gingerly.

- Salad dressing is served on the side. There's no need for a special request.
- More fruits and vegetables are creeping into menus in response to health concerns. You'll see baby carrots, apple slices, fresh fruit cups, and more.
- Choose healthier cold drinks: low-fat (1%) or fat-free (skim) milk, fruit juice, water, unsweetened ice tea, diet soft drinks.
- Low-fat, low-calorie, and fat-free salad dressings are now common. Remember that these salad dressings are not calorie free. They can also be high in sodium.

Healthy Tips

- ★ Zero in on the words "regular," "junior," "small," or "single." These mean small portions.
- ★ Try lower-calorie ketchup, mustard, or barbecue sauce as a substitute for higher-fat mayonnaise or mayonnaise-based special sauces.
- ★ Walk in rather than drive through. If you eat and drive, you hardly realize how much food you've eaten.
- ★ Order less food from the beginning. Remember, you can go back and get more in a flash.
- ★ Want fries? Go ahead, but split a small or medium order and enjoy a few while they're hot.

- Healthier dessert options include low-fat frozen yogurt in a cone or dish and low-fat milkshakes.
- Honesty is their policy. Full disclosure of nutrition information is there for the asking.
- You know the menu well. You can plan what to order before you walk in the door.

NUTRITION CONS

- Many menu items are high in fat. Cheese, cheese sauce, bacon, special sauces, and mayonnaise add fat.
- Large portions are all too frequent. "Large," "jumbo," "double," and "triple" are a few words to watch out for.
- Sodium can skyrocket from added salt in special sauces and in salad dressings. Also, some prepared menu items, such as chicken breasts, can be high in sodium.
- Chicken and fish start off healthy, but they are often buried in a crisp, golden, high-fat coating.
- Some of the salad toppings and dressings can undo the healthiness of entrée salads.
- Biscuits are loaded with fat to begin with. Tuck sausage, bacon, egg, and/or cheese in the middle and you've just downed your fat grams for the day in one fell swoop.
- Fruit is still not plentiful, but easier to find lately.
- French fries and onion rings—deep fried, of course—are still the traditional sides.
- The meal deals can push you to eat larger portions because you buy more food (most often fried items and drinks) for less money. Don't get caught up in this unhealthy mentality.

Get It Your Way

- ★ Avoid busy times. This way, you'll get your food your way with a smile.
- ★ Be ready to wait. Fast-food restaurants are not set up for special requests, so limit them to only reasonable changes.
- ★ Ask for simple changes. Leave off the special sauce or mayonnaise; hold the pickles, bacon, or cheese; or hold the salt on the French fries.

Exclusive Web Content

Be sure to visit the following restaurants online at http://www.diabetes.org/healthyrestaurant

Carvel
Del Taco
El Pollo Loco
Frëshens
Godfather's
Jersey Mike's
Jimmy John's
Tim Hortons
Whataburger
Wienerschnitzel
Zaxby's

Burger King
(www.burgerking.com)

Light 'n Lean Choice

Tendergrill Chicken Garden Salad
Ken's Light Italian Dressing *(1 oz, 2 Tbsp)*
Onion Rings *(small)*

Calories	440	Cholesterol (mg)	80
Fat (g)	22	Sodium (mg)	1,150
% calories from fat	45	Carbohydrate (g)	29
Saturated fat (g)	6	Fiber (g)	6
Trans fat (g)	1	Protein (g)	35

Exchanges: 1 starch, 2 veg, 4 lean meat, 2 fat

Healthy 'n Hearty Choice

Flame Broiled Cheeseburger
French Fries *(small)*
Strawberry Applesauce

Calories	650	Cholesterol (mg)	55
Fat (g)	29	Sodium (mg)	1,160
% calories from fat	40	Carbohydrate (g)	80
Saturated fat (g)	10	Fiber (g)	3
Trans fat (g)	3.5	Protein (g)	19

Exchanges: 4 starch, 1 fruit, 1 1/2 medium-fat meat, 4 1/2 fat

(*Continued*)

Burger King

	Amount	Cal.	Fat (g)	% Cal. Fat	Sat. Fat (g)	Trans Fat (g)	Chol. (mg)	Sod. (mg)	Carb. (g)	Fiber (g)	Pro. (g)	Choices/Exchanges
BREAKFAST SANDWICHES												
✔Croissan'wich Bacon, Egg & Cheese	1	340	20	5	7	2	155	890	26	0	15	1 1/2 starch, 1 medium-fat meat, 2 1/2 fat
✔Croissan'wich Egg & Cheese	1	300	17	5	6	2	145	740	26	0	12	1 1/2 starch, 1 medium-fat meat, 2 1/2 fat
Croissan'wich Ham, Egg & Cheese	1	340	18	5	6	2	160	1230	26	1	18	1 1/2 starch, 2 medium-fat meat, 2 fat
Croissan'wich Sausage & Cheese	1	370	25	6	9	2	50	810	23	0	14	1 1/2 starch, 2 high-fat meat, 1 fat
Croissan'wich Sausage, Egg & Cheese	1	470	32	6	11	2.5	180	1060	26	0	19	1 1/2 starch, 3 high-fat meat, 1 fat
Double Croissan'wich Bacon, Egg & Cheese	1	430	27	6	10	2	175	1250	27	0	21	2 starch, 2 medium-fat meat, 3 fat
Double Croissan'wich Ham, Bacon, Egg & Cheese	1	420	24	5	9	2	180	1600	27	1	24	2 starch, 3 medium-fat meat, 2 fat

Double Croissan'wich Ham, Egg & Cheese	1	420	23	5	9	2	185	2210	27	1	27	2 starch, 3 medium-fat meat, 1 1/2 fat
Double Croissan'wich Ham, Sausage, Egg & Cheese	1	550	37	6	15	2.5	205	2040	27	1	28	2 starch, 3 medium-fat meat, 4 fat
Double Croissan'wich Sausage, Bacon, Egg & Cheese	1	550	39	6	14	2.5	200	1420	27	1	25	2 starch, 3 medium-fat meat, 5 fat
Double Croissan'wich Sausage, Egg & Cheese	1	680	51	7	18	3	220	1590	26	1	29	1 1/2 starch, 4 high-fat meat, 3 1/2 fat
Enormous Omelet Sandwich	1	730	45	6	16	1	330	1940	44	2	37	3 starch, 4 medium-fat meat, 5 fat
✔Ham Omelet Sandwich	1	290	13	4	4.5	0	85	870	33	1	13	2 starch, 1 medium-fat meat, 1 1/2 fat
Sausage , Egg & Cheese Biscuit	1	530	37	6	12	6	175	1490	31	1	20	2 starch, 3 high-fat meat, 3 fat
Sausage Biscuit	1	390	26	6	8	5	35	1020	28	1	12	2 starch, 2 high-fat meat, 2 fat

✔ = Healthiest Bets

(*Continued*)

	Amount	Cal.	Fat (g)	% Cal. Fat	Sat. Fat (g)	Trans Fat (g)	Chol. (mg)	Sod. (mg)	Carb. (g)	Fiber (g)	Pro. (g)	Choices/Exchanges
BREAKFAST SIDES												
✔Breakfast Syrup	2 oz	80	0	0	0	0	0	0	20	0	0	1 starch
Cini-minis	1 order	390	18	4	5	4	20	560	51	2	7	3 1/2 starch, 3 fat
French Toast Kid's Meal w/ syrup	1 order	680	24	3	6	3	10	590	100	3	15	6 1/2 starch, 4 fat
French Toast Sticks	3 pc	240	13	5	2.5	2	0	260	26	1	4	1 1/2 starch, 2 1/2 fat
French Toast Sticks	5 pc	390	22	5	4.5	3	0	440	43	2	7	3 starch, 4 fat
✔Grape Jam	1 oz	30	0	0	0	0	0	0	7	0	0	1/2 starch
Hash Browns	sm	260	17	6	4.5	5	0	500	25	2	2	1 1/2 starch, 3 1/2 fat
Hash Browns	med	430	28	6	8	9	0	830	42	4	4	3 starch, 5 1/2 fat
Hash Browns	lg	620	40	6	11	13	0	1200	60	6	5	4 starch, 8 fat
✔Strawberry Jam	1 oz	30	0	0	0	0	0	0	7	0	0	1/2 starch
Vanilla Icing for Cini-minis	1 order	110	3	2	0.5	0.5	0	40	21	0	0	1 1/2 starch, 1/2 fat

CHICKEN, FISH, AND VEGGIE												
BK Big Fish Sandwich - no tartar sauce	1	470	13	2	3	2	50	1240	65	3	23	4 starch, 2 lean meat, 1 1/2 fat
✔BK Chicken Fries	6 pc	260	15	5	3.5	3	35	650	18	2	12	1 starch, 1 lean meat, 2 1/2 fat
BK Chicken Fries	9 pc	390	23	5	5	1.5	50	980	26	3	18	1 1/2 starch, 2 lean meat, 3 1/2 fat
BK Chicken Fries	12 pc	520	31	5	7	6	65	1300	35	4	25	2 1/2 starch, 3 lean meat, 4 1/2 fat
✔BK Veggie Burger - no mayo	1	340	8	2	1	0	0	1030	46	7	23	3 starch, 2 lean meat, 1/2 fat
BK Veggie Burger w/ cheese	1	470	20	4	5	0	20	1320	47	7	25	3 starch, 2 lean meat, 2 1/2 fat
✔Chicken Tenders	5 pc	210	12	5	3	2	35	600	13	0	12	1 starch, 1 lean meat, 1 1/2 fat

✔ = Healthiest Bets

(*Continued*)

CHICKEN, FISH, AND VEGGIE *(Continued)*	Amount	Cal.	Fat (g)	% Cal. Fat	Sat. Fat (g)	Trans Fat (g)	Chol. (mg)	Sod. (mg)	Carb. (g)	Fiber (g)	Pro. (g)	Choices/Exchanges
✔Chicken Tenders	8 pc	340	20	5	5	3	55	960	21	0	19	1 1/2 starch, 2 lean meat, 2 1/2 fat
✔Chicken Tenders - Big Kids Meal	6 pc	250	15	5	3.5	2.5	40	720	16	0	14	1 starch, 2 lean meat, 2 fat
✔Chicken Tenders - Kids Meal	4 pc	170	10	5	2.5	1.5	25	180	11	0	9	1/2 starch, 1 lean meat, 1 1/2 fat
Original Chicken Sandwich - no mayo	1	450	17	3	4	2	50	1205	52	4	23	3 1/2 starch, 2 lean meat, 2 1/2 fat
✔Spicy Chick'n Crisp Sandwich - no mayo	1	320	13	4	2.5	1.5	30	730	36	1	15	2 1/2 starch, 1 lean meat, 2 fat
Tendercrisp Crisp Chicken Sandwich	1	790	44	5	8	4	70	1640	68	5	33	4 1/2 starch, 3 lean meat, 6 1/2 fat
Tendergrill Chicken Sandwich - no mayo	1	400	7	2	1.5	0	70	1090	49	4	36	3 starch, 3 lean meat

COLD BEVERAGES												
Icee Coca Cola	16 oz	110	0	0	0	0	0	10	31	0	0	2 carb
Icee Coca Cola	22 oz	140	0	0	0	0	0	10	40	0	0	2 1/2 carb
Icee Minute Maid Cherry	16 oz	110	0	0	0	0	0	10	31	0	0	2 carb
Mocha BK Joe Iced Coffee	1	380	10	2	6	0	40	290	66	1	6	4 carb, 2 fat
DESSERTS												
Dutch Apple Pie	1	300	13	4	3	3	0	270	45	1	2	3 carb, 2 1/2 fat
Hershey's Sundae Pie	1	310	19	6	12	0	10	220	32	1	2	2 carb, 4 fat
FLAME BROILED BURGERS												
BK Double Stacker	1	610	39	6	16	1.5.	125	1100	32	2	34	2 starch, 4 medium-fat meat, 4 fat
BK Quad Stacker	1	1000	68	6	30	3	240	1800	34	1	62	2 1/2 starch, 8 medium-fat meat, 5 1/2 fat
BK Triple Stacker	1	800	54	6	23	2	185	1450	33	1	48	2 starch, 6 medium-fat meat, 5 fat

✓ = Healthiest Bets

(*Continued*)

FLAME BROILED BURGERS *(Continued)*	Amount	Cal.	Fat (g)	% Cal. Fat	Sat. Fat (g)	Trans Fat (g)	Chol. (mg)	Sod. (mg)	Carb. (g)	Fiber (g)	Pro. (g)	Choices/Exchanges
✔Cheeseburger	1	330	16	4	7	0.5	55	780	31	1	17	2 starch, 2 medium-fat meat, 1 1/2 fat
Double Cheeseburger	1	500	29	5	14	1.5	105	1030	31	1	30	2 starch, 3 medium-fat meat, 2 1/2 fat
Double Hamburger	1	410	21	5	9	1	85	600	30	1	25	2 starch, 3 medium-fat meat, 1 1/2 fat
✔Hamburger	1	290	12	4	4.5	0	40	560	30	1	15	2 starch, 1 medium-fat meat, 1 fat
The Angus Steak Burger	1	640	33	5	10	1.5	185	1260	55	3	33	3 1/2 starch, 3 medium-fat meat, 3 1/2 fat
SALAD DRESSINGS, SAUCES, AND CONDIMENTS												
Bacon for Whopper Sandwiches	4 strips	50	4	7	1.5	0	10	290	0	0	4	1 fat
✔Dipping Sauce - Barbecue	1 oz	40	0	0	0	0	0	310	11	0	0	1 carb

✔Dipping Sauce - Buffalo	1 oz	80	8	9	1.5	0	5	350	2	0	0	1 1/2 fat
✔Dipping Sauce - Honey Mustard	1 oz	90	6	6	1	0	10	180	8	0	0	1/2 carb, 1 fat
Dipping Sauce - Ranch	1 oz	140	15	10	2.5	0	5	95	1	0	1	3 fat
✔Dipping Sauce - Sweet and Sour	1 oz	45	0	0	0	0	0	55	11	0	0	1 carb
✔Garlic Parmesan Croutons	1 pkg	60	2	3	0	0	0	120	9	0	1	1/2 carb, 1/2 fat
Ken's Creamy Caesar Dressing	2 oz	210	21	9	4	0	25	610	4	0	3	4 fat
✔Ken's Fat Free Ranch Dressing	2 oz	60	0	0	0	0	0	740	15	2	0	1 carb
Ken's Honey Mustard Dressing	2 oz	270	23	8	3	0	20	520	15	0	1	1 carb, 4 1/2 fat
✔Ken's Light Italian Dressing	2 oz	120	11	8	1.5	0	0	440	5	0	0	2 fat
✔Ken's Ranch Dressing	2 oz	190	20	9	3	0	20	560	2	0	1	4 fat

✔ = Healthiest Bets

(Continued)

SALAD DRESSINGS, SAUCES, AND CONDIMENTS *(Continued)*	Amount	Cal.	Fat (g)	% Cal. Fat	Sat. Fat (g)	Trans Fat (g)	Chol. (mg)	Sod. (mg)	Carb. (g)	Fiber (g)	Pro. (g)	Choices/Exchanges
Zesty Onion Ring Dipping Sauce	1 oz	150	15	9	2.5	0	15	210	3	0	0	3 fat
SALADS												
✔Garden Salad - no chicken	1	90	5	5	2.5	0	15	125	7	3	5	2 veg
✔Side Garden Salad	1	15	0	0	0	0	0	0	3	0	1	Free
Tendercrisp Chicken Garden Salad	1	410	22	5	6	3.5	70	1080	26	5	29	1 starch, 2 veg, 4 lean meat, 2 fat
✔Tendergrill Chicken Garden Salad	1	240	9	3	3.5	0	80	720	8	4	33	2 veg, 4 lean meat
SHAKES												
Chocolate - large	32 oz	950	29	3	19	0.5	115	640	151	2	16	10 carb, 6 fat
Chocolate - medium	22 oz	690	20	3	12	0	75	480	114	2	11	7 1/2 carb, 4 fat
Chocolate - small	16 oz	470	14	3	9	0	55	320	75	1	8	5 carb, 2 1/2 fat

Chocolate - value	12 oz	370	11	3	7	0	42	30	61	1	6	4 carb, 1 1/2 fat
Oreo Sundae Shake Chocolate - medium	22 oz	960	32	3	20	0.5	75	720	154	3	13	10 1/2 carb, 6 1/2 fat
Oreo Sundae Shake Chocolate - small	16 oz	680	24	3	15	0.5	55	480	105	2	9	7 carb, 5 fat
Oreo Sundae Shake Strawberry - medium	22 oz	940	31	3	19	0.5	75	55	151	2	12	10 carb, 6 fat
Oreo Sundae Shake Strawberry - small	16 oz	660	23	3	15	0.5	55	380	103	1	9	7 carb, 4 1/2 fat
Oreo Sundae Shake Vanilla - medium	22 oz	830	33	4	20	1	85	570	119	2	13	8 carb, 6 1/2 fat
Oreo Sundae Shake Vanilla - small	16 oz	610	24	4	16	0.5	60	400	87	1	9	6 carb, 5 fat
Strawberry - large	32 oz	930	28	3	18	0.5	115	490	148	0	15	10 carb, 5 1/2 fat
Strawberry - medium	22 oz	660	19	3	12	0	75	330	111	0	10	7 1/2 carb, 4 fat

✔ = Healthiest Bets

(*Continued*)

SHAKES *(Continued)*	Amount	Cal.	Fat (g)	% Cal. Fat	Sat. Fat (g)	Trans Fat (g)	Chol. (mg)	Sod. (mg)	Carb. (g)	Fiber (g)	Pro. (g)	Choices/Exchanges
Strawberry - small	16 oz	460	14	3	9	0	55	240	73	0	7	5 carb, 3 fat
Strawberry - value	12 oz	360	10	3	7	0	40	180	60	0	6	4 carb, 2 fat
Vanilla - large	32 oz	820	30	3	19	1	125	490	117	0	16	8 carb, 5 1/2 fat
Vanilla - medium	22 oz	560	21	3	13	0.5	85	330	79	0	11	5 1/2 carb, 3 1/2 fat
Vanilla - small	16 oz	400	15	3	9	0	60	240	57	0	8	4 carb, 3 fat
Vanilla - value	12 oz	310	11	3	7	0	45	180	44	0	6	3 carb, 2 fat
SIDE ORDERS												
Cheesy Tots Potatoes	6 pc	210	12	5	4.5	2	20	650	20	2	7	1 1/2 starch, 2 1/2 fat
Cheesy Tots Potatoes	9 pc	320	18	5	7	3	30	970	30	2	10	2 starch, 1 high-fat meat, 2 1/2 fat
Cheesy Tots Potatoes	12 pc	430	24	5	9	4	40	1300	40	3	14	2 1/2 starch, 1 high-fat meat, 1 fat

French Fries, no added salt	sm	230	13	5	3	3	0	240	26	2	2	1 1/2 starch, 2 1/2 fat
French Fries, no added salt	med	360	20	5	4.5	4.5	0	380	41	4	4	2 1/2 starch, 4 fat
French Fries, no added salt	lg	500	28	5	6	6	0	530	57	5	5	4 starch, 5 fat
French Fries, no added salt	king	600	33	5	8	7	0	640	69	6	6	4 1/2 starch, 6 fat
French Fries, salted	sm	230	13	5	3	3	0	380	26	2	2	1 1/2 starch, 2 1/2 fat
French Fries, salted	med	360	20	5	4.5	4.5	0	590	41	4	4	2 1/2 starch, 4 fat
French Fries, salted	lg	500	28	5	6	6	0	820	57	5	5	3 1/2 starch, 5 1/2 fat
French Fries, salted	king	600	33	5	8	7	0	990	69	6	6	4 1/2 starch, 6 fat
✔Mott's Strawberry Flavored Apple Sauce	4 oz	90	0	0	0	0	0	0	23	0	0	1 1/2 carb

✔ = Healthiest Bets

(*Continued*)

SIDE ORDERS *(Continued)*	Amount	Cal.	Fat (g)	% Cal. Fat	Sat. Fat (g)	Trans Fat (g)	Chol. (mg)	Sod. (mg)	Carb. (g)	Fiber (g)	Pro. (g)	Choices/Exchanges
Onion Rings	sm	140	7	5	1.5	1	0	210	18	2	2	1 starch, 1 1/2 fat
Onion Rings	med	310	15	4	3.5	2.5	0	440	37	3	4	2 1/2 starch, 3 fat
Onion Rings	lg	440	22	5	4.5	4	0	620	53	5	6	3 1/2 starch, 4 1/2 fat
WHOPPER SANDWICHES												
Double Whopper - no mayo	1	740	39	5	17	2	160	950	51	3	47	3 1/2 starch, 5 medium-fat meat, 2 1/2 fat
Double Whopper w/ cheese - no mayo	1	830	47	5	22	2	180	1380	52	3	52	3 1/2 starch, 6 medium-fat meat, 3 1/2 fat
Triple Whopper - no mayo	1	980	57	5	24	2.5	240	1020	51	3	66	3 1/2 starch, 8 medium-fat meat, 3 1/2 fat
Triple Whopper w/ cheese - no mayo	1	1070	65	5	29	3	260	1450	52	3	71	3 1/2 starch, 9 medium-fat meat, 4 1/2 fat

Whopper - no mayo	1	510	22	4	9	1	80	880	51	3	28	3 1/2 starch, 3 medium-fat meat, 2 fat
WHOPPER JR. - NO MAYO												
✔Whopper Jr. - no mayo	1	290	12	4	4.5	0	40	490	31	2	15	2 starch, 1 medium-fat meat, 1 fat
✔Whopper Jr. w/ cheese - no mayo	1	330	16	4	7	0.5	55	710	31	2	17	2 starch, 2 medium-fat meat, 1 1/2 fat
Whopper w/ cheese - no mayo	1	600	30	5	14	1.5	100	1310	52	3	32	3 1/2 starch, 3 medium-fat meat, 3 fat

✔ = Healthiest Bets

Carl's Jr.

(www.carlsjr.com)

Light 'n Lean Choice

Charbroiled BBQ Chicken Sandwich
Side Salad
Low-Fat Balsamic Dressing *(1 packet, 4 Tbsp)*

Calories	445	Cholesterol (mg)	65
Fat (g)	10	Sodium (mg)	1,190
% calories from fat	20	Carbohydrate (g)	58
Saturated fat (g)	2.5	Fiber (g)	6
Trans fat (g)	na	Protein (g)	37

Exchanges: 3 1/2 starch, 1 veg, 3 1/2 lean meat

Healthy 'n Hearty Choice

Big Hamburger
French Fries *(1/2 serving)*
Side Salad
House Dressing *(1/2 of 2-oz packet, 2 Tbsp)*

Calories	720	Cholesterol (mg)	70
Fat (g)	32	Sodium (mg)	1,320
% calories from fat	40	Carbohydrate (g)	79
Saturated fat (g)	10	Fiber (g)	7
Trans fat (g)	na	Protein (g)	30

Exchanges: 5 starch, 1 veg, 2 medium-fat meat, 5 fat

Carl's Jr.

	Amount	Cal.	Fat (g)	% Cal. Fat	Sat. Fat (g)	Trans Fat (g)	Chol. (mg)	Sod. (mg)	Carb. (g)	Fiber (g)	Pro. (g)	Choices/Exchanges
BREAKFAST												
Bacon and Egg Burrito	1	570	33	5	11	na	515	990	37	1	30	2 1/2 starch, 3 medium-fat meat, 3 1/2 fat
Breakfast Burger	1	830	47	5	15	na	275	1580	65	3	37	4 1/2 starch, 3 medium-fat meat, 6 fat
French Toast Dips - no syrup	5 pcs	430	18	4	2.5	na	0	530	58	1	9	4 starch, 3 1/2 fat
Hash Brown Nuggets	1	330	21	6	4.5	na	0	460	32	3	3	2 starch, 4 fat
Loaded Breakfast Burrito	1	820	51	6	16	na	6+5	1530	52	2	38	3 1/2 starch, 4 medium-fat meat, 6 1/2 fat

✓ = Healthiest Bets; na - not available

(*Continued*)

BREAKFAST *(Continued)*	Amount	Cal.	Fat (g)	% Cal. Fat	Sat. Fat (g)	Trans Fat (g)	Chol. (mg)	Sod. (mg)	Carb. (g)	Fiber (g)	Pro. (g)	Choices/Exchanges
Sourdough Breakfast Sandwich	1	460	21	4	9	na	280	1050	39	2	28	2 1/2 starch, 3 medium-fat meat, 1 1/2 fat
Steak and Egg Burrito	1	660	36	5	13	na	545	1690	44	2	40	3 starch, 4 medium-fat meat, 2 1/2 fat
Sunrise Croissant	1	560	41	7	15	na	290	970	27	1	20	2 starch, 2 medium-fat meat, 6 fat
CHARBROILED BURGERS												
The Bacon Cheese Six Dollar Burger	1	1070	76	6	30	na	170	1910	50	3	46	3 1/2 starch, 5 medium-fat meat, 10 fat
Big Hamburger	1	470	17	3	6	na	60	1060	54	3	24	3 1/2 starch, 2 medium-fat meat, 1 1/2 fat
Double Western Cheeseburger	1	970	52	5	21	na	155	1820	71	3	52	4 1/2 starch, 5 medium-fat meat, 5 fat

Famous Star w/ Cheese	1	660	39	5	12	na	85	1260	53	3	27	3 1/2 starch, 2 medium-fat meat, 5 1/2 fat
The Guacamole Bacon Six Dollar Burger	1	1140	85	7	29	na	160	2010	54	6	43	3 1/2 starch, 5 medium-fat meat, 12 fat
Jalapeno Burger	1	720	45	6	8	na	90	1320	50	3	27	3 1/2 starch, 2 medium-fat meat, 6 1/2 fat
The Jalapeno Six Dollar Burger	1	1030	74	6	37	na	150	2050	52	3	39	3 1/2 starch, 4 medium-fat meat, 10 1/2 fat
Kid's Burger	1	460	17	3	6	na	60	1060	53	2	24	3 1/2 starch, 2 medium-fat meat, 1 1/2 fat
The Low Carb Six Dollar Burger	1	490	37	7	15	na	130	1290	6	2	33	1/2 starch, 5 medium-fat meat, 3 fat
The Original Six Dollar Burger	1	1010	68	6	27	na	150	1980	60	3	40	4 starch, 4 medium-fat meat, 9 1/2 fat
Super Star w/ Cheese	1	930	59	6	32	na	160	1600	54	3	47	3 1/2 starch, 5 medium fat meat, 6 1/2 fat

✓ = Healthiest Bets; na - not available

(*Continued*)

CHARBROILED BURGERS *(Continued)*	Amount	Cal.	Fat (g)	% Cal. Fat	Sat. Fat (g)	Trans Fat (g)	Chol. (mg)	Sod. (mg)	Carb. (g)	Fiber (g)	Pro. (g)	Choices/Exchanges
Teriyaki Burger	1	660	34	5	11	na	80	1070	61	3	28	4 starch, 2 medium-fat meat, 4 1/2 fat
Western Bacon Cheeseburger	1	710	33	4	12	na	85	1480	70	3	32	4 1/2 starch, 3 medium-fat meat, 4 fat
The Western Bacon Six Dollar Burger	1	1130	66	5	28	na	150	2540	83	4	47	5 1/2 starch, 4 medium-fat meat, 8 1/2 fat
CHICKEN AND OTHER CHOICES												
Bacon Swiss Crispy Chicken Sandwich	1	720	35	4	8	na	85	1750	64	3	35	4 1/2 starch, 3 medium-fat meat, 4 fat
Carl's Catch Fish Sandwich	1	660	31	4	5	na	60	1290	75	3	22	5 starch, 1 lean meat, 5 fat
Charbroiled BBQ Chicken Sandwich	1	360	5	1	1	na	60	1150	48	4	34	3 starch, 3 lean meat, 1 fat

Charbroiled Chicken Club Sandwich	1	550	25	4	7	na	95	1410	43	4	40	3 starch, 4 lean meat, 2 1/2 fat
Charbroiled Santa Fe Chicken Sandwich	1	610	32	5	8	na	100	1540	43	4	37	3 starch, 4 lean meat, 4 fat
Chicken Breast Strips	5 pcs	710	41	5	6	na	80	2020	46	2	38	3 starch, 4 lean meat, 5 1/2 fat
Chicken Breast Strips	3 pcs	420	25	5	3.5	na	60	1210	28	1	23	2 starch, 2 lean meat, 3 1/2 fat
Spicy Chicken Sandwich	1	560	30	5	6	na	40	1480	59	2	15	4 starch, 0 lean meat, 5 1/2 fat
DESSERTS												
Chocolate Cake	1	300	12	4	3	na	30	350	48	1	3	3 carb, 2 fat
Chocolate Chip Cookie	1	350	18	5	7	na	20	330	46	1	3	3 carb, 3 fat
Strawberry Swirl Cheesecake	1	290	17	5	9	na	55	130	30	0	6	2 carb, 3 1/2 fat

✔ = Healthiest Bets; na - not available

(Continued)

	Amount	Cal.	Fat (g)	% Cal. Fat	Sat. Fat (g)	Trans Fat (g)	Chol. (mg)	Sod. (mg)	Carb. (g)	Fiber (g)	Pro. (g)	Choices/Exchanges
HAND-SCOOPED ICE CREAM SHAKES & MALTS												
Chocolate Malt	1	780	35	4	24	na	105	360	98	1	17	6 1/2 carb, 6 fat
Chocolate Shake	1	710	33	4	23	na	100	290	85	1	14	5 1/2 carb, 6 1/2 fat
Oreo Cookie Malt	1	790	39	4	25	na	105	42	91	1	18	6 carb, 7 fat
Oreo Cookie Shake	1	720	37	5	24	na	100	250	79	1	16	5 1/2 carb, 7 1/2 fat
Strawberry Malt	1	770	35	4	24	na	105	310	97	0	17	6 1/2 carb, 6 fat
Strawberry Shake	1	700	33	4	23	na	100	240	84	0	14	5 1/2 carb, 6 1/2 fat
Vanilla Malt	1	780	35	4	24	na	105	300	99	0	17	6 1/2 carb, 6 fat
Vanilla Shake	1	710	33	4	23	na	100	230	86	0	14	5 1/2 carb, 6 fat
SALAD DRESSING												
Blue Cheese Dressing	2 oz pkt	320	34	10	7	na	20	410	1	0	2	7 fat
House Dressing	2 oz pkt	220	22	9	3.5	na	20	440	2	0	1	4 1/2 fat

Low-Fat Balsamic Dressing	2 oz pkt	35	2	5	0	na	0	480	5	0	0	1/2 starch, 1/2 fat
Thousand Island Dressing	2 oz pkt	240	23	9	3.5	na	20	460	7	0	0	1/2 starch, 4 1/2 fat
SALADS - NO DRESSING												
✔Charbroiled Chicken Salad	1	260	7	2	3.4	na	75	710	16	5	34	1/2 starch, 2 veg, 4 lean meat
✔Side Salad	1	50	3	5	1.5	na	5	60	5	2	3	1 veg, 1 fat
SIDES												
✔Chicken Stars	4 pcs	170	11	6	3	na	25	320	10	1	9	1/2 starch, 1 lean meat, 1 1/2 fat
Chicken Stars	9 pcs	380	14	3	6	na	55	710	21	1	20	1 1/2 starch, 2 lean meat, 1 1/2 fat
Chicken Stars	6 pcs	260	16	6	4	na	35	470	14	1	13	1 starch, 1 lean meat, 2 1/2 fat
Cris Cut Fries	1	410	24	5	5	na	0	950	43	4	5	3 starch, 5 fat

✔ = Healthiest Bets; na - not available

(*Continued*)

SIDES ***(Continued)***	**Amount**	**Cal.**	**Fat (g)**	**% Cal. Fat**	**Sat. Fat (g)**	**Trans Fat (g)**	**Chol. (mg)**	**Sod. (mg)**	**Carb. (g)**	**Fiber (g)**	**Pro. (g)**	**Choices/Exchanges**
Fish and Chips	1	630	28	4	5	na	10	99	68	3	26	4 1/2 starch, 2 lean meat, 4 1/2 fat
French Fries, kids	1	250	12	4	2.5	na	0	150	32	3	4	2 starch, 2 1/2 fat
French Fries, large	1	620	29	4	6	na	0	380	80	7	10	5 1/2 starch, 5 fat
French Fries, medium	1	460	22	4	4.5	na	0	280	59	5	7	4 starch, 4 fat
French Fries, small	1	290	14	4	3	na	0	180	37	3	5	2 1/2 starch, 3 fat
Fried Zucchini	1	320	19	5	5	na	0	850	31	0	6	2 starch, 4 fat
Onion Rings	1	430	21	4	4	na	0	550	53	2	6	3 1/2 starch, 4 fat

✔ = Healthiest Bets; na - not available

Dairy Queen/Brazier
(www.dairyqueen.com)

Light 'n Lean Choice

DQ Original Burger
Vanilla Cone *(small)*

Calories	590	Cholesterol (mg)	52
Fat (g)	21	Sodium (mg)	790
% calories from fat	32	Carbohydrate (g)	65
Saturated fat (g)	12	Fiber (g)	1
Trans fat (g)	0.5	Protein (g)	23

Exchanges: 2 starch, 2 carb, 1 1/2 lean meat, 3 fat

Healthy 'n Hearty Choice

Grilled Chicken Sandwich
DQ Chocolate Soft Serve *(4 oz)*
DQ Fries *(small, 1/2 order)*

Calories	695	Cholesterol (mg)	70
Fat (g)	28	Sodium (mg)	1,175
% calories from fat	36	Carbohydrate (g)	74
Saturated fat (g)	7	Fiber (g)	3
Trans fat (g)	1	Protein (g)	29

Exchanges: 3 1/2 starch, 1 1/2 carb, 2 lean meat, 4 fat

(*Continued*)

Dairy Queen/Brazier

	Amount	Cal.	Fat (g)	&& Cal. Fat	Sat. Fat (g)	Trans Fat (g)	Chol. (mg)	Sod. (mg)	Carb. (g)	Fiber (g)	Pro. (g)	Choices/Exchanges
BLIZZARD TREATS												
Choc. Chip Cookie Dough Blizzard	sm	720	28	4	14	3	50	370	105	1	12	7 carb, 4 1/2 fat
Choc. Chip Cookie Dough Blizzard	med	1030	40	3	20	4.5	70	530	151	1	17	10 carb, 6 fat
Choc. Chip Cookie Dough Blizzard	lg	1320	52	4	27	6	90	680	193	2	21	13 carb, 8 fat
Oreo Cookies Blizzard	sm	560	21	3	10	0	40	430	83	1	11	5 1/2 carb, 3 1/2 fat
Oreo Cookies Blizzard	med	690	26	3	12	0.5	45	560	103	1	13	7 carb, 4 fat
Oreo Cookies Blizzard	lg	1000	37	3	18	0.5	70	770	148	2	19	10 carb, 6 fat
Reese's Peanut Butter Cups Blizzard	sm	550	22	4	12	0	45	280	76	1	12	5 carb, 4 fat

Reese's Peanut Butter Cups Blizzard	med	770	32	4	16	0.5	55	400	104	2	17	7 carb, 5 1/2 fat
Reese's Peanut Butter Cups Blizzard	lg	1080	46	4	23	0.5	75	570	144	3	24	9 1/2 carb, 8 fat
CONES												
Chocolate Dipped Cone	sm	340	16	4	10	1	20	120	36	0	6	2 1/2 carb, 3 fat
Chocolate Dipped Cone	med	490	23	4	15	1.5	30	170	61	0	8	4 carb, 4 fat
Chocolate Dipped Cone	lg	670	31	4	21	2.5	40	210	83	0	13	5 1/2 carb, 5 1/2 fat
✔DQ Chocolate Soft Serve	1/2 cup	150	5	3	3.5	0	15	75	22	0	4	1 1/2 carb, 1 fat
✔DQ Vanilla Soft Serve	1/2 cup	150	5	3	3	0	15	70	22	0	3	1 1/2 carb, 1 fat
Vanilla Cone	sm	240	7	3	4.5	0	2	110	32	0	6	2 carb, 1 1/2 fat
Vanilla Cone	med	340	10	3	6	0	30	160	54	0	8	3 1/2 carb, 2 fat
Vanilla Cone	lg	480	15	3	9	0.5	45	230	76	0	11	5 carb, 2 1/2 fat

✔ = Healthiest Bets

(*Continued*)

	Amount	Cal.	Fat (g)	% Cal. Fat	Sat. Fat (g)	Trans Fat (g)	Chol. (mg)	Sod. (mg)	Carb. (g)	Fiber (g)	Pro. (g)	Choices/Exchanges
FRIES AND ONION RINGS												
DQ Small Fries	1	290	13	4	2.5	2	0	620	40	4	3	2 1/2 starch, 2 1/2 fat
DQ Medium Fries	1	370	17	4	3	2.5	0	780	51	5	4	3 1/2 starch, 3 fat
DQ Large Fries	1	480	21	4	4	3	0	1000	66	7	5	4 1/2 starch, 3 1/2 fat
Regular Onion Rings	1	470	30	6	6	7	0	740	45	3	6	3 starch, 6 fat
GRILL BURGERS												
1/4 lb. Chili Meltdown Grill Burger	1	600	34	5	12	2.5	70	1060	41	3	29	2 1/2 starch, 3 medium-fat meat, 4 fat
1/4 lb. Flame Thrower Grill Burger	1	840	59	6	16	3	105	1490	41	2	34	2 1/2 starch, 4 medium-fat meat, 8 fat
Bacon Cheddar Grill Burger	1	710	42	5	15	2.5	95	1450	41	2	36	2 1/2 starch, 4 medium-fat meat, 4 1/2 fat
✓DQ Original Burger	1	350	14	4	7	0.5	50	680	33	1	17	2 starch, 1 medium-fat meat, 1 1/2 fat

✔DQ Original Cheese Burger	1	400	18	4	9	0.5	65	920	34	1	19	2 1/2 starch, 2 medium-fat meat, 2 fat
DQ Original Double Bacon Cheeseburger	1	730	41	5	21	1	150	1550	35	1	41	2 1/2 starch, 5 medium-fat meat, 3 1/2 fat
DQ Original Double Cheeseburger	1	640	34	5	18	1	125	1230	34	1	34	2 1/2 starch, 4 medium-fat meat, 3 fat
DQ Ultimate Burger	1	780	48	6	22	1.5	155	1390	33	1	41	2 starch, 5 medium-fat meat, 4 1/2 fat
Mushroom Swiss Burger	1	680	42	6	13	2.5	75	950	39	2	29	2 1/2 starch, 3 medium-fat meat, 5 1/2 fat
HOT DOGS												
All-Beef Chili Cheese Dog	1	430	23	5	10	0	45	990	39	2	18	2 1/2 starch, 1 high-fat meat, 2 1/2 fat
✔All-Beef Hot Dog	1	250	14	5	5	0	25	770	21	1	9	1 1/2 starch, 1 high-fat meat, 1 1/2 fat

✔ = Healthiest Bets

(Continued)

	Amount	Cal.	Fat (g)	% Cal. Fat	Sat. Fat (g)	Trans Fat (g)	Chol. (mg)	Sod. (mg)	Carb. (g)	Fiber (g)	Pro. (g)	Choices/Exchanges
MALTS, SHAKES, AND ARCTIC RUSH												
Arctic Rush Slush	sm	240	0	0	0	0	0	0	48	0	0	3 carb
Arctic Rush Slush	med	310	0	0	0	0	0	0	63	0	0	4 carb
Chocolate Malt	sm	650	15	2	10	0	50	330	112	0	14	7 1/2 carb, 2 fat
Chocolate Malt	med	900	21	2	13	0.5	65	460	157	0	19	10 1/2 carb, 3 fat
Chocolate Malt	lg	1300	31	2	20	1	95	670	224	0	28	15 carb, 3 fat
Vanilla Shake	sm	560	14	2	9	0	45	220	96	0	12	6 1/2 carb, 2 fat
Vanilla Shake	med	780	20	2	13	0.5	60	300	136	0	17	9 carb, 2 1/2 fat
Vanilla Shake	lg	1130	29	2	19	1	90	450	192	0	25	13 carb, 2 1/2 fat
MOOLATTE FROZEN BLENDED COFFEE												
Cappuccino Moolatte	16 oz	500	19	3	15	0	30	180	73	0	7	5 carb, 3 1/2 fat
Cappuccino Moolatte	24 oz	700	24	3	18	0.5	45	260	105	0	11	7 carb, 4 1/2 fat

Caramel Moolatte	16 oz	630	19	3	16	0	35	260	103	0	8	7 carb, 2 1/2 fat
Caramel Moolatte	24 oz	880	25	3	20	0.5	55	380	146	0	12	9 1/2 carb, 3 fat
French Vanilla Moolatte	16 oz	570	18	3	14	0	30	170	90	0	7	6 carb, 3 fat
French Vanilla Moolatte	24 oz	770	24	3	18	0.5	45	260	123	0	11	8 carb, 3 1/2 fat
Mocha Moolatte	16 oz	590	23	4	15	0	30	200	84	0	8	5 1/2 carb, 4 fat
Mocha Moolatte	24 oz	840	31	3	20	0.5	45	300	121	1	7	8 carb, 5 fat
NOVELTIES												
Buster Bar	1	480	31	6	15	0	20	220	45	2	11	3 carb, 6 fat
Chocolate Dilly Bar	1	240	15	6	9	0	15	70	24	1	4	1 1/2 carb, 3 fat
✓DQ Fudge Bar - no added sugar	1	50	0	0	0	0	0	70	12	6	4	1 carb
✓DQ Sandwich	1	190	5	2	2.5	0.5	10	105	32	1	4	2 carb, 1 fat
✓DQ Vanilla Orange Bar - no added sugar	1	60	0	0	0	0	0	45	18	6	2	1 carb

✓ = Healthiest Bets

(Continued)

NOVELTIES (Continued)	Amount	Cal.	Fat (g)	% Cal. Fat	Sat. Fat (g)	Trans Fat (g)	Chol. (mg)	Sod. (mg)	Carb. (g)	Fiber (g)	Pro. (g)	Choices/Exchanges
✔Starkiss	1	80	0	0	0	0	0	10	21	0	0	1 1/2 carb
ROYAL TREATS												
Banana Split	1	530	14	2	10	0	30	180	98	3	8	5 1/2 carb, 2 fruit, 1 fat
Brownie Earth Quake	1	740	28	3	15	0	60	370	149	1	10	10 carb, 3 fat
Peanut Buster Parfait	1	710	30	4	16	0	30	380	96	2	16	6 1/2 carb, 5 fat
SALADS												
Crispy Chicken Salad - no dressing	1	420	22	5	7	2	70	960	30	6	28	1 starch, 3 veg, 4 lean meat, 2 fat
✔Grilled Salad - no dressing	1	320	11	3	5	0	75	890	14	4	31	3 veg, 4 lean meat
✔Side Salad - no dressing	1	45	0	0	0	0	0	50	11	2	1	2 veg
SANDWICHES/BASKETS												
Chicken Strip Basket, 4 pc w/ BBQ Hot Dip	1	1090	48	4	7	7.5	75	2680	129	9	37	8 1/2 starch, 2 lean meat, 7 fat

Chicken Strip Basket, 4 pc w/ Country Gravy	1	1030	54	5	9	10	75	2400	105	8	37	7 starch, 2 lean meat, 8 fat
Chicken Strip Basket, 4 pc w/ Wild Buffalo	1	1340	96	6	18	11	90	4820	82	9	36	5 1/2 starch, 3 lean meat, 17 fat
Crispy Chicken Sandwich	1	530	29	5	4.5	3	55	1020	47	5	22	3 starch, 2 lean meat, 4 1/2 fat
Fish Sandwich	1	420	20	4	3	2.5	30	1070	54	1	17	3 1/2 starch, 1 lean meat, 3 fat
✔Grilled Chicken Sandwich	1	400	16	4	2.5	0	55	790	32	1	23	2 starch, 2 lean meat, 2 fat
Grilled Flame Thrower Chicken Sandwich	1	630	36	5	9	0	100	1580	34	2	34	2 1/2 starch, 4 lean meat, 5 fat
SUNDAES												
Chocolate Sundae	sm	280	7	2	4.5	0	20	130	49	0	5	3 1/2 carb, 1 fat
Chocolate Sundae	med	410	10	2	7	0	30	190	72	0	7	5 carb, 1 1/2 fat
Chocolate Sundae	lg	580	15	2	9	0.5	45	260	100	0	10	6 1/2 carb, 2 fat

✔ = Healthiest Bets

(*Continued*)

SUNDAES *(Continued)*	Amount	Cal.	Fat (g)	% Cal. Fat	Sat. Fat (g)	Trans Fat (g)	Chol. (mg)	Sod. (mg)	Carb. (g)	Fiber (g)	Pro. (g)	Choices/Exchanges
Strawberry Sundae	sm	280	7	2	4.5	0	20	130	50	1	5	3 1/2 carb, 1 fat
Strawberry Sundae	med	370	10	2	7	0	30	170	63	1	7	4 carb, 1 1/2 fat
Strawberry Sundae	lg	510	15	3	9	0.5	45	240	83	1	10	5 1/2 carb, 2 1/2 fat
WAFFLE TREATS												
Chocolate Coated Waffle Cone with Soft Serve	1	550	22	4	10	2.5	40	190	79	1	9	5 1/2 carb, 3 1/2 fat
Chocolate Covered Strawberry Waffle Bowl Sundae	1	800	40	5	24	3.5	35	200	100	2	9	6 1/2 carb, 6 1/2 fat
Fab Fudge Waffle Bowl	1	730	29	4	19	2	35	250	106	1	10	7 carb, 4 1/2 fat
Plain Waffle Cone w/ Soft Serve	1	430	13	3	7	0.5	35	160	68	0	9	4 1/2 carb, 4 1/2 fat
Turtle Waffle Bowl Sundae	1	820	35	4	16	2	40	330	117	2	11	8 carb, 4 1/2 fat

✔ = Healthiest Bets

Hardee's

(www.hardees.com)

Light 'n Lean Choice

Regular Roast Beef Sandwich
Natural Cut French Fries *(kid's size)*

Calories	530	Cholesterol (mg)	40
Fat (g)	25	Sodium (mg)	1,310
% calories from fat	42	Carbohydrate (g)	57
Saturated fat (g)	9	Fiber (g)	4
Trans fat (g)	0	Protein (g)	21

Exchanges: 4 starch, 2 medium-fat meat, 3 fat

Healthy 'n Hearty Choice

Regular Roast Beef Sandwich
Mashed Potatoes *(1 serving)*
Side Salad with Ranch
Dressing *(1/2 portion, 1 Tbsp)*

Calories	620	Cholesterol (mg)	68
Fat (g)	33	Sodium (mg)	1,550
% calories from fat	48	Carbohydrate (g)	54
Saturated fat (g)	14	Fiber (g)	4
Trans fat (g)	0	Protein (g)	27

Exchanges: 3 starch, 1 veg, 2 medium-fat meat, 5 1/2 fat

(*Continued*)

Hardee's

	Amount	Cal.	Fat (g)	% Cal. Fat	Sat. Fat (g)	Trans Fat (g)	Chol. (mg)	Sod. (mg)	Carb. (g)	Fiber (g)	Pro. (g)	Choices/Exchanges
BREAKFAST												
Bacon Biscuit	1	430	28	6	7	na	10	1110	35	0	8	2 1/2 starch, 1 high-fat meat, 4 fat
Bacon, Egg & Cheese Biscuit	1	560	38	6	44	na	225	1360	37	0	16	2 1/2 starch, 1 medium-fat meat, 6 1/2 fat
Big Country Breakfast Platter - Bacon	1	980	56	5	13	na	435	2080	90	3	28	6 starch, 4 high-fat meat, 3 fat
Big Country Breakfast Platter - Breaded Pork Chop	1	1220	68	5	13	na	465	2230	105	4	48	7 starch, 4 medium-fat meat, 9 fat
Big Country Breakfast Platter - Chicken	1	1140	61	5	13	na	480	2580	105	4	44	7 starch, 3 lean meat, 9 fat

Big Country Breakfast Platter - Country Ham	1	970	53	5	12	na	460	2600	90	3	33	6 starch, 2 lean meat, 9 fat
Big Country Breakfast Platter - Country Steak	1	1150	68	5	16	na	455	2260	98	4	36	6 1/2 starch, 2 medium-fat meat, 11 fat
Big Country Breakfast Platter - Sausage	1	1060	64	5	15	na	455	2140	91	4	30	6 starch, 4 high-fat meat, 4 fat
Biscuit Gravy	1 srvg	160	11	6	3	na	10	660	12	0	3	1 starch, 2 fat
Biscuit 'N' Gravy	1	530	34	6	8	na	10	1550	47	0	8	3 starch, 7 fat
✔Breaded Chicken Fillet	1 srvg	230	11	4	2	na	55	790	15	1	19	1 starch, 2 lean meat, 1 fat
Breaded Chicken Fillet Biscuit	1	600	34	5	7	na	55	1680	50	1	24	3 1/2 starch, 2 lean meat, 5 1/2 fat
Breaded Country Steak	1 srvg	240	18	7	5	na	30	470	9	0	11	1/2 starch, 1 medium-fat meat, 2 1/2 fat
Breaded Country Steak Biscuit	1	620	41	6	11	na	35	1360	44	0	16	3 starch, 1 medium-fat meat, 7 fat

✔ = Healthiest Bets

(*Continued*)

BREAKFAST *(Continued)*	Amount	Cal.	Fat (g)	% Cal. Fat	Sat. Fat (g)	Trans Fat (g)	Chol. (mg)	Sod. (mg)	Carb. (g)	Fiber (g)	Pro. (g)	Choices/Exchanges
Breaded Pork Chop Biscuit	1	690	42	5	8	na	40	1330	48	1	29	3 starch, 3 medium-fat meat, 5 1/2 fat
Butter Blend Packet	1 srvg	25	3	11	1	na	0	45	0	0	0	1/2 fat
Cinnamon 'N' Raisin Biscuit	1	280	12	4	3	na	0	650	40	0	3	3 starch, 2 1/2 fat
✔Country Ham (slice)	1 srvg	60	3	5	2	na	35	810	1	0	9	1 lean meat
Country Ham Biscuit	1	440	26	5	6	na	35	1710	36	0	14	2 1/2 starch, 1 lean meat, 4 1/2 fat
Country Steak & Egg Biscuit	1	690	47	6	11	na	235	1800	44	0	22	3 starch, 2 medium-fat meat, 7 1/2 fat
Egg Biscuit	1	450	29	6	6	na	205	940	35	0	11	2 1/2 starch, 1 medium-fat meat, 5 fat
✔Folded Egg	1 srvg	80	6	7	2	na	205	50	10	0	6	1 medium-fat meat
Frisco Breakfast Sandwich	1	420	20	4	7	na	240	1340	38	2	24	2 1/2 starch, 2 medium-fat meat, 1 1/2 fat

✓Grape Jam	1 srvg	10	0	0	0	na	0	0	2	0	0	Free
✓Grits	1 srvg	110	5	4	1	na	0	480	16	0	2	1 starch, 1 fat
Ham, Egg & Cheese Biscuit	1	560	35	6	10	na	245	1800	37	0	23	2 1/2 starch, 2 medium-fat meat, 5 fat
Hash Rounds	sm	260	16	6	4	na	0	360	25	2	3	2 starch, 3 fat
Hash Rounds	med	350	22	6	5	na	0	490	34	3	4	2 starch, 4 1/2 fat
Hash Rounds	lg	460	29	6	6	na	0	650	45	4	5	3 starch, 6 fat
Loaded Biscuit 'N' Gravy	1	770	54	6	14	na	245	1950	49	1	2	3 1/2 starch, 10 1/2 fat
BREAKFAST BOWL												
Loaded Breakfast Burrito	1	780	51	6	20	na	195	1620	38	2	40	2 1/2 starch, 5 medium-fat meat, 5 1/2 fat
Loaded Omelet	1 srvg	270	21	7	9	na	245	620	2	0	16	2 medium-fat meat, 2 fat
Loaded Omelet Biscuit	1	640	44	6	14	na	245	1510	37	0	21	2 1/2 starch, 2 medium-fat meat, 7 fat

✓ = Healthiest Bets

(*Continued*)

BREAKFAST BOWL ***(Continued)***	Amount	Cal.	Fat (g)	% Cal. Fat	Sat. Fat (g)	Trans Fat (g)	Chol. (mg)	Sod. (mg)	Carb. (g)	Fiber (g)	Pro. (g)	Choices/Exchanges
Low Carb Breakfast Bowl	1	620	50	7	21	na	325	1380	6	2	36	1/2 starch, 5 high-fat meat, 2 fat
Monster Biscuit	1	710	51	6	17	na	70	2250	37	0	24	2 1/2 starch, 2 medium-fat meat, 8 fat
Pancake Platter	1	300	5	2	1	na	25	830	55	2	8	4 starch, 1 fat
Pancake Syrup	1 srvg	90	0	0	0	na	0	0	21	0	0	1 carb
Sausage & Egg Biscuit	1	610	44	6	11	na	256	1290	36	0	17	2 1/2 starch, 2 high-fat meat, 5 fat
Sausage Biscuit	1	530	38	6	10	na	30	1240	36	0	11	2 1/2 starch, 2 high-fat meat, 5 fat
Sausage Patty	1 srvg	150	14	8	5	na	30	350	1	0	6	1 high-fat meat, 1 1/2 fat
Scrambled Egg	1 srvg	160	12	7	3	na	405	100	1	0	12	2 medium-fat meat
Scratch Biscuit	1	370	23	6	5	na	0	890	35	0	5	2 starch, 5 fat

✔Strawberry Jam	1 srvg	35	0	0	0	na	0	0	9	0	0	1/2 carb
✔Sunrise Croissant	1	210	10	4	4	na	5	200	26	0	4	2 starch, 2 fat
Sunrise Croissant w/ Bacon	1	450	29	6	12	na	240	900	28	0	19	2 starch, 3 high-fat meat, 1 1/2 fat
Sunrise Croissant w/ Ham	1	430	26	5	10	na	250	1050	28	0	23	2 starch, 2 lean meat, 3 1/2 fat
Sunrise Croissant w/ Sausage	1	550	38	6	15	na	265	1060	29	0	22	2 starch, 3 high-fat meat, 2 1/2 fat
KID'S MEAL												
Cheeseburger	1	600	27	4	6	na	45	930	68	4	21	4 1/2 starch, 1 medium-fat meat, 4 1/2 fat
Chicken Strips	2 pcs	500	25	5	5	na	35	1050	50	3	19	3 1/2 starch, 1 lean meat, 4 fat
Hamburger	1	560	24	4	6	na	35	710	67	4	18	4 1/2 starch, 1 medium-fat meat, 4 fat

✔ = Healthiest Bets

(*Continued*)

	Amount	Cal.	Fat (g)	% Cal. Fat	Sat. Fat (g)	Trans Fat (g)	Chol. (mg)	Sod. (mg)	Carb. (g)	Fiber (g)	Pro. (g)	Choices/Exchanges
LUNCH & DINNER												
1/4 lb Double Cheese Burger	1	510	26	5	5	na	90	1120	38	1	28	2 1/2 starch, 3 medium-fat meat, 2 1/2 fat
✔1/4 lb Double Hamburger	1	420	19	4	5	na	70	670	37	1	23	2 1/2 starch, 2 medium-fat meat, 1 1/2 fat
1/3 lb Bacon Cheese Thickburger	1	910	64	6	24	na	115	1550	50	3	33	3 1/2 starch, 3 medium-fat meat, 9 1/2 fat
1/3 lb Cheeseburger	1	680	39	5	19	na	90	1450	52	2	29	3 1/2 starch, 3 medium-fat meat, 5 fat
1/3 lb Low Carb Thickburger	1	420	31	7	12	na	115	1010	5	2	30	1/2 starch, 4 medium-fat meat, 2 fat
1/3 lb Mushroom 'N' Swiss Thickburger	1	720	42	5	21	na	100	1570	48	2	35	3 starch, 4 medium-fat meat, 5 fat

1/3 lb Thickburger	1	910	64	6	21	na	110	1560	53	3	30	3 1/2 starch, 3 medium-fat meat, 10 fat
1/2 lb Grilled Sourdough Thickburger	1	1030	77	7	28	na	155	1910	42	3	42	3 starch, 5 medium-fat meat, 10 1/2 fat
1/2 lb Six Dollar Burger	1	1060	73	6	28	na	150	1950	58	3	40	4 starch, 4 medium-fat meat, 10 1/2 fat
2/3 lb Double Bacon Cheese Burger	1	1300	97	7	38	na	205	2200	50	3	54	3 1/2 starch, 6 medium-fat meat, 13 fat
2/3 lb Double Thickburger	1	1250	90	6	35	na	195	2160	54	3	51	3 1/2 starch, 6 medium-fat meat, 12 1/2 fat
2/3 lb Monster Thickburger	1	1420	108	7	43	na	230	2770	46	2	60	3 starch, 7 medium-fat meat, 14 1/2 fat
BBQ Chicken Sandwich	1	320	6	2	1	na	50	1200	43	3	33	3 starch, 2 lean meat
Big Chicken Fillet Sandwich	1	800	37	4	6	na	90	1890	76	3	41	5 starch, 4 lean meat, 5 fat

✔ = Healthiest Bets

(*Continued*)

LUNCH & DINNER *(Continued)*	**Amount**	**Cal.**	**Fat (g)**	**% Cal. Fat**	**Sat. Fat (g)**	**Trans Fat (g)**	**Chol. (mg)**	**Sod. (mg)**	**Carb. (g)**	**Fiber (g)**	**Pro. (g)**	**Choices/Exchanges**
Big Hot Ham 'N' Cheese	1	520	24	4	13	na	85	2190	40	2	40	2 1/2 starch, 5 lean meat, 2 fat
Big Roast Beef Sandwich	1	470	23	4	10	na	60	1290	38	2	29	2 1/2 starch, 3 medium-fat meat, 1 1/2 fat
Charbroiled Chicken Club Sandwich	1	550	30	5	8	na	80	1560	35	2	28	2 1/2 starch, 3 lean meat, 4 fat
✔Cheeseburger	1	350	16	4	4	na	45	780	35	1	17	2 1/2 starch, 1 medium-fat meat, 2 fat
Chicken Strips	3 pcs	380	21	5	4	na	55	1360	27	1	22	2 starch, 2 lean meat, 3 fat
Chicken Strips	5 pcs	630	34	5	6	na	90	2260	45	2	37	3 starch, 4 lean meat, 4 1/2 fat
✔Hamburger	1	310	12	3	4	na	35	560	36	1	14	2 1/2 starch, 1 medium-fat meat, 1 1/2 fat

Hot Dog	1	420	30	6	12	na	55	1200	22	1	16	1 1/2 starch, 2 high-fat meat, 2 1/2 fat
Hot Ham 'N' Cheese	1	420	18	4	10	na	55	1600	39	2	30	2 1/2 starch, 3 lean meat, 1 1/2 fat
Low Carb Charbroiled Chicken Club Sandwich	1	370	21	5	7	na	90	1170	10	2	35	1/2 starch, 4 medium-fat meat
✔Regular Roast Beef Sandwich	1	330	16	4	7	na	40	860	29	2	19	2 starch, 2 medium-fat meat, 1 1/2 fat
Spicy Chicken Sandwich	1	470	21	4	5	na	50	1220	46	3	11	3 starch, 4 fat
SALAD DRESSINGS & SAUCES												
✔BBQ Sauce	1 srvg	45	0	0	0	na	0	290	10	1	1	1/2 carb
Buttermilk Ranch Dressing	1 srvg	240	25	9	4	na	20	360	2	0	1	5 fat
✔Fat Free Italian Dressing	1 srvg	10	0	0	0	na	0	420	3	0	0	Free

✔ = Healthiest Bets

(*Continued*)

SALAD DRESSINGS & SAUCES *(Continued)*	Amount	Cal.	Fat (g)	% Cal. Fat	Sat. Fat (g)	Trans Fat (g)	Chol. (mg)	Sod. (mg)	Carb. (g)	Fiber (g)	Pro. (g)	Choices/Exchanges
✔Honey Mustard Dipping sauce	1 srvg	110	9	7	2	na	10	220	6	0	0	1/2 carb, 2 fat
Ranch Dressing	1 srvg	160	16	9	3	na	15	240	2	0	0	3 fat
✔Sweet 'N' Sour Dipping Sauce	1 srvg	45	0	0	0	na	0	85	10	0	0	1/2 carb
SIDES & ADD-ONS												
✔American Cheese - large	1 slice	60	5	8	4	na	15	260	1	0	3	1 fat
✔American Cheese - small	1 slice	50	4	7	3	na	10	200	1	0	2	1 fat
✔Au Jus Sauce	1 srvg	10	0	0	0	na	0	320	2	0	0	Free
Bacon	2 strips	45	4	8	1	na	10	150	0	0	3	1 fat
✔Chicken Gravy	1 srvg	20	1	5	0	na	0	220	3	0	0	Free
Cole Slaw	1 srvg	170	10	5	2	na	10	140	20	2	1	1 starch, 2 veg, 2 fat
Crispy Curls	sm	340	17	5	4	na	0	840	43	4	4	3 starch, 3 fat

Crispy Curls	med	410	20	4	5	na	0	1020	52	4	5	3 starch, 4 fat
Crispy Curls	lg	480	23	4	6	na	0	1190	60	5	6	4 starch, 4 fat
Fried Chicken Breast	1	370	15	4	4	na	75	1190	29	0	29	2 starch, 3 lean meat, 1 fat
Fried Chicken Leg	1	330	15	4	4	na	60	1000	30	0	19	2 starch, 2 lean meat, 2 fat
Fried Chicken Wing	1	200	8	4	2	na	30	740	23	0	10	1 1/2 starch, 1 lean meat, 1 fat
✔Mashed Potatoes	1 srvg	90	2	2	0	na	0	410	17	0	1	1 starch, 1/2 fat
✔Natural Cut French Fries	kid's	200	9	4	2	na	0	450	28	2	2	2 starch, 2 fat
Natural Cut French Fries	sm	320	14	4	3	na	0	710	45	3	4	3 starch, 2 1/2 fat
Natural Cut French Fries	med	430	19	4	4	na	5	960	60	4	5	4 starch, 3 fat
Natural Cut French Fries	lg	470	21	4	4	na	5	1640	65	5	5	4 starch, 3 fat
Peach Cobbler	1 srvg	280	7	2	2	na	0	230	56	1	1	4 starch, 1 fat

✔ = Healthiest Bets

(*Continued*)

SIDES & ADD-ONS *(Continued)*	Amount	Cal.	Fat (g)	% Cal. Fat	Sat. Fat (g)	Trans Fat (g)	Chol. (mg)	Sod. (mg)	Carb. (g)	Fiber (g)	Pro. (g)	Choices/Exchanges
✔Side Salad - no dressing	1	120	7	5	5	na	20	160	7	2	7	1 veg, 2 fat
✔Swiss Cheese	1 slice	50	4	7	3	na	15	230	0	0	4	1 high-fat meat

✔ = Healthiest Bets

Exclusive Web Content

Be sure to visit the following restaurants online at http://www.diabetes.org/healthyrestaurant

Carvel	**Frëshens**	**Jimmy John's**	**Wienerschnitzel**
Del Taco	**Godfather's**	**Tim Hortons**	**Zaxby's**
El Pollo Loco	**Jersey Mike's**	**Whataburger**	

Jack in the Box

(www.jackinthebox.com)

Light 'n Lean Choice

Hamburger
Side Salad with Lite Ranch Dressing *(1/2 serving, 2 Tbsp)*

Calories	368	Cholesterol (mg)	41
Fat (g)	19	Sodium (mg)	780
% calories from fat	46	Carbohydrate (g)	3
Saturated fat (g)	6.5	Fiber (g)	3
Trans fat (g)	0.5	Protein (g)	18

Exchanges: 2 1/2 starch, 1 veg, 1 medium-fat meat, 2 fat

Healthy 'n Hearty Choice

Chicken Fajita Pita *(on whole-grain pita bread)* with Cilantro-Lime Dressing *(1/2 serving, 2 Tbsp)*

Calories	310	Cholesterol (mg)	0
Fat (g)	1	Sodium (mg)	920
% calories from fat	9	Carbohydrate (g)	66
Saturated fat (g)	0	Fiber (g)	2
Trans fat (g)	0	Protein (g)	9

Exchanges: 4 1/2 starch, 1 veg, 2 1/2 lean meat, 3 fat

(*Continued*)

Jack in the Box

	Amount	Cal.	Fat (g)	% Cal. Fat	Sat. Fat (g)	Trans Fat (g)	Chol. (mg)	Sod. (mg)	Carb. (g)	Fiber (g)	Pro. (g)	Choices/Exchanges
BREAKFAST												
✔Bacon Breakfast Jack	1	300	14	4	5	0.5	215	730	29	1	16	2 starch, 3 fat
Bacon, Egg and Cheese Biscuit	1	430	25	5	8	5	220	1100	34	1	17	2 1/2 starch, 1 medium-fat meat, 3 1/2 fat
✔Breakfast Jack	1	290	12	4	4.5	0	220	760	29	1	17	2 starch, 2 medium-fat meat, 1 fat
Ciabatta Breakfast Sandwich	1	710	36	5	10	1	440	1730	63	3	36	4 starch, 3 medium-fat meat, 4 fat
Extreme Sausage Sandwich	1	670	48	6	17	1.5	290	1300	31	2	29	2 starch, 4 high-fat meat, 2 fat
Hash Brown Sticks	5	230	16	6	4	4.5	0	330	20	2	2	1 1/2 starch, 3 fat

Meaty Breakfast Burrito	1	610	36	5	14	0.5	450	1400	39	5	32	2 1/2 starch, 3 medium-fat meat, 3 1/2 fat
Meaty Breakfast Burrito w/ Fire Roasted Salsa	1	620	36	5	14	0.5	450	1520	40	5	33	2 1/2 starch, 4 medium-fat meat, 3 1/2 fat
Original French Toast Sticks	4	470	23	4	5	5	25	450	58	4	7	4 starch, 4 fat
Sausage Biscuit	1	440	29	6	8	5	35	870	32	2	12	2 starch, 2 high-fat meat, 2 fat
Sausage Breakfast Jack	1	450	28	6	10	1	245	840	29	1	20	2 starch, 2 medium-fat meat, 3 1/2 fat
Sausage Croissant	1	580	29	5	13	4	255	770	37	2	21	2 1/2 starch, 3 high-fat meat, 2 fat
Sausage, Egg & Cheese Biscuit	1	740	55	7	17	6	280	1430	35	2	27	2 1/2 starch, 3 medium-fat meat, 8 fat
Sirloin Steak & Egg Burrito - no salsa	1	790	48	5	15	3.5	450	1320	52	6	37	3 1/2 starch, 4 medium-fat meat, 4 1/2 fat

✔ = Healthiest Bets

(*Continued*)

BREAKFAST (Continued)	Amount	Cal.	Fat (g)	% Cal. Fat	Sat. Fat (g)	Trans Fat (g)	Chol. (mg)	Sod. (mg)	Carb. (g)	Fiber (g)	Pro. (g)	Choices/Exchanges
Sirloin Steak & Egg Burrito w/ Fire Roasted Tomato Salsa	1	790	48	5	15	3.5	450	1440	54	6	37	3 1/2 starch, 4 medium-fat meat, 4 1/2 fat
Sourdough Breakfast Sandwich	1	420	24	5	8	2	23	980	21	2	20	1 1/2 starch, 2 medium-fat meat, 3 fat
Spicy Chicken Biscuit	1	460	22	4	5	7	40	1020	44	2	21	3 starch, 2 lean meat, 3 1/2 fat
Supreme Croissant	1	450	25	5	9	3.4	235	860	36	1	18	2 1/2 starch, 2 medium-fat meat, 4 fat
Ultimate Breakfast Sandwich	1	570	27	4	10	1	445	1700	49	2	34	3 1/2 starch, 3 medium-fat meat, 2 fat
Warm Cinnamon Roll	1	460	19	4	9	0	5	340	66	1	6	4 1/2 starch, 3 fat
BURGERS AND MORE												
Bacon Ultimate Cheeseburger	1	1090	77	6	30	3	140	2040	53	2	46	3 1/2 starch, 5 medium-fat meat, 10 1/2 fat

Big Cheeseburger	1	640	38	5	15	1.5	70	1180	50	2	24	3 1/2 starch, 2 medium-fat meat, 5 1/2 fat
Double Bacon & Cheese Ciabatta Burger	1	1120	76	6	28	3	135	1670	66	4	45	4 1/2 starch, 5 medium-fat meat, 10 fat
✔Hamburger	1	280	12	4	4.5	0.5	30	580	30	1	14	2 starch, 1 medium-fat meat, 1 1/2 fat
✔Hamburger Deluxe	1	350	18	5	6	1	40	600	32	2	15	2 starch, 1 medium-fat meat, 2 1/2 fat
Hamburger Deluxe w/ Cheese	1	440	25	5	10	1	65	970	34	2	19	2 1/2 starch, 2 medium-fat meat, 3 1/2 fat
✔Hamburger w/ Cheese	1	330	15	4	7	1	45	770	31	1	16	2 starch, 1 medium-fat meat, 1 1/2 fat
Jumbo Jack	1	600	35	5	12	1.5	45	940	51	3	21	3 1/2 starch, 2 medium-fat meat, 5 1/2 fat
Jumbo Jack w/ Cheese	1	690	42	5	16	1.5	70	1310	54	3	25	3 1/2 starch, 2 medium-fat meat, 6 1/2 fat

✔ = Healthiest Bets

(*Continued*)

BURGERS AND MORE *(Continued)*	Amount	Cal.	Fat (g)	% Cal. Fat	Sat. Fat (g)	Trans Fat (g)	Chol. (mg)	Sod. (mg)	Carb. (g)	Fiber (g)	Pro. (g)	Choices/Exchanges
Junior Bacon Cheeseburger	1	400	23	5	8	1	55	860	31	1	18	2 starch, 2 medium-fat meat, 3 fat
Single Bacon & Cheese Ciabatta Burger	1	870	54	6	18	1.5	90	1550	66	4	31	4 1/2 starch, 3 medium-fat meat, 8 1/2 fat
Sirloin Steak & Cheddar Ciabatta	1	770	38	4	8	0	110	1310	65	4	43	4 1/2 starch, 4 medium-fat meat, 3 fat
Sirloin Steak Melt	1	880	51	5	15	3.5	95	1850	63	5	43	4 starch, 4 medium-fat meat, 5 1/2 fat
Sourdough Jack	1	710	51	6	18	3	75	1230	36	3	27	2 1/2 starch, 3 medium-fat meat, 7 1/2 fat
Sourdough Ultimate Jack	1	950	73	7	29	4.5	125	1360	36	2	38	2 1/2 starch, 4 medium-fat meat, 10 fat
Ultimate Cheeseburger	1	1010	71	6	28	3	125	1580	53	2	40	3 1/2 starch, 4 medium-fat meat, 10 fat

CHICKEN AND FISH

Chicken Fajita Pita w/ whole grain and no salsa	1	300	9	3	3.5	0	60	1090	33	4	23	2 starch, 2 lean meat, 1/2 fat
✓Chicken Sandwich	1	400	21	5	4.5	2.5	35	730	38	2	15	2 1/2 starch, 1 lean meat, 3 1/2 fat
Chicken Sandwich w/ Bacon	1	440	24	5	6	2.5	40	970	39	2	19	2 1/2 starch, 2 lean meat, 4 fat
Chipotle Chicken Ciabatta w/ Grilled Chicken	1	690	28	4	9	0	105	1850	65	4	44	4 1/2 starch, 4 lean meat, 3 fat
Chipotle Chicken Ciabatta w/ Spicy Crispy Chicken	1	750	34	4	10	3	80	1650	75	5	37	5 starch, 3 lean meat, 4 1/2 fat
Crispy Chicken Strips	4	500	25	5	6	6	80	1260	36	3	35	2 1/2 starch, 4 lean meat, 2 1/2 fat
Fish and Chips	sm	570	30	5	7	9	35	1100	58	4	17	4 starch, 1 lean meat, 5 1/2 fat

✓ = Healthiest Bets

(*Continued*)

CHICKEN AND FISH *(Continued)*	Amount	Cal.	Fat (g)	% Cal. Fat	Sat. Fat (g)	Trans Fat (g)	Chol. (mg)	Sod. (mg)	Carb. (g)	Fiber (g)	Pro. (g)	Choices/Exchanges
Fish and Chips	med	660	34	5	8	10	35	1250	70	5	18	4 1/2 starch, 1 lean meat, 6 1/2 fat
Fish and Chips	lg	830	42	5	10	12	35	1530	92	6	21	6 starch, 7 1/2 fat
✔Grilled Chicken Strips	4	180	2	1	0.5	0	125	700	3	0	37	5 lean meat
Jack's Spicy Chicken	1	620	31	5	6	3	50	1100	61	4	25	4 starch, 2 lean meat, 5 fat
Jack's Spicy Chicken w/ Cheese	1	700	37	5	10	3	70	1410	62	4	29	4 starch, 2 lean meat, 6 fat
Sourdough Grilled Chicken Club	1	530	28	5	7	2	85	1430	34	3	36	2 1/2 starch, 4 lean meat, 3 fat
KID'S MEALS												
✔Apple Sauce	1 cup	100	0	0	0	0	0	0	25	1	0	1 fruit
✔Chicken Breast Strips	2 pcs	250	12	4	3	3	40	630	18	2	17	1 starch, 2 lean meat

✔Grilled Cheese	1	330	18	5	6	1.5	25	730	31	2	11	2 starch, 1 medium-fat meat, 3 fat
✔Hamburger	1	280	12	4	4.5	0.5	30	580	30	1	14	2 starch, 1 medium-fat meat, 1 1/2 fat
✔Hamburger w/ Cheese	1	330	15	4	7	1	45	770	31	1	16	2 starch, 1 medium-fat meat, 1 1/2 fat
Natural Cut Fries	1 kids portion	220	11	5	2.5	3.5	0	410	27	3	3	2 starch, 2.2 fat
SALADS - NO DRESSING												
Acapulco Chicken Salad w/ Spicy Bites	1	440	24	5	8	3	70	930	36	7	27	1 starch, 3 veg, 3 lean meat, 2 fat
Acapulco Chicken Salad w/ Crispy Chicken Strips	1	410	22	5	8	3	65	900	32	6	26	1 starch, 3 veg, 3 lean meat, 2 fat
✔Acapulco Chicken Salad w/ Grilled Chicken Strips	1	250	11	4	5	0	90	620	15	5	27	3 veg, 4 lean meat

✔ = Healthiest Bets

(*Continued*)

SALADS - NO DRESSING *(Continued)*	Amount	Cal.	Fat (g)	% Cal. Fat	Sat. Fat (g)	Trans Fat (g)	Chol. (mg)	Sod. (mg)	Carb. (g)	Fiber (g)	Pro. (g)	Choices/Exchanges
✔Asian Chicken Salad w/ Crispy Chicken Strips	1	330	13	4	3	3	40	660	34	7	21	1 starch, 3 veg, 3 lean meat, 1 fat
✔Asian Chicken Salad w/ Grilled Chicken Strips	1	160	1.5	1	0	0	65	380	18	5	22	3 veg, 3 lean meat
✔Asian Chicken Salad w/ Spicy Bites	1	360	15	4	3	3	45	680	38	8	21	1 starch, 3 veg, 3 lean meat, 1 fat
Chicken Club Salad w/ Crispy Chicken Strips	1	490	28	5	10	3.5	75	1060	28	6	33	1 starch, 3 veg, 4 lean meat, 2 fat
Chicken Club Salad w/ Grilled Chicken Strips	1	520	30	5	10	3	80	1090	32	7	34	1 starch, 3 veg, 4 lean meat, 3 1/2 fat
✔Chicken Club Salad w/ Spicy Bites	1	320	16	5	7	0	100	780	12	4	34	3 veg, 4 lean meat, 1 fat
✔Side Salad	1	50	3	5	1.5	0	10	60	5	2	3	1 veg, 1/2 fat

Southwest Chicken Salad w/ Crispy Chicken Strips	1	470	23	4	8	3	65	1120	44	9	30	2 starch, 3 veg, 3 lean meat, 1 1/2 fat
✔Southwest Chicken Salad w/ Grilled Chicken Strips	1	310	12	3	5	0	90	810	28	7	31	1 starch, 3 veg, 3 lean meat
Southwest Chicken Salad w/ Spicy Bites	1	510	25	4	8	3	70	1140	48	10	30	2 starch, 3 veg, 3 lean meat, 2 fat
SAUCES & DRESSINGS												
✔Asian Sesame Dressing	2 oz	190	14	7	2	0	0	630	16	0	1	Free
Bacon Ranch Dressing	2 oz	260	26	9	4	0.5	30	700	3	0	2	Free
✔Barbecue Dipping Sauce	1 oz	45	0	0	0	0	0	330	11	0	0	Free
Buttermilk House Dipping Sauce	1 oz	130	13	9	2	0	10	210	3	0	0	Free
Chipotle Sauce	1 oz	110	12	10	2	0	10	230	1	0	0	2 1/2 fat
Cilantro Lime Dressing	2 oz	250	24	9	4	1	20	580	9	0	1	Free

✔ = Healthiest Bets

(Continued)

SAUCES & DRESSINGS *(Continued)*	Amount	Cal.	Fat (g)	% Cal. Fat	Sat. Fat (g)	Trans Fat (g)	Chol. (mg)	Sod. (mg)	Carb. (g)	Fiber (g)	Pro. (g)	Choices/Exchanges
Creamy Southwest Dressing	2 oz	220	22	9	3.5	0	20	850	3	0	1	4 1/2 fat
Frank's Red Hot Buffalo Dipping Sauce	1 oz	10	0	0	0	0	0	840	2	0	0	Free
Hollandaise Sauce	1 oz	60	0	0	0	0	0	460	13	0	1	1 carb
✔Honey Mustard Dipping Sauce	1 oz	60	0	0	0	0	0	220	11	0	0	1/2 carb
✔Lite Ranch Dressing	2 oz	150	15	9	2.5	0	20	560	3	0	1	3 fat
✔Log Cabin Syrup	3 oz	190	0	0	0	0	0	35	49	0	0	3 1/2 carb
✔Low Fat Balsamic Dressing	2.5 oz	35	1.5	4	0	0	0	480	5	0	0	1/2 carb, 1/2 fat
Mayo-Onion Sauce	.5 oz	90	10	10	1.5	0	5	85	1	0	0	2 fat
Ranch Dressing	2 oz	310	33	10	5	1	20	470	3	0	1	6 1/2 fat
✔Sweet and Sour Dipping Sauce	1 oz	45	0	0	0	0	0	160	11	0	0	1/2 carb

✔Taco Sauce	.25 oz	0	0	0	0	0	0	80	0	0	0	Free
Tartar Dipping Sauce	1.5 oz	210	22	9	3.5	0	20	370	2	0	0	4 1/2 fat
✔Teriyaki Dipping Sauce	1 oz	60	0	0	0	0	0	460	13	0	1	1 carb
✔Zesty Marinara Dipping Sauce	1 oz	15	0	0	0	0	0	200	4	0	0	1/2 carb
SELECTED BEVERAGES												
✔Caramel Iced Coffee	16 oz	90	2	2	1	0	10	55	17	0	4	1 carb, 1/2 fat
✔Caramel Iced Coffee	24 oz	150	3	2	2	0	15	95	25	0	6	1 1/2 carb, 1/2 fat
Lemonade	20 oz	160	0	0	0	0	0	65	42	0	0	3 carb
Mango Smoothie	16 oz	280	0	0	0	0	0	75	71	0	3	4 1/2 carb
Mango Smoothie	24 oz	43	0	0	0	0	5	115	106	0	4	7 carb
Orange Sunrise Smoothie	16 oz	280	0	0	0	0	0	75	68	0	3	4 1/2 carb
Orange Sunrise Smoothie	24 oz	42	0	0	0	0	5	115	102	0	5	7 carb

✔ = Healthiest Bets

(*Continued*)

SELECTED BEVERAGES *(Continued)*	Amount	Cal.	Fat (g)	% Cal. Fat	Sat. Fat (g)	Trans Fat (g)	Chol. (mg)	Sod. (mg)	Carb. (g)	Fiber (g)	Pro. (g)	Choices/Exchanges
✔Original Iced Coffee	16 oz	100	2	2	1	0	10	55	17	0	4	1 carb, 1/2 fat
✔Original Iced Coffee	24 oz	150	3	2	2	0	15	95	26	0	6	1 1/2 carb, 1/2 fat
Strawberry Banana Smoothie	16 oz	280	0	0	0	0	0	75	68	1	3	4 1/2 carb
Strawberry Banana Smoothie	24 oz	420	0	0	0	0	5	115	102	2	4	6 1/2 carb
✔Vanilla Iced Coffee	16 oz	100	2	2	1	0	10	55	18	0	4	1 carb, 1/2 fat
✔Vanilla Iced Coffee	24 oz	150	3	2	2	0	15	95	26	0	6	1 1/2 carb, 1/2 fat
SHAKES AND DESSERTS												
Cheesecake	1 pc	310	16	5	9	1	55	220	34	0	7	2 1/2 carb, 3 fat
Chocolate Ice Cream Shake	16 oz	720	35	4	22	1.5	130	270	89	1	12	6 carb, 7 fat
Chocolate Ice Cream Shake	24 oz	1230	58	4	39	2.5	190	470	159	2	19	10 1/2 carb, 11 1/2 fat

Chocolate Overload Cake	1 pc	300	7	2	1.5	0	40	350	57	2	4	4 carb, 1 fat
Egg Nog Shake	16 oz	730	35	4	24	1.5	115	240	90	0	11	6 carb, 6 1/2 fat
Egg Nog Shake	24 oz	1210	57	4	39	2.5	190	390	152	1	18	10 carb, 10 fat
Oreo Cookie Ice Cream Shake	16 oz	770	40	5	26	1.5	115	370	88	1	12	6 carb, 7 1/2 fat
Oreo Cookie Ice Cream Shake	24 oz	1290	67	5	42	2.5	190	650	148	2	20	10 carb, 11 1/2 fat
Strawberry Ice Cream Shake	16 oz	730	35	4	24	1.5	115	240	91	0	11	6 carb, 5 1/2 fat
Strawberry Ice Cream Shake	24 oz	1210	57	4	39	2.5	190	390	155	1	18	10 1/2 carb, 9 fat
Vanilla Ice Cream Shake	16 oz	650	35	5	24	1.5	115	230	70	0	11	4 1/2 carb, 7 fat
Vanilla Ice Cream Shake	24 oz	1050	57	5	19	2.5	190	380	112	1	18	7 1/2 carb, 11 1/2 fat

✔ = Healthiest Bets

(*Continued*)

	Amount	Cal.	Fat (g)	% Cal. Fat	Sat. Fat (g)	Trans Fat (g)	Chol. (mg)	Sod. (mg)	Carb. (g)	Fiber (g)	Pro. (g)	Choices/Exchanges
SNACKS & EXTRAS												
Bacon Cheddar Potato Wedges	1 order	720	48	6	15	12	45	1360	52	4	21	3 1/2 starch, 9 1/2 fat
Beef Monster Taco	1	240	14	5	5	2	20	390	20	3	8	1 1/2 starch, 1 medium-fat meat, 2 fat
Egg Rolls	3	400	19	4	6	3	15	920	44	6	14	3 starch, 4 fat
✔Fruit Cup	1 order	90	0	0	0	0	0	20	22	2	1	1 1/2 fruit
Mozzarella Cheese Sticks	3	240	12	5	5	2	25	420	21	1	11	1 1/2 starch, 2 1/2 fat
Mozzarella Cheese Sticks	6	483	27	5	11	4	46	1018	39	2	20	2 1/2 starch, 5 1/2 fat
Natural Cut Fries	sm	340	17	5	4	5	0	620	41	5	5	2 1/2 starch, 3 1/2 fat
Natural Cut Fries	med	450	23	5	5	7	0	830	54	6	6	3 1/2 starch, 4 fat
Natural Cut Fries	lg	640	33	5	8	10	0	1180	77	9	9	5 starch, 6 fat

Onion Rings	1 order	500	30	5	6	10	0	420	51	3	6	3 1/2 starch, 5 1/2 fat
✔Regular Beef Taco	1	160	8	5	3	1	15	270	15	2	5	1 starch, 1 1/2 fat
Sampler Trio	1 order	750	39	5	14	7	85	1760	65	5	35	4 1/2 starch, 3 medium-fat meat, 4 fat
Seasoned Curly Fries	sm	270	15	5	3	5	0	590	30	3	4	2 starch, 3 fat
Seasoned Curly Fries	med	400	23	5	5	7	0	890	45	5	6	3 starch, 4 fat
Seasoned Curly Fries	lg	550	31	5	6	10	0	1200	60	6	8	4 starch, 5 1/2 fat
Spicy Chicken Bites	7	290	14	4	3	3	45	660	21	3	18	1 1/2 starch, 2 lean meat, 1 1/2 fat
Spicy Chicken Bites	16	650	33	5	7	7	100	1500	49	6	41	3 1/2 starch, 4 lean meat, 4 fat
Stuffed Jalapenos	3	230	13	5	6	2	20	690	22	2	7	1 1/2 starch, 2 1/2 fat
Stuffed Jalapenos	7	530	30	5	13	4.5	45	1600	51	4	15	3 1/2 starch, 6 fat

✔ = Healthiest Bets

McDonald's

(www.mcdonalds.com)

Light 'n Lean Choice

Premium Asian Salad with Grilled Chicken
Newman's Own Low-Fat Balsamic Vinaigrette *(1.5 oz, 3 Tbsp)*
Fruit and Yogurt Parfait with granola

Calories	500	Cholesterol (mg)	70
Fat (g)	15	Sodium (mg)	1,705
% calories from fat	27	Carbohydrate (g)	58
Saturated fat (g)	2	Fiber (g)	6
Trans fat (g)	0	Protein (g)	36

Exchanges: 2 veg, 1/2 starch, 1 1/2 carb, 1 fruit, 3 lean meat, 1 fat

Healthy 'n Hearty Choice

Hamburger
French Fries *(small)*
Premium Southwest Salad (no chicken) with Newman's Own Low-Fat Family Italian Recipe *(1.5 oz, 3 Tbsp)*

Calories	660	Cholesterol (mg)	35
Fat (g)	26	Sodium (mg)	1,310
% calories from fat	35	Carbohydrate (g)	86
Saturated fat (g)	7	Fiber (g)	11
Trans fat (g)	1	Protein (g)	22

Exchanges: 4 starch, 1 carb, 2 veg, 1 medium-fat meat, 4 fat

McDonald's

	Amount	Cal.	Fat (g)	% Cal. Fat	Sat. Fat (g)	Trans Fat (g)	Chol. (mg)	Sod. (mg)	Carb. (g)	Fiber (g)	Pro. (g)	Choices/Exchanges
BREAKFAST												
Bacon, Egg & Cheese Biscuit	reg	430	24	5	12	0	240	1230	37	2	16	2 1/2 starch, 1 medium-fat meat, 3 1/2 fat
Bacon, Egg & Cheese Biscuit	lg	520	30	5	13	0	256	1520	43	3	19	3 starch, 1 medium-fat meat, 4 1/2 fat
Bacon, Egg & Cheese McGriddles	1	420	19	4	9	0	240	1190	48	2	16	3 starch, 1 medium-fat meat, 3 fat
Big Breakfast, large biscuit	1	800	52	6	18	0	555	1680	56	4	28	3 1/2 starch, 2 medium-fat meat, 8 fat
Big Breakfast, regular biscuit	1	740	48	6	17	0	555	1560	51	3	28	3 1/2 starch, 3 medium-fat meat, 7 fat

✓ = Healthiest Bets

(*Continued*)

BREAKFAST *(Continued)*	Amount	Cal.	Fat (g)	% Cal. Fat	Sat. Fat (g)	Trans Fat (g)	Chol. (mg)	Sod. (mg)	Carb. (g)	Fiber (g)	Pro. (g)	Choices/Exchanges
Biscuit	reg	260	12	4	7	0	0	740	33	2	5	2 carb, 2 1/2 fat
Biscuit	lg	320	16	5	8	0	0	850	39	3	5	2 1/2 carb, 3 fat
Deluxe Breakfast - reg biscuit, no syrup or margarine	1	1090	56	5	19	0	575	2150	111	6	36	7 1/2 starch, 2 medium-fat meat, 8 fat
Deluxe Breakfast, lg biscuit, no syrup or margarine	1	1150	60	5	20	0	575	2260	116	7	36	7 1/2 starch, 2 medium-fat meat, 9 fat
✔Egg McMuffin	1	300	12	4	5	0	260	820	30	2	18	2 starch, 2 medium-fat meat, 1/2 fat
✔English Muffin	1	160	3	2	0.5	0	0	280	27	2	5	2 carb, 1/2 fat
✔Grape Jam	.5 oz	35	0	0	0	0	0	0	9	0	0	1/2 carb
✔Hash Brown	1	150	9	5	1.5	0	0	310	15	2	1	1 starch, 2 fat
Hotcake syrup	1 pkg	180	0	0	0	0	0	20	45	0	0	3 carb
Hotcakes - no syrup or margarine	1 order	350	9	2	2	0	20	590	60	3	8	4 starch, 2 fat

Hotcakes and Sausage - no syrup or margarine	1 order	520	24	4	7	0	50	930	61	3	15	4 starch, 2 high-fat meat, 1 fat
McSkillet Burrito w/ Sausage	1	610	36	5	14	0.5	410	1390	44	3	27	3 starch, 3 medium-fat meat, 4 1/2 fat
McSkillet Burrito w/ Steak	1	570	30	5	12	1	430	1470	44	3	32	3 starch, 3 medium-fat meat, 2 1/2 fat
Sausage Biscuit	reg	410	20	4	8	0	30	1180	41	2	17	2 1/2 starch, 1 medium-fat meat, 2 1/2 fat
Sausage Biscuit	lg	480	31	6	13	0	30	1190	39	3	11	2 1/2 starch, 5 1/2 fat
Sausage Biscuit w/ Egg	reg	430	27	6	12	0	30	1080	34	2	11	2 1/2 starch, 1 medium-fat meat, 5 fat
Sausage Biscuit w/ Egg	lg	570	37	6	15	0	250	1280	42	3	18	3 starch, 1 medium-fat meat, 6 fat
✔Sausage Burrito	1	300	16	5	7	0.5	130	830	26	1	12	1 1/2 starch, 2 high-fat meat, 1/2 fat

✔ = Healthiest Bets

(*Continued*)

BREAKFAST *(Continued)*	Amount	Cal.	Fat (g)	% Cal. Fat	Sat. Fat (g)	Trans Fat (g)	Chol. (mg)	Sod. (mg)	Carb. (g)	Fiber (g)	Pro. (g)	Choices/Exchanges
Sausage McGriddles	1	420	22	5	8	0	35	1030	44	2	11	3 starch, 4 fat
Sausage McMuffin	1	370	22	5	8	0	45	850	29	2	14	2 starch, 1 medium-fat meat, 3 fat
Sausage McMuffin w/ Egg	1	450	27	5	40	0	285	920	30	2	21	2 starch, 2 medium-fat meat, 3 1/2 fat
Sausage Patty	1	170	15	8	5	0	30	340	1	0	7	1 high-fat meat, 1 fat
Sausage, Egg & Cheese McGriddles	1	560	32	5	12	0	265	1360	48	2	20	3 starch, 1 medium-fat meat, 5 fat
✔Scrambled Eggs - 2	1 order	170	11	6	4	0	520	180	1	0	15	2 medium-fat meat
Southern Style Chicken Biscuit	reg	410	20	4	8	0	30	1180	41	2	17	2 1/2 starch, 1 lean meat, 3 fat
Southern Style Chicken Biscuit	lg	470	24	5	9	0	30	1290	46	3	17	3 starch, 1 lean meat, 4 fat
✔Strawberry Preserves	.5 oz	35	0	0	0	0	0	0	9	0	0	1/2 carb

✔Whipped Margarine	1 pat	40	5	11	1.5	0	0	55	0	0	0	1 fat
CHICKEN MCNUGGET AND SELECTS SAUCES												
✔Barbeque Sauce	1 oz	50	0	0	0	0	0	260	12	0	0	1 starch
Creamy Ranch Sauce	1.5 oz	200	22	10	3.4	0	10	320	2	0	0	4.4 fat
✔Honey	1 oz	50	0	0	0	0	0	260	12	0	0	1 starch
✔Hot Mustard	1 oz	60	2.5	4	0	0	5	250	9	2	1	1/2 starch, 1/2 fat
✔Southwestern Chipotle Barbeque Sauce	1.5 oz	70	0	0	0	0	0	260	18	1	0	1 starch
Spicy Buffalo Sauce	1.5 oz	70	7	9	1	0	0	960	1	2	0	1.4 fat
✔Sweet 'N Sour Sauce	1 oz	50	0	0	0	0	0	150	12	0	0	1 starch
✔Tangy Honey Mustard	1.5 oz	70	2.5	3	0	0	5	170	13	0	1	1 starch, 1/2 fat
CHICKEN MCNUGGETS & SELECTS STRIPS												
✔Chicken McNuggets	6 pcs	280	17	5	3	0	40	600	16	0	14	1 starch, 2 lean meat, 2 1/2 fat

✔ = Healthiest Bets

(*Continued*)

CHICKEN MCNUGGETS & SELECTS STRIPS *(Continued)*	Amount	Cal.	Fat (g)	% Cal. Fat	Sat. Fat (g)	Trans Fat (g)	Chol. (mg)	Sod. (mg)	Carb. (g)	Fiber (g)	Pro. (g)	Choices/Exchanges
✔Chicken McNuggets	4 pcs	190	12	6	2	0	30	400	11	0	10	1/2 starch, 1 lean meat, 1 1/2 fat
Chicken McNuggets	10 pcs	460	29	6	5	0	70	1000	27	0	24	2 starch, 3 lean meat, 4 fat
Chicken Selects Premium Breast Strips	3 pcs	400	24	5	3.5	0	50	1010	23	0	23	1 1/2 starch, 3 lean meat, 3 fat
Chicken Selects Premium Breast Strips	5 pcs	660	40	5	6	0	85	1680	39	0	37	2 1/2 starch, 4 lean meat, 5 1/2 fat
DESSERTS AND SHAKES												
✔Apple Dippers	1 order	35	0	0	0	0	0	0	8	0	0	1/2 fruit
Baked Apple Pie	1	270	12	4	3.5	5	0	190	36	4	3	2 1/2 carb, 2 1/2 fat
✔Chocolate Chip Cookie	1	160	7	4	2.5	1.5	10	90	22	1	2	1 1/2 carb, 1 1/2 fat
Chocolate Triple Thick Shake	21 oz	770	18	2	11	1	70	330	134	1	18	9 carb, 3 fat

Chocolate Triple Thick Shake	16 oz	580	14	2	8	1	50	250	102	1	13	7 carb, 2 fat
Chocolate Triple Thick Shake	12 oz	440	10	2	6	0.5	40	190	76	1	10	5 carb, 2 fat
Chocolate Triple Thick Shake	32 oz	1160	27	2	16	2	100	510	203	2	27	13 1/2 carb, 4 fat
Cinnamon Melts	1 order	460	19	4	9	0	15	370	66	3	6	4 1/2 carb, 3 fat
✔Fruit and Yogurt Parfait	1	160	2	1	1	0	5	85	31	1	4	1 carb, 1 milk
✔Fruit and Yogurt Parfait - no Granola	1	130	2	1	1	0	5	55	25	0	4	1/2 carb, 1 milk
Hot Caramel Sundae	1	340	8	2	5	0	30	160	60	1	7	4 carb, 1 1/2 fat
Hot Fudge Sundae	1	330	10	3	7	0	25	180	54	2	8	3 1/2 carb, 2 fat
✔Kiddie Cone	1	45	1	2	0.5	0	5	20	8	0	1	1/2 carb
✔Low Fat Caramel Dip	1 order	70	1	1	0	0	5	35	15	0	0	1 carb

✔ = Healthiest Bets

(Continued)

DESSERTS AND SHAKES *(Continued)*	Amount	Cal.	Fat (g)	% Cal. Fat	Sat. Fat (g)	Trans Fat (g)	Chol. (mg)	Sod. (mg)	Carb. (g)	Fiber (g)	Pro. (g)	Choices/Exchanges
McDonaldland Cookies	1 pkg	250	8	3	2	0	0	260	42	1	4	3 carb, 1 1/2 fat
McFlurry w/ M&M's Candies	12 oz	620	20	3	12	1	55	190	96	1	14	6 1/2 carb, 3 1/2 fat
McFlurry w/ Oreo Cookies	12 oz	550	17	3	9	1	50	250	88	1	13	6 carb, 3 fat
✔Oatmeal Raisin Cookie	1	150	6	4	1.5	1.5	10	135	22	1	2	1 1/2 carb, 1 fat
✔Peanuts (for Sundaes)	1 pkg	45	4	8	0.5	0	0	0	2	1	2	1 fat
Strawberry Sundae	1	280	6	2	4	0	25	95	49	1	6	3 1/2 carb, 1 fat
Strawberry Triple Thick Shake	12 oz	420	10	2	6	0.5	40	130	73	0	10	5 carb, 2 fat
Strawberry Triple Thick Shake	16 oz	560	13	2	8	1	50	170	97	0	13	6 1/2 carb, 2 fat
Strawberry Triple Thick Shake	21 oz	740	18	2	11	1	70	230	128	0	17	8 1/2 carb, 3 fat
Strawberry Triple Thick Shake	32 oz	1110	26	2	16	2	100	350	194	0	25	13 carb, 4 fat

✔Sugar Cookie	1	150	6	4	1.5	2	5	110	21	0	2	1 1/2 carb, 1 fat
✔Vanilla Reduced Fat Ice Cream Cone	1	150	4	2	2	0	15	60	24	0	4	1 1/2 carb, 1/2 fat
Vanilla Triple Thick Shake	12 oz	420	10	2	6	0.5	40	140	72	0	9	5 carb, 1 1/2 fat
Vanilla Triple Thick Shake	16 oz	550	13	2	8	1	50	190	96	0	13	6 1/2 carb, 2 fat
Vanilla Triple Thick Shake	21 oz	740	18	2	11	1	70	250	128	0	17	8 1/2 carb, 3 fat
Vanilla Triple Thick Shake	32 oz	1110	26	2	16	2	100	370	193	0	25	13 carb, 4 fat
FRENCH FRIES												
French Fries	sm	230	11	4	1.5	0	0	160	29	3	3	2 starch, 2 fat
French Fries	med	380	19	5	2.5	0	0	270	48	5	4	3 starch, 4 fat
French Fries	lg	500	25	5	3.5	0	0	350	63	6	6	4 starch, 4 1/2 fat
ICED COFFEE												
✔Caramel Iced Coffee	16 oz	130	5	3	3.5	0	20	80	21	0	1	1 1/2 carb, 1 fat

✔ = Healthiest Bets

(Continued)

ICED COFFEE *(Continued)*	Amount	Cal.	Fat (g)	% Cal. Fat	Sat. Fat (g)	Trans Fat (g)	Chol. (mg)	Sod. (mg)	Carb. (g)	Fiber (g)	Pro. (g)	Choices/Exchanges
Caramel Iced Coffee	22 oz	190	8	4	5	0	30	115	27	0	1	2 carb, 1 1/2 fat
Caramel Iced Coffee	32 oz	270	11	4	7	0	40	160	41	0	2	2 1/2 carb, 1 1/2 fat
✓Hazelnut Iced Coffee	16 oz	130	5	3	3.5	0	20	40	21	0	1	1 1/2 carb, 1 1/2 fat
Hazelnut Iced Coffee	22 oz	190	8	4	5	0	30	60	29	0	1	2 carb, 1 1/2 fat
Hazelnut Iced Coffee	32 oz	270	11	4	7	0	40	80	43	0	2	3 carb, 1 1/2 fat
✓Regular Iced Coffee	16 oz	140	5	3	3.5	0	20	40	22	0	1	1 1/2 carb, 1 fat
Regular Iced Coffee	22 oz	200	8	4	5	0	30	60	30	0	1	2 carb, 1 1/2 fat
Regular Iced Coffee	32 oz	280	11	4	7	0	40	80	45	0	2	3 carb, 1 1/2 fat
✓Sugar Free Vanilla Iced Coffee	16 oz	60	5	8	3.5	0	20	70	8	0	1	1/2 carb
Sugar Free Vanilla Iced Coffee	22 oz	90	8	8	5	0	30	95	11	0	1	1/2 carb

Sugar Free Vanilla Iced Coffee	32 oz	120	11	8	7	0	40	140	16	0	2	1 carb
✔Vanilla Iced Coffee	16 oz	130	5	3	3.5	0	20	40	21	0	1	1 1/2 carb, 1 fat
Vanilla Iced Coffee	22 oz	190	8	4	5	0	30	60	29	0	1	2 carb, 1 1/2 fat
Vanilla Iced Coffee	32 oz	270	11	4	7	0	40	80	43	0	2	3 carb, 1 1/2 fat
SALAD DRESSING												
✔Newman's Own Creamy Caesar Dressing	2 oz	190	18	9	2.4	0	20	500	4	0	2	1/2 carb, 3 1/2 fat
✔Newman's Own Creamy Southwest Dressing	1.5 oz	100	6	5	1	0	20	340	11	0	1	1/2 carb, 1 fat
✔Newman's Own Low Fat Balsamic Vinaigrette	1.5 oz	40	3	7	0	0	0	730	4	0	0	1/2 carb, 1/2 fat
✔Newman's Own Low Fat Family Italian Recipe	1.5 oz	60	2.5	4	0	0	0	730	8	0	1	1/2 carb, 1/2 fat

✔ = Healthiest Bets

(Continued)

SALAD DRESSING *(Continued)*	Amount	Cal.	Fat (g)	% Cal. Fat	Sat. Fat (g)	Trans Fat (g)	Chol. (mg)	Sod. (mg)	Carb. (g)	Fiber (g)	Pro. (g)	Choices/Exchanges
✔Newman's Own Ranch Dressing	2 oz	170	15	8	2.5	0	20	530	9	0	1	1/2 carb, 3 fat
SALADS												
✔Butter Garlic Croutons	.5 oz	60	1.5	2	0	0	0	140	10	1	2	1/2 starch
✔Premium Asian Salad - no Chicken	1	150	7	4	0.5	0	0	35	15	5	8	1 starch, 1.4 fat
✔Premium Asian Salad w/ Crispy Chicken	1	410	20	4	2.5	0	45	850	31	5	28	1 starch, 3 veg, 3 lean meat, 2 fat
✔Premium Asian Salad w/ Grilled Chicken	1	300	10	3	1	0	65	890	23	5	32	1/2 starch, 3 veg, 3 lean meat
✔Premium Bacon Ranch Salad w/ Crispy Chicken	1	370	20	5	6	0	75	970	20	3	29	3 veg, 4 lean meat, 1 1/2 fat

✔Premium Bacon Ranch Salad w/ Grilled Chicken	1	260	9	3	4	0	90	1010	12	3	33	3 veg, 4 lean meat
✔Premium Bacon Salad - no Chicken	1	140	7	5	3.5	0	25	300	10	3	9	2 veg, 1 medium-fat meat
✔Premium Caesar Salad - no Chicken	1	90	4	4	2.5	0	10	180	9	3	7	3 veg, 1/2 fat
✔Premium Caesar Salad w/ Crispy Chicken	1	330	17	5	4.5	0	60	840	20	3	26	3 veg, 3 lean meat, 1 1/2 fat
✔Premium Caesar Salad w/ Grilled Chicken	1	220	6	2	3	0	75	890	12	3	30	3 veg, 3 lean meat
✔Premium Southwest Salad - no Chicken	1	140	4.5	3	2	0	10	150	20	6	6	4 veg, 1 medium-fat meat
✔Premium Southwest Salad w/ Crispy Chicken	1	430	20	4	4	0	55	920	38	6	26	1 starch, 3 veg, 3 lean meat, 2 fat
✔Premium Southwest Salad w/ Grilled Chicken	1	320	9	3	3	0	70	960	30	6	30	1 starch, 3 veg, 3 lean meat

✔ = Healthiest Bets

(*Continued*)

SALADS *(Continued)*	Amount	Cal.	Fat (g)	% Cal. Fat	Sat. Fat (g)	Trans Fat (g)	Chol. (mg)	Sod. (mg)	Carb. (g)	Fiber (g)	Pro. (g)	Choices/Exchanges
✔Side Salad	1	20	0	0	0	0	0	10	4	1	1	1 veg
Snack Size Fruit and Walnut Salad	1	210	8	3	1.5	0	5	60	31	2	4	2 fruit, 1 1/2 fat
SANDWICHES												
Big Mac	1	540	29	5	10	1.5	75	1040	45	3	25	3 starch, 2 medium-fat meat, 3 1/2 fat
Big N' Tasty	1	460	24	5	8	1.5	70	710	37	3	24	2 1/2 starch, 2 medium-fat meat, 2 1/2 fat
Big N' Tasty w/ Cheese	1	510	28	5	11	1.5	85	960	38	3	27	2 1/2 starch, 3 medium-fat meat, 3 fat
✔Cheeseburger	1	300	12	4	6	0.5	40	750	33	2	15	2 starch, 1 medium-fat meat, 1 fat
✔Chipotle BBQ Snack Wrap (Crispy)	1	330	15	4	4.5	0	30	810	35	1	14	2 1/2 starch, 1 lean meat, 2 1/2 fat

✔Chipotle BBQ Snack Wrap (Grilled)	1	260	9	3	3.5	0	45	830	28	1	18	2 starch, 2 lean meat, 1/2 fat
Double Cheeseburger	1	440	23	5	11	1.5	80	1150	34	2	25	2 1/2 starch, 3 medium-fat meat, 2 fat
Double Quarter Pounder w/ Cheese	1	740	42	5	19	2.5	155	1380	40	3	48	2 1/2 starch, 6 medium-fat meat, 2 1/2 fat
Filet-O-Fish	1	380	18	4	3.5	0	40	640	38	2	15	2 1/2 starch, 1 lean meat, 3 fat
✔Hamburger	1	250	9	3	3.5	0.5	25	520	31	2	12	2 starch, 1 medium-fat meat, 1 fat
✔Honey Mustard Snack Wrap (Crispy)	1	330	16	4	4.5	0	30	780	34	1	14	2 1/2 starch, 1 lean meat, 2 1/2 fat
✔Honey Mustard Snack Wrap (Grilled)	1	260	9	3	3.5	0	45	800	27	1	18	2 starch, 2 lean meat, 1/2 fat
✔McChicken	1	360	16	4	3	0	35	830	40	2	14	2 1/2 starch, 1 lean meat, 2 1/2 fat

✔ = Healthiest Bets

(*Continued*)

SANDWICHES *(Continued)*	Amount	Cal.	Fat (g)	% Cal. Fat	Sat. Fat (g)	Trans Fat (g)	Chol. (mg)	Sod. (mg)	Carb. (g)	Fiber (g)	Pro. (g)	Choices/Exchanges
McRib	1	500	26	5	10	0	70	980	44	3	22	3 starch, 2 lean meat, 4 fat
Premium Crispy Chicken Classic	1	530	20	3	3.5	0	50	1150	59	3	28	4 starch, 2 lean meat, 2 1/2 fat
Premium Crispy Chicken Club	1	630	28	4	7	0	75	1420	60	4	36	4 starch, 3 lean meat, 3 1/2 fat
Premium Crispy Chicken Ranch BLT	1	580	23	4	4.5	0	60	1460	61	3	32	4 starch, 3 lean meat, 3 fat
Premium Grilled Chicken Classic	1	420	10	2	2	0	70	1190	51	3	32	3 1/2 starch, 3 lean meat
Premium Grilled Chicken Club	1	530	17	3	6	0	90	1470	52	4	40	3 1/2 starch, 4 lean meat, 1 fat
Premium Grilled Chicken Ranch BLT	1	470	12	2	3	0	80	1500	53	3	36	3 1/2 starch, 4 lean meat

✔Quarter Pounder	1	410	19	4	7	1	65	730	37	2	24	2 1/2 starch, 2 medium-fat meat, 1 1/2 fat
Quarter Pounder w/ Cheese	1	510	26	5	12	1.5	90	1190	40	3	29	2 1/2 starch, 3 medium-fat meat, 2 fat
✔Ranch Snack Wrap (Crispy)	1	340	17	5	4.5	0	30	810	33	1	14	2 starch, 1 lean meat, 3 fat
✔Ranch Snack Wrap (Grilled)	1	270	10	3	4	0	45	830	26	4	17	1 1/2 starch, 2 lean meat, 1 fat
Southern Style Crispy Chicken	1	400	17	4	3	0	45	1030	39	1	24	2 1/2 starch, 2 lean meat, 2 fat

✔ = Healthiest Bets

Sonic, America's Drive-In

(www.sonicdrivein.com)

Light 'n Lean Choice

Junior Burger
Tater Tots *(1/2 regular order)*
Low-Fat Milk *(8 oz)*

Calories	530	Cholesterol (mg)	45
Fat (g)	25	Sodium (mg)	1,120
% calories from fat	42	Carbohydrate (g)	69
Saturated fat (g)	8	Fiber (g)	5
Trans fat (g)	2	Protein (g)	24

Exchanges: 3 starch, 1 milk, 1 medium-fat meat, 4 fat

Healthy 'n Hearty Choice

Grilled Chicken Wrap
Onion Rings *(1/2 regular order)*
Vanilla Shake *(1/2 regular order)*

Calories	900	Cholesterol (mg)	118
Fat (g)	35	Sodium (mg)	1,570
% calories from fat	35	Carbohydrate (g)	113
Saturated fat (g)	11	Fiber (g)	6
Trans fat (g)	5	Protein (g)	35

Exchanges: 5 starch, 3 carb, 3 lean meat, 5 fat

Sonic, America's Drive-In

	Amount	Cal.	Fat (g)	% Cal. Fat	Sat. Fat (g)	Trans Fat (g)	Chol. (mg)	Sod. (mg)	Carb. (g)	Fiber (g)	Pro. (g)	Choices/Exchanges
ADD INS												
✔Apple Juice	lg	50	0	0	0	0	0	5	13	0	0	1 carb
Blue Coconut Syrup	lg	60	0	0	0	0	0	10	14	0	0	1 carb
Cherry Syrup	lg	70	0	0	0	0	0	10	20	0	0	1 1/2 carb
Chocolate Topping	lg	150	0	0	0	0	0	120	35	0	0	2 1/2 carb
✔Cranberry Juice	lg	60	0	0	0	0	0	5	15	0	0	1 carb
✔Diet Cherry	lg	10	0	0	0	0	0	5	2	0	0	Free
Grape Syrup	lg	60	0	0	0	0	0	15	14	0	0	1 carb
HI-C	lg	80	0	0	0	0	0	5	21	0	0	1 1/2 carb

✔ = Healthiest Bets

(Continued)

ADD INS *(Continued)*	Amount	Cal.	Fat (g)	% Cal. Fat	Sat. Fat (g)	Trans Fat (g)	Chol. (mg)	Sod. (mg)	Carb. (g)	Fiber (g)	Pro. (g)	Choices/Exchanges
✔Lemon	lg	5	0	0	0	0	0	0	2	0	0	Free
✔Lime	lg	5	0	0	0	0	0	0	2	0	0	Free
Orange	lg	60	0	0	0	0	0	10	15	0	0	1 carb
Pineapple Topping	lg	90	0	0	0	0	0	15	21	0	0	1 1/2 carb
✔Powerade	lg	70	0	0	0	0	0	60	19	0	0	1 1/2 carb
Strawberry Topping	lg	100	0	0	0	0	0	15	25	1	0	1 1/2 carb
Vanilla Syrup	lg	60	0	0	0	0	0	0	16	0	0	1 carb
ADD ONS												
Bacon	1 srvg	70	5	6	2	0	15	260	0	0	4	1 high-fat meat
Cheese	1 srvg	60	5	8	3	0	20	310	2	0	3	1 medium-fat meat
✔Chili	1 srvg	50	4	7	1.5	0	10	160	2	1	3	1 medium-fat meat
✔Green Chilies	1 srvg	5	0	0	0	0	0	5	1	0	0	Free

✔Grilled Onions	1 srvg	25	2	7	0	0	0	500	5	1	0	1/2 carb
✔Jalapeno	1 srvg	5	0	0	0	0	0	280	1	1	0	Free
Ranch Dressing	2 oz	260	28	10	5	0	20	490	0	0	0	5 1/2 fat
✔Slaw	1 srvg	45	3	6	0.5	0	5	45	4	1	0	1/2 carb
BREAKFAST COMBOS												
Bacon Egg & Cheese Breakfast Burrito	1	450	27	5	10	1.5	320	1140	38	3	20	2 1/2 starch, 2 medium-fat meat, 3 fat
Bacon Egg & Cheese Toaster	1	540	30	5	10	1.5	325	1440	46	2	22	3 starch, 2 medium-fat meat, 4 fat
Ham Egg & Cheese Breakfast Burrito	1	440	23	5	8	1.5	330	1530	37	3	25	2 1/2 starch, 3 lean meat, 3 fat
Ham Egg & Cheese Toaster	1	500	23	4	7	1.5	325	1700	46	2	26	3 starch, 2 medium-fat meat, 2 fat
Sausage Egg & Cheese Breakfast Burrito	1	470	30	6	11	1.5	325	1040	38	3	19	2 1/2 starch, 2 medium-fat meat, 4 fat

✔ = Healthiest Bets

(*Continued*)

BREAKFAST COMBOS *(Continued)*	Amount	Cal.	Fat (g)	% Cal. Fat	Sat. Fat (g)	Trans Fat (g)	Chol. (mg)	Sod. (mg)	Carb. (g)	Fiber (g)	Pro. (g)	Choices/Exchanges
Sausage Egg & Cheese Toaster	1	630	39	6	13	1.5	340	1380	46	2	23	3 starch, 2 medium-fat meat, 6 fat
Super Sonic Breakfast Burrito	1	550	35	6	11	2.5	325	1240	47	4	19	3 starch, 1 medium-fat meat, 5 fat
BREAKFAST TOASTER SANDWICHES												
Breakfast Bistro - Bacon, Egg & Cheese	1	470	27	5	9	1	320	1370	35	2	21	2 1/2 starch, 2 medium-fat meat, 3 1/2 fat
Breakfast Bistro - Ham, Egg & Cheese	1	430	21	4	7	1	325	1640	35	2	25	2 1/2 starch, 3 medium-fat meat, 1 1/2 fat
Breakfast Bistro - Sausage, Egg & Cheese	1	560	37	6	12	1.5	360	1320	35	2	22	2 1/2 starch, 2 medium-fat meat, 5 1/2 fat
Breakfast Toaster - Bacon, Egg & Cheese	1	540	30	5	10	1.5	325	1440	46	2	22	3 starch, 2 medium-fat meat, 4 fat

Breakfast Toaster - Ham, Egg & Cheese	1	500	23	4	7	1.5	325	1700	46	2	26	3 starch, 2 medium-fat meat, 2 fat
Breakfast Toaster - Sausage, Egg & Cheese	1	630	39	6	13	1.5	340	1380	46	2	23	3 starch, 2 medium-fat meat, 6 fat
French Toast Sticks	4	500	26	5	5	4.5	25	580	49	2	8	3 1/2 starch, 5 fat
Syrup	1 oz	80	0	0	0	0	0	0	21	0	0	1 1/2 carb
BURGERS												
Bacon Cheeseburger	1	780	48	6	16	1.5	100	1300	57	5	33	4 starch, 3 medium-fat meat, 6 fat
California Burger	1	690	39	5	13	1.5	80	1060	57	5	29	4 starch, 3 medium-fat meat, 5 1/2 fat
Chili Cheeseburger	1	660	35	5	14	1.5	85	990	56	5	31	3 1/2 starch, 3 medium-fat meat, 4 fat
Dixie Burger	1	660	37	5	10	1	70	810	55	5	26	3 1/2 starch, 2 medium-fat meat, 5 1/2 fat

✔ = Healthiest Bets

(Continued)

BURGERS *(Continued)*	Amount	Cal.	Fat (g)	% Cal. Fat	Sat. Fat (g)	Trans Fat (g)	Chol. (mg)	Sod. (mg)	Carb. (g)	Fiber (g)	Pro. (g)	Choices/Exchanges
Dixie Cheeseburger	1	720	42	5	14	1.5	90	1120	56	5	29	3 1/2 starch, 3 medium-fat meat, 6 fat
Double Cheeseburger	1	570	35	6	16	1.5	110	1290	33	3	30	2 starch, 3 medium-fat meat, 3 1/2 fat
Green Chili Cheeseburger	1	630	31	4	12	1.5	75	4070	56	5	29	3 1/2 starch, 3 medium-fat meat, 3 1/2 fat
Hamburger w/ Ketchup	1	560	26	4	9	1	60	750	54	5	26	3 1/2 starch, 2 medium-fat meat, 3 fat
Hickory Cheeseburger	1	640	31	4	12	1.5	75	1170	61	5	28	4 starch, 2 medium-fat meat, 4 fat
Jalapeno Burger	1	550	26	4	9	1	60	610	52	5	25	3 1/2 starch, 2 medium-fat meat, 3 fat
Jalapeno Cheese Burger	1	610	31	5	12	1.5	75	930	53	5	28	3 1/2 starch, 2 medium-fat meat, 3 1/2 fat

✔Jr. Burger	1	310	15	4	5	0.5	35	610	30	3	15	2 starch, 1 medium-fat meat, 1 1/2 fat
✔Jr. Cheeseburger	1	380	20	5	9	1	55	930	31	3	18	2 starch, 2 medium-fat meat, 2 1/2 fat
Sonic Cheeseburger w/Ketchup	1	630	31	4	12	1.5	75	1140	59	5	29	4 starch, 2 medium-fat meat, 3 1/2 fat
Super Sonic Cheeseburger w/ Ketchup	1	900	53	5	22	2.5	155	1460	57	5	46	4 starch, 5 medium-fat meat, 5 1/2 fat
Super Sonic Jalapeno Cheeseburger	1	890	53	5	22	2.5	155	1600	56	5	46	3 1/2 starch, 5 medium-fat meat, 5 1/2 fat
Thousand Island Cheeseburger	1	680	38	5	13	1.5	85	1130	58	5	29	4 starch, 2 medium-fat meat, 4 1/2 fat
Thousand Island Jr. Cheeseburger	1	430	27	6	10	4	60	700	30	3	18	2 starch, 2 medium-fat meat, 3 1/2 fat

✔ = Healthiest Bets

(*Continued*)

	Amount	Cal.	Fat (g)	% Cal. Fat	Sat. Fat (g)	Trans Fat (g)	Chol. (mg)	Sod. (mg)	Carb. (g)	Fiber (g)	Pro. (g)	Choices/Exchanges
CHICKEN												
Breaded Chicken Sandwich	1	670	33	4	6	3	55	1290	66	6	49	4 1/2 starch, 5 lean meat, 2 fat
Chicken Strip Dinner	1	920	43	4	8	8	70	1730	97	9	36	6 1/2 starch, 2 lean meat, 6 1/2 fat
✔Grilled Chicken Sandwich	1	340	12	3	2.5	0.5	75	990	32	2	27	2 starch, 3 lean meat, 1/2 fat
Jumbo Popcorn Chicken, large	1	560	32	5	6	6	65	1910	41	3	28	2 1/2 starch, 3 lean meat, 4 1/2 fat
Jumbo Popcorn Chicken, snack	1	370	21	5	4	4	40	1270	27	2	19	2 starch, 2 lean meat, 3 fat
CONEYS												
✔Corn Dog	1	250	15	5	4	1.5	15	80	12	2	5	1 starch, 1 medium-fat meat, 2 fat

Extra Long Slaw Dog	1	670	36	5	12	0	80	1770	60	4	24	4 starch, 2 medium-fat meat, 5 1/2 fat
Extra Long Cheese Coney	1	600	33	5	11	1	75	1700	54	4	24	3 1/2 starch, 2 medium-fat meat, 4 1/2 fat
CREAM SLUSH												
Blue Coconut	reg	430	13	3	8	0	45	160	76	0	5	5 carb, 1 1/2 fat
Cherry	reg	440	13	3	8	0	45	160	77	0	5	5 carb, 1 1/2 fat
Grape	reg	430	13	3	8	0	45	160	76	0	5	5 carb, 1 1/2 fat
Lemon-Berry	reg	460	12	2	7	0	45	150	80	1	5	5 1/2 carb, 1 1/2 fat
Lime	reg	430	13	3	8	0	45	160	77	0	5	5 carb, 1 1/2 fat
Orange	reg	430	13	3	8	0	45	160	77	0	5	5 carb, 1 1/2 fat
FAVES & CRAVES SIDE ORDERS												
✔French Fries	reg	210	10	4	2	2	0	260	28	4	3	2 starch, 2 fat

✔ = Healthiest Bets

(*Continued*)

FAVES & CRAVES SIDE ORDERS *(Continued)*	**Amount**	**Cal.**	**Fat (g)**	**% Cal. Fat**	**Sat. Fat (g)**	**Trans Fat (g)**	**Chol. (mg)**	**Sod. (mg)**	**Carb. (g)**	**Fiber (g)**	**Pro. (g)**	**Choices/Exchanges**
French Fries w/ Cheese	reg	280	15	5	5	2.5	20	570	29	4	6	2 starch, 1 high-fat meat, 1 1/2 fat
French Fries w/ Chili & Cheese	reg	300	18	5	6	2.5	25	530	31	5	9	2 starch, 1 high-fat meat, 1 fat
Fritos Chili Pie	1 order	940	64	6	18	1	65	1540	72	6	25	5 starch, 4 high-fat meat, 6 fat
Mozzarella Sticks	1 order	410	21	5	9	2.5	40	1040	35	2	19	2 1/2 starch, 3 high-fat meat
Onion Rings	reg	500	28	5	5	6	0	210	55	4	6	4 starch, 5 1/2 fat
Tater Tots	reg	220	14	6	2.5	3	0	600	23	3	2	2 starch, 3 fat
Tater Tots w/ Cheese	reg	290	19	6	6	3	20	910	25	3	5	1 1/2 starch, 1 high-fat meat, 2 1/2 fat

Tater Tots w/ Chili & Cheese	reg	310	21	6	7	3	25	860	26	3	8	1 1/2 starch, 1 high-fat meat, 2 fat
FLOATS												
Barq's Root Beer	reg	300	8	2	5	0	30	110	56	0	3	3 1/2 carb, 1 fat
Coca-Cola	reg	290	8	2	5	0	30	95	54	0	3	3 1/2 carb, 1 fat
Diet Coke	reg	220	8	3	5	0	30	100	33	0	3	2 carb, 1 1/2 fat
Diet Dr. Pepper	reg	220	8	3	5	0	30	130	33	0	3	2 carb, 1 1/2 fat
Dr. Pepper	reg	310	8	2	5	0	30	120	58	0	3	4 carb, 1 fat
ICE CREAM												
Banana Split	1	450	12	2	8	0	30	150	82	2	5	3 1/2 carb, 2 fruit, 2 fat
Chocolate Sundae	1	410	13	3	9	0	35	190	67	0	4	4 1/2 carb, 2 fat
Hot Fudge Sundae	1	440	18	4	13	0	35	170	63	1	4	4 carb, 3 fat
Nuts added to sundae	1 srvg	20	1.5	7	0	0	0	0	1	0	1	Free

✔ = Healthiest Bets

(*Continued*)

ICE CREAM *(Continued)*	Amount	Cal.	Fat (g)	% Cal. Fat	Sat. Fat (g)	Trans Fat (g)	Chol. (mg)	Sod. (mg)	Carb. (g)	Fiber (g)	Pro. (g)	Choices/Exchanges
Pineapple Sundae	1	370	13	3	9	0	35	135	58	0	4	4 carb, 2 fat
Strawberry Sundae	1	380	13	3	9	0	35	120	61	1	4	4 carb, 2 fat
✔Vanilla Cone	1	180	6	3	4	0	25	80	30	0	2	2 carb, 1 fat
Vanilla Dish	1	240	9	3	5	0	35	100	36	0	3	2 1/2 carb, 2 fat
KID'S MEAL												
✔Chicken Strips	2	210	11	5	2	2	35	430	13	1	14	1 starch, 2 lean meat, 1 fat
✔Corn Dog	1	250	15	5	4	1.5	15	80	23	2	6	1 1/2 starch, 1 high-fat meat, 1 1/2 fat
Grilled Cheese	1	390	17	4	8	1.5	35	1010	45	2	14	3 starch, 1 medium-fat meat, 2 1/2 fat
✔Jr. Burger	1	320	16	5	5	1	35	610	29	2	15	2 starch, 1 medium-fat meat, 2 fat

Jr. Cheeseburger	1	380	21	5	9	1.5	55	930	30	2	18	2 starch, 2 medium-fat meat, 2 1/2 fat
LIMEADES												
Apple Juice	sm	160	0	0	0	0	0	35	42	0	0	3 carb
Cherry	sm	170	0	0	0	0	0	35	45	0	0	3 carb
Cranberry	sm	150	0	0	0	0	0	35	41	0	0	3 carb
✔Diet Cherry	sm	10	0	0	0	0	0	10	2	0	0	Free
✔Diet Limeade	sm	5	0	0	0	0	0	10	1	0	0	Free
Limeade	sm	140	0	0	0	0	0	30	38	0	0	2 1/2 carb
Strawberry	sm	170	0	0	0	0	0	35	45	0	0	3 carb
MALTS												
Banana	reg	560	20	3	12	0.5	70	230	89	1	8	6 carb, 3 fat
Chocolate	reg	630	20	3	12	0.5	70	310	102	0	8	7 carb, 3 fat

✔ = Healthiest Bets

(Continued)

MALTS *(Continued)*	Amount	Cal.	Fat (g)	% Cal. Fat	Sat. Fat (g)	Trans Fat (g)	Chol. (mg)	Sod. (mg)	Carb. (g)	Fiber (g)	Pro. (g)	Choices/Exchanges
Pineapple	reg	590	20	3	12	0.5	70	240	93	0	8	6 carb, 3 fat
Strawberry	reg	590	20	3	12	0.5	70	230	96	1	8	6 1/2 carb, 3 fat
Vanilla	reg	550	21	3	13	1	75	240	84	0	8	5 1/2 carb, 3 fat
REAL FRUIT SLUSHES												
Lemon Berry Slush	sm	210	0	0	0	0	0	30	55	0	0	3 1/2 carb
Lemon Slush	sm	200	0	0	0	0	0	30	53	0	0	3 1/2 carb
Lime Slush	sm	200	0	0	0	0	0	30	52	0	0	3 1/2 carb
SALADS AND DRESSING												
Fat Free Golden Italian Dressing	2 oz	50	0	0	0	0	0	600	13	0	0	1 carb
Grilled Chicken Salad	1 srvg	310	14	4	6	1	100	1090	19	4	30	4 veg, 3 lean meat, 2 fat
Honey Mustard Dressing	1 srvg	240	21	8	3	0	15	300	14	0	0	1 carb, 4 fat

Jumbo Popcorn Chicken Salad	1 srvg	490	28	5	9	4	60	1440	39	5	22	1 starch, 4 veg, 3 lean meat, 4 fat
✔Light Original Ranch Dressing	2 oz	120	7	5	1	0	15	740	14	0	1	1 carb, 1 1/2 fat
Santa Fe Chicken Salad	1 srvg	380	15	4	7	1	100	1180	29	6	32	1 starch, 3 veg, 4 lean meat, 1/2 fat
✔Southwest Ranch Dressing	2 oz	120	7	5	1	0	0	770	15	0	1	1 carb, 1 1/2 fat
Thousand Island Dressing	2 oz	250	25	9	4	0	30	590	9	0	1	1/2 carb, 5 fat
SANDWICHES AND TOASTER SANDWICHES												
Bacon Cheeseburger	1	690	37	5	14	3	90	1410	58	3	31	4 starch, 3 medium-fat meat, 4 1/2 fat
Breaded Pork Fritter Sandwich	1	640	33	5	6	0	30	840	66	7	22	4 1/2 starch, 1 medium-fat meat, 5 1/2 fat
✔Burrito	1	370	18	4	6	0	15	480	10	6	10	1 starch, 1 high-fat meat, 2 fat

✔ = Healthiest Bets

(Continued)

SANDWICHES AND TOASTER SANDWICHES *(Continued)*	Amount	Cal.	Fat (g)	% Cal. Fat	Sat. Fat (g)	Trans Fat (g)	Chol. (mg)	Sod. (mg)	Carb. (g)	Fiber (g)	Pro. (g)	Choices/Exchanges
Burrito Deluxe	1	420	22	5	7	0.5	25	640	43	6	13	3 starch, 1 medium-fat meat, 4 fat
Chicken Club	1	690	35	5	10	3	80	1900	64	4	32	4 1/2 starch, 3 lean meat, 5 1/2 fat
Fish Sandwich	1	650	31	4	5	0	40	1160	71	7	22	4 1/2 starch, 1 lean meat, 5 1/2 fat
✔Tacos	1 order	340	20	5	6	0.5	25	360	35	4	8	2 1/2 starch, 4 fat
SHAKES												
Banana	reg	550	19	3	12	0.5	70	220	87	1	8	6 carb, 3 fat
Banana Cream Pie	reg	690	23	3	15	1	65	230	113	1	8	7 1/2 carb, 3 1/2 fat
Chocolate	reg	610	19	3	12	0.5	70	300	101	0	11	6 1/2 carb, 3 fat
Chocolate Cream Pie	reg	750	23	3	15	1	65	310	127	1	8	8 1/2 carb, 3 1/2 fat

Coconut Cream Pie	reg	680	24	3	15	1	70	240	108	1	8	7 carb, 4 fat
Pineapple	reg	570	19	3	12	0.5	70	230	92	0	7	6 carb, 3 fat
Strawberry	reg	580	19	3	12	0.5	70	220	94	1	8	6 1/2 carb, 3 fat
Strawberry Cream Pie	reg	720	23	3	15	1	65	240	120	1	8	8 carb, 3 1/2 fat
Vanilla	reg	540	20	3	12	1	75	230	82	0	8	5 1/2 carb, 3 fat
SLUSHES												
Blue Coconut Slush	sm	190	0	0	0	0	0	30	52	0	0	3 1/2 carb
Bubble Gum	sm	190	0	0	0	0	0	35	53	0	0	3 1/2 carb
Cherry Slush	sm	200	0	0	0	0	0	30	53	0	0	3 1/2 carb
Grape Slush	sm	190	0	0	0	0	0	35	52	0	0	3 1/2 carb
Green Apple	sm	200	0	0	0	0	0	30	54	0	0	3 1/2 carb
SMOOTHIES												
Strawberry	reg	460	0	0	0	0	0	180	113	8	1	7 1/2 carb

✔ = Healthiest Bets

(Continued)

SMOOTHIES *(Continued)*	Amount	Cal.	Fat (g)	% Cal. Fat	Sat. Fat (g)	Trans Fat (g)	Chol. (mg)	Sod. (mg)	Carb. (g)	Fiber (g)	Pro. (g)	Choices/Exchanges
Strawberry - Banana	reg	440	0	0	0	0	0	160	108	3	1	7 carb
Tropical Fruit	reg	500	0	0	0	0	0	170	124	4	1	8 1/2 carb
SONIC BLASTS												
Butterfinger	reg	670	31	4	19	1	60	250	89	1	9	6 carb, 5 fat
M&M's	reg	660	28	4	18	1	60	220	95	1	8	6 1/2 carb, 5 fat
Oreo	reg	660	28	4	18	1	60	220	94	1	8	6 1/2 carb, 5 fat
Reese's Peanut Butter Cup	reg	620	22	3	14	0.5	65	270	96	1	10	6 1/2 carb, 3 1/2 fat
WRAPS												
Chicken Strip Wrap	1	480	20	4	4	6	40	1170	56	5	20	3 1/2 starch, 1 lean meat, 3 fat
Fritos Chili Cheese Wrap	1	670	38	5	12	1.5	50	1260	66	6	22	4 1/2 starch, 3 high-fat meat, 2 fat

Grilled Chicken Wrap	1	380	11	3	2.5	1	80	1350	44	4	28	3 starch, 3 lean meat, 1/2 fat

✔ = Healthiest Bets

Exclusive Web Content

Be sure to visit the following restaurants online at http://www.diabetes.org/healthyrestaurant

Carvel | **Frëshens** | **Jimmy John's** | **Wienerschnitzel**

Carvel	**Frëshens**	**Jimmy John's**	**Wienerschnitzel**
Del Taco	**Godfather's**	**Tim Hortons**	**Zaxby's**
El Pollo Loco	**Jersey Mike's**	**Whataburger**	

Wendy's

(www.wendys.com)

Light 'n Lean Choice

Mandarin Chicken Salad with
Roasted Almonds *(1 packet)*
Low-Fat Honey Mustard *(1/2 packet, 2 Tbsp)*
Jr. Chocolate Frosty

Calories	570	Cholesterol (mg)	100
Fat (g)	22	Sodium (mg)	1,055
% calories from fat	35	Carbohydrate (g)	59
Saturated fat (g)	5	Fiber (g)	5
Trans fat (g)	0	Protein (g)	34

Exchanges: 1/2 starch, 2 1/2 carb, 2 veg, 3 lean meat, 4 fat

Healthy 'n Hearty Choice

Baked Potato, plain
Chili *(large)*
Side Salad with Light Classic
Ranch Dressing *(1 serving)*

Calories	675	Cholesterol (mg)	80
Fat (g)	35	Sodium (mg)	1,650
% calories from fat	47	Carbohydrate (g)	102
Saturated fat (g)	17	Fiber (g)	16
Trans fat (g)	5	Protein (g)	30

Exchanges: 6 starch, 1 veg, 2 medium-fat meat, 1 1/2 fat

Wendy's

	Amount	Cal.	Fat (g)	% Cal. Fat	Sat. Fat (g)	Trans Fat (g)	Chol. (mg)	Sod. (mg)	Carb. (g)	Fiber (g)	Pro. (g)	Choices/Exchanges
CHICKEN NUGGETS AND SAUCES												
✔Barbecue Sauce	1 order	45	0	0	0	0	0	160	11	0	1	1/2 carb
✔Chicken Nuggets	4 pcs	190	12	6	2	0	30	430	10	0	10	1/2 starch, 1 lean meat, 1 1/2 fat
✔Chicken Nuggets	5 pcs	230	15	6	3	0	35	420	12	0	12	1 starch, 1 lean meat, 2 fat
Chicken Nuggets	10 pcs	460	30	6	6	0	70	1040	24	0	24	1 1/2 starch, 3 lean meat, 4 1/2 fat
Heartland Ranch	1 order	160	17	10	2.5	0	15	220	1	0	0	3 1/2 fat
✔Honey Mustard	1 order	130	12	8	2	0	10	220	6	0	0	1/2 carb, 2 1/2 fat
✔Sweet & Sour	1 order	50	0	0	0	0	0	150	13	0	0	1 carb

✔ = Healthiest Bets

(Continued)

CHICKEN NUGGETS AND SAUCES *(Continued)*	Amount	Cal.	Fat (g)	% Cal. Fat	Sat. Fat (g)	Trans Fat (g)	Chol. (mg)	Sod. (mg)	Carb. (g)	Fiber (g)	Pro. (g)	Choices/Exchanges
FROSTY												
✔Chocolate	jr	160	4	2	2.5	0	15	75	26	0	4	1 1/2 carb, 1 fat
Chocolate	sm	320	8	2	5	0	35	150	52	0	9	3 1/2 carb, 1 1/2 fat
Chocolate	med	410	11	2	7	0.5	45	200	68	0	11	4 1/2 carb, 1 1/2 fat
Chocolate	lg	530	14	2	9	0.5	55	260	86	0	14	5 1/2 carb, 2 1/2 fat
Chocolate Fudge	sm	410	11	2	7	0.5	35	230	69	1	8	4 1/2 carb, 1 1/2 fat
Chocolate Fudge	lg	540	13	2	8	0.5	45	310	94	1	11	6 1/2 carb, 2 fat
Chocolate Twisted w/ M&M's	1	560	19	3	12	0.5	40	180	86	1	10	5 1/2 carb, 3 fat
Chocolate Twisted w/ Oreo	1	450	14	3	7	0	30	300	72	1	10	5 carb, 2 1/2 fat
Chocolate Twisted w/ Toll House Cookie Dough	1	480	16	3	10	0.5	35	220	77	1	10	5 carb, 2 1/2 fat

Strawberry	sm	390	11	3	7	0.5	35	170	67	0	7	4 1/2 carb, 1 1/2 fat
Strawberry	lg	520	13	2	8	0.5	45	220	91	0	9	6 carb, 2 fat
✔Vanilla	jr	150	4	2	2.5	0	20	90	26	0	4	1 1/2 carb, 1 fat
Vanilla	sm	310	8	2	5	0	35	180	52	0	8	3 1/2 carb, 1 1/2 fat
Vanilla	med	410	10	2	6	0.5	45	240	68	0	11	4 1/2 carb, 2 fat
Vanilla	lg	520	13	2	8	1	60	300	86	0	14	5 1/2 carb, 2 fat
Vanilla Bean	sm	380	11	3	7	0.5	35	170	65	0	7	4 1/2 carb, 1 1/2 fat
Vanilla Bean	lg	500	12	2	8	0.5	45	220	89	0	9	6 carb, 2 fat
Vanilla Float w/ Coca-Cola	1	380	7	2	4.5	0	30	160	75	0	7	5 carb, 1 fat
Vanilla Twisted w/ M&M's	1	550	19	3	12	0.5	40	210	86	1	10	5 1/2 carb, 3 fat
Vanilla Twisted w/ Oreo	1	440	14	3	6	0.5	35	320	72	1	9	5 carb, 2 1/2 fat
Vanilla Twisted w/ Toll House Cookie Dough	1	480	16	3	10	0.5	40	240	77	1	9	5 carb, 2 1/2 fat

✔ = Healthiest Bets

(*Continued*)

	Amount	Cal.	Fat (g)	% Cal. Fat	Sat. Fat (g)	Trans Fat (g)	Chol. (mg)	Sod. (mg)	Carb. (g)	Fiber (g)	Pro. (g)	Choices/Exchanges
SALAD DRESSINGS												
✓Balsamic Vinaigrette	1 srvg	90	6	6	1	0	0	380	8	0	0	1/2 carb, 1 fat
Chunky Blue Cheese	1 srvg	230	24	9	5	0	35	370	2	0	2	5 fat
Classic Ranch	1 srvg	200	20	9	3	0	15	340	3	0	1	4 fat
✓Fat Free French	1 srvg	70	0	0	0	0	0	170	17	1	0	1 carb
Italian Vinaigrette	1 srvg	130	11	8	1.5	0	0	320	8	0	6	1/2 carb, 2 fat
✓Light Classic Ranch	1 srvg	90	8	8	1.5	0	20	360	4	0	1	1/2 carb, 1 1/2 fat
Light Honey Dijon	1 srvg	100	5	5	1	0	20	280	13	1	1	1 carb, 1 fat
Thousand Island	1 srvg	290	28	9	4.5	0	30	530	9	0	1	1/2 carb, 5 1/2 fat
SALADS												
✓Caesar Salad	1	70	4	5	2	0	10	170	4	2	6	1 veg, 1 fat
✓Caesar Salad - Dressing	1 srvg	120	13	10	2	0	10	200	1	0	1	2 fat

Caesar Salad - Garlic Croutons	1 srvg	70	2.5	3	0	0	0	125	9	0	2	1/2 starch, 1/2 fat
Chicken BLT Salad	1	470	27	5	10	0	85	1280	23	3	35	1 starch, 3 veg, 5 lean meat, 2 fat
Chicken BLT Salad - Garlic Croutons	1 srvg	250	24	9	3.5	0	20	330	9	0	1	1/2 starch, 5 fat
✔Chicken BLT Salad - Honey Dijon Dressing	1 srvg	70	3	4	0	0	0	125	9	0	2	1/2 carb, 1/2 fat
✔Mandarin Chicken Salad	1	180	2	1	0.5	0	65	630	16	2	24	1/2 starch, 2 veg, 3 lean meat
✔Mandarin Chicken Salad - Crispy Noodles	1 srvg	70	3	4	0	0	0	190	10	0	1	1/2 starch, 1 fat
✔Mandarin Chicken Salad - Oriental Sesame Dressing	1 srvg	170	10	5	1.5	0	0	360	19	0	1	1 carb, 2 fat

✔ = Healthiest Bets

(*Continued*)

SALADS *(Continued)*	Amount	Cal.	Fat (g)	% Cal. Fat	Sat. Fat (g)	Trans Fat (g)	Chol. (mg)	Sod. (mg)	Carb. (g)	Fiber (g)	Pro. (g)	Choices/Exchanges
✔Mandarin Chicken Salad - Roasted Almonds	1 srvg	130	11	8	1	0	0	70	4	2	5	2 fat
✔Side Salad	1	35	0	0	0	0	0	25	8	2	1	1 veg
Southwest Taco Salad	1	400	22	5	12	1	85	1140	26	7	27	1 starch, 3 veg, 3 lean meat, 2 fat
✔Southwest Taco Salad - Ancho Chipotle Dressing	1 srvg	90	8	8	2	0	10	240	3	0	1	1 1/2 fat
✔Southwest Taco Salad - Sour Cream	1 srvg	45	4	8	2	0	10	25	2	0	1	1 fat
Southwest Taco Salad - Tortilla Strips	1 srvg	110	5	4	1	0	0	160	13	1	2	1 starch, 1 fat
SANDWICHES												
Baconator	1	840	51	5	23	2.5	195	1880	38	1	56	2 1/2 starch, 7 medium-fat meat, 3 1/2 fat

✔Cheeseburger, Kid's Meal	1	270	11	4	5	0.5	40	70	27	1	15	2 starch, 1 medium-fat meat, 1 fat
✔Crispy Chicken Sandwich	1	330	14	4	2.5	0	35	680	34	1	15	2 1/2 starch, 1 lean meat, 2 fat
Double w/ Everything and Cheese	1	710	40	5	17	2	160	1440	41	2	47	2 1/2 starch, 6 medium-fat meat, 2 1/2 fat
✔Grilled Chicken Go Wrap	1	260	11	4	3.5	0	45	760	23	1	17	1 1/2 starch, 2 lean meat, 1 fat
✔Hamburger, Kid's Meal	1	220	8	3	3	0	43	490	26	1	12	1 1/2 starch, 1 medium-fat meat, 1/2 fat
✔Homestyle Chicken Fillet Sandwich	1	430	16	3	2.5	0	45	1120	48	2	25	3 starch, 2 lean meat, 2 fat
✔Homestyle Chicken Go Wrap	1	320	15	4	4.5	0	35	860	29	1	15	2 starch, 1 lean meat, 2 fat
✔Jr. Bacon Cheeseburger	1	320	16	5	6	0.5	50	670	26	1	17	1 1/2 starch, 2 medium-fat meat, 1 1/2 fat

✔ = Healthiest Bets

(*Continued*)

SANDWICHES *(Continued)*	**Amount**	**Cal.**	**Fat (g)**	**% Cal. Fat**	**Sat. Fat (g)**	**Trans Fat (g)**	**Chol. (mg)**	**Sod. (mg)**	**Carb. (g)**	**Fiber (g)**	**Pro. (g)**	**Choices/Exchanges**
✔Jr. Cheeseburger	1	270	11	4	5	0.5	10	360	27	1	15	2 starch, 1 medium-fat meat, 1 fat
✔Jr. Cheeseburger Deluxe	1	300	14	4	6	0.5	45	730	29	2	15	2 starch, 1 medium-fat meat, 1 1/2 fat
✔Jr. Hamburger	1	230	5	2	3	0	30	490	27	1	13	2 starch, 1 medium-fat meat
✔Single w/ Everything	1	430	20	4	7	1	75	870	39	2	25	2 1/2 starch, 2 medium-fat meat, 1 1/2 fat
Spicy Chicken Filet Sandwich	1	440	16	3	2.5	0	60	1300	46	3	28	3 starch, 3 lean meat, 1 1/2 fat
✔Spicy Chicken Go Wrap	1	320	16	5	4.5	0	43	960	28	2	17	2 starch, 2 lean meat, 2 fat
✔Stack Attack	1	380	20	5	9	1	75	750	27	1	23	2 starch, 3 medium-fat meat, 1 1/2 fat

Triple w/ Everything and Cheese	1	980	60	6	27	3.5	245	2010	43	2	69	3 starch, 9 medium-fat meat, 3 1/2 fat
✔Ultimate Chicken Grill Sandwich	1	320	7	2	1.5	0	70	952	36	2	28	2 1/2 starch, 3 lean meat
SIDE SELECTIONS												
✔Baked Potato - Plain	1	270	0	0	0	0	0	25	61	7	7	4 starch
✔Baked Potato - Sour Cream & Chive	1	320	4	1	2	0	10	50	63	7	8	4 starch, 1 fat
Chili	sm	190	6	3	2.5	0	40	830	19	5	14	1 1/2 starch, 1 medium-fat meat
Chili	lg	280	9	3	3.5	0.5	60	1240	29	7	21	2 starch, 2 medium-fat meat
✔Chili - Saltine Crackers	1 order	25	1	4	0	0	0	95	4	0	0	Free
✔Chili - Seasoning	1 order	5	0	0	0	0	0	270	1	0	0	Free

✔ = Healthiest Bets

(Continued)

SIDE SELECTIONS *(Continued)*	Amount	Cal.	Fat (g)	% Cal. Fat	Sat. Fat (g)	Trans Fat (g)	Chol. (mg)	Sod. (mg)	Carb. (g)	Fiber (g)	Pro. (g)	Choices/Exchanges
Chili - Shredded Cheddar Cheese	1 order	70	6	8	3.5	0	15	110	1	0	4	1 fat
✔French Fries	kid's	210	10	4	1.5	0	0	180	28	3	3	2 starch, 2 fat
French Fries	small	340	16	4	2.5	0	0	290	45	4	4	3 starch, 3 fat
French Fries	med	430	20	4	3	0	0	370	56	5	6	4 starch, 3 1/2 fat
French Fries	lg	550	26	4	4	0	0	480	72	7	7	5 starch, 4 fat
✔Mandarin Orange Cup	1	80	0	0	0	0	0	15	19	1	1	1 fruit

✔ = Healthiest Bets

Chicken—Fried, Roasted, or Grilled

RESTAURANTS

Chick-fil-A

Church's Chicken

KFC

Popeyes Louisiana Kitchen

EXCLUSIVE WEB CONTENT

El Pollo Loco (http://www.diabetes.org/healthyrestaurant)

NUTRITION PROS

- No foods greet you at the table. What you order is what you eat. This puts you in the driver's seat.
- There's no waiting for food. You order and then eat.
- You can be in the know. Most large chicken chains provide full disclosure of their nutrition information.
- You know the menu well, so you can know what to order before you walk through the door.
- Order à la carte. Doing so makes it easier for you to order and eat smaller quantities.
- Fried entrees are not the only option in some chicken chains. A few have mastered roasting or grilling.
- Healthier side items can fill your plate—corn, green beans, baked beans, rice, potatoes—but make sure they're not swimming in butter, sweet sauces, or gravy.
- You can sometimes get a salad. But take control: you pour the dressing.

NUTRITION CONS

- Portions are often enough for two people or two meals.
- Some chicken chains stick to the tried and true: high-fat battered and fried chicken.
- Some side items are sure candidates for the high-fat column: French fries, fried okra, potato salad, coleslaw, and biscuits.
- Some side items may hide their fat grams well: coleslaw, mashed potatoes, corn, and pasta salad.
- Unadulterated cooked vegetables don't appear often.
- Fruit is usually not available unless it's part of a high-fat, high-sugar dessert.

Exclusive Web Content

Be sure to visit the following restaurants online at http://www.diabetes.org/healthyrestaurant

Carvel	**Godfather's**	**Whataburger**
Del Taco	**Jersey Mike's**	**Wienerschnitzel**
El Pollo Loco	**Jimmy John's**	**Zaxby's**
Frëshens	**Tim Hortons**	

Healthy Tips

- ★ You are better off without the skin. If the chicken is served with skin, take it off and save yourself some fat grams. You'll also lighten up on cholesterol and saturated fat.
- ★ Skip the wing, especially if it's fried.
- ★ If there's enough for two meals, ask for a take-out container and split the meal into two before you dig in.
- ★ To keep fat grams and calories down, go with the quarter white meat. Wings and thighs have the most fat.
- ★ If you are going to eat the meal at home, a better buy (price and health wise) is a whole chicken and several sides. That way you—rather than the server—can decide on your portions.
- ★ Split a quarter of a chicken meal and add an extra side or two. This keeps the protein portion where it should be, at about 2–3 ounces.

Get It Your Way

- ★ Ask to have the skin removed if you can't trust yourself to do it.
- ★ Ask the server to take the wing off the breast.
- ★ Ask for the gravy, butter, or salad dressing on the side.

Chick-fil-A

(www.chickfila.com)

Light 'n Lean Choice

Spicy Chicken Cool Wrap
Waffle Potato Fries *(1/2 small order)*
Fruit Cup *(medium)*

Calories	615	Cholesterol (mg)	60
Fat (g)	19	Sodium (mg)	1,378
% calories from fat	28	Carbohydrate (g)	79
Saturated fat (g)	6	Fiber (g)	13
Trans fat (g)	0	Protein (g)	37

Exchanges: 4 starch, 1 fruit, 4 lean meat, 1 fat

Healthy 'n Hearty Choice

Chargrilled Chicken Club Sandwich
Carrot & Raisin Salad
Icedream *(small cone)*

Calories	800	Cholesterol (mg)	110
Fat (g)	27	Sodium (mg)	1,470
% calories from fat	30	Carbohydrate (g)	104
Saturated fat (g)	8.5	Fiber (g)	8
Trans fat (g)	0	Protein (g)	42

Exchanges: 2 1/2 starch, 2 veg, 1 fruit, 2 carb, 4 lean meat, 3 fat

Chick-fil-A

	Amount	Cal.	Fat (g)	% Cal. Fat	Sat. Fat (g)	Trans Fat (g)	Chol. (mg)	Sod. (mg)	Carb. (g)	Fiber (g)	Pro. (g)	Choices/Exchanges
BREAKFAST												
Bacon, Egg, & Cheese Biscuit	1	470	27	5	10	3	270	1190	39	1	19	2 1/2 starch, 2 medium-fat meat, 4 fat
Chicken Biscuit	1	420	19	4	4.5	3	35	1270	44	2	18	3 starch, 1 lean meat, 3 fat
✔Chicken Breakfast Burrito	1	420	18	4	7	0	245	880	40	4	22	2 1/2 starch, 2 lean meat, 2 1/2 fat
Chicken, Egg, & Cheese on Sunflower Multigrain Bagel	1	500	20	4	7	0	290	1260	49	3	31	3 1/2 starch, 3 lean meat, 2 fat
✔Chick-n-Minis	3-count	280	11	4	3.5	1	45	580	29	2	14	2 starch, 1 lean meat, 1 1/2 fat

✔ = Healthiest Bets

(*Continued*)

BREAKFAST *(Continued)*	Amount	Cal.	Fat (g)	% Cal. Fat	Sat. Fat (g)	Trans Fat (g)	Chol. (mg)	Sod. (mg)	Carb. (g)	Fiber (g)	Pro. (g)	Choices/Exchanges
✔Chick-n-Minis	4-count	370	15	4	5	1	60	770	38	3	19	2 1/2 starch, 2 lean meat, 2 fat
Cinnamon Cluster	1 srvg	400	15	3	6	0	35	280	61	3	8	4 starch, 2 fat
Hash Browns	1 srvg	260	17	6	3.5	0	5	380	25	3	2	2 starch, 3 fat
Hot Buttered Biscuit	1	270	12	4	3	3	0	660	38	1	4	3 starch, 2 fat
Sausage & Egg Biscuit	1	570	37	6	11	3	285	1130	39	2	19	2 1/2 starch, 2 medium-fat meat, 6 fat
Sausage Breakfast Burrito	1	450	24	5	10	0	250	800	37	4	20	2 1/2 starch, 2 medium-fat meat, 3 fat
✔Sunflower Multigrain Bagel	1	220	3	1	0	0	0	350	41	2	7	3 starch, 1/2 fat
CLASSICS												
Chargrilled Chicken Club Sandwich	1	380	11	3	5	0	90	1230	37	4	36	2 1/2 starch, 4 lean meat

✔Chargrilled Chicken Sandwich	1	280	3	1	1	0	65	940	36	4	28	2 starch, 3 lean meat
Chicken Salad Sandwich	1	500	20	4	3.5	0	95	1220	53	4	29	3 1/2 starch, 3 lean meat, 2 fat
Chicken Sandwich	1	410	16	4	3.5	0	60	1300	38	1	28	2 1/2 starch, 3 lean meat, 1 1/2 fat
Chick-n-Strips	3-count	350	17	4	3.5	0	95	1040	17	2	33	1 starch, 4 lean meat, 1 fat
Nuggets	8-count	260	13	5	2.5	0	70	840	10	2	27	1/2 starch, 4 lean meat, 1/2 fat
COOL WRAP												
Chargrilled Chicken Cool Wrap	1	410	12	3	4	0	65	1250	47	9	33	3 starch, 3 lean meat
Chicken Caesar Cool Wrap	1	480	16	3	7	0	80	1560	44	8	40	3 starch, 4 lean meat
Spicy Chicken Cool Wrap	1	410	12	3	4	0	60	1320	45	9	34	3 starch, 4 lean meat

✔ = Healthiest Bets

(*Continued*)

	Amount	Cal.	Fat (g)	% Cal. Fat	Sat. Fat (g)	Trans Fat (g)	Chol. (mg)	Sod. (mg)	Carb. (g)	Fiber (g)	Pro. (g)	Choices/Exchanges
DESSERTS												
Cheesecake	1 srvg	330	24	7	14	0.5	125	290	23	0	6	1 1/2 carb, 5 fat
Chocolate Milkshake	18 oz.	760	28	3	16	0	95	530	113	1	16	7 1/2 carb, 4 fat
Cookies & Cream Milkshake	18 oz.	790	33	4	18	0	95	660	111	1	17	7 1/2 carb, 5 fat
Fudge Nut Brownie	1	370	19	5	6	0	25	180	45	3	4	3 carb, 4 fat
✓Icedream - cone	1 sm	160	4	2	2	0	15	80	28	0	4	2 carb, 1 fat
Icedream - cup	1 sm	240	6	2	3.5	0	25	105	41	0	6	2 1/2 carb, 1 fat
Lemon Pie	1 srvg	350	11	3	5	0	20	250	59	1	6	4 carb, 1 fat
Strawberry Milkshake	19 oz.	730	27	3	16	0	95	550	132	1	16	9 carb, 3 fat
Vanilla Milkshake	17 oz.	660	27	4	16	0	95	510	90	0	16	6 carb, 4 fat
DRESSINGS & SAUCES												
✓Barbecue Sauce	1 oz.	45	0	0	0	0	0	180	11	0	0	1/2 carb

✔Blue Cheese Dressing	2 T	150	16	10	3	0	20	300	1	0	1	3 fat
✔Buffalo Sauce	0.75 oz.	15	1.5	9	0	0	0	410	1	0	0	Free
Buttermilk Ranch Dressing	2 T	160	16	9	2.5	0	5	270	1	0	0	3 fat
Buttermilk Ranch Sauce	0.75 oz.	110	12	10	2	0	5	200	1	0	0	2 1/2 fat
Caesar Dressing	2 T	160	17	10	2.5	0	30	240	1	0	1	3 1/2 fat
Chick-fil-A Sauce	1 oz.	140	13	8	2	0	10	170	6	0	0	1/2 carb, 2 1/2 fat
✔Fat Free Honey Mustard Dressing	2 T	60	0	0	0	0	0	200	14	0	0	1 carb
✔Honey Mustard Sauce	1 oz.	45	0	0	0	0	0	150	10	0	0	1/2 carb
✔Honey Roasted BBQ Sauce	0.4 oz.	60	6	9	1	0	5	90	2	0	0	1 fat
Light Italian Dressing	2 T	15	0.5	3	0	0	0	570	2	0	0	Free
✔Polynesian Sauce	1 oz.	110	6	5	1	0	0	210	13	0	0	1 carb, 1 fat
✔Reduced Fat Berry Balsamic Vinaigrette	2 T	70	2	3	0	0	0	150	12	0	0	1 carb, 1/2 fat

✔ = Healthiest Bets

(*Continued*)

DRESSINGS & SAUCES *(Continued)*	Amount	Cal.	Fat (g)	% Cal. Fat	Sat. Fat (g)	Trans Fat (g)	Chol. (mg)	Sod. (mg)	Carb. (g)	Fiber (g)	Pro. (g)	Choices/Exchanges
Spicy Dressing	2 T	140	14	9	2	0	5	130	2	0	0	3 fat
Thousand Island Dressing	2 T	150	14	8	2	0	10	250	5	0	0	1/2 carb, 3 fat
SALADS												
✔Chargrilled & Fruit Salad	1 srvg	220	6	2	3.5	0	65	610	20	5	22	1 fruit, 3 lean meat
✔Chargrilled Chicken Garden Salad	1 srvg	180	6	3	3.5	0	65	610	10	4	23	2 veg, 3 lean meat
Chick-n-Strips Salad	1 srvg	450	22	4	6	0	105	1170	25	6	39	1 starch, 3 veg, 5 lean meat, 1 fat
✔Garlic & Butter Croutons	1 srvg	60	2	3	0	0	0	150	9	0	2	1 starch, 1/2 fat
✔Harvest Nut Granola	1 srvg	60	2	3	0	0	0	10	10	1	1	1 starch, 1/2 fat
Honey Roasted Sunflower Kernels	1 srvg	80	7	8	1	0	0	38	3	1	2.5	1 1/2 fat

✔Southwest Chargrilled Salad	1 srvg	240	9	3	4	0	60	750	17	5	25	3 veg, 4 lean meat
✔Tortilla Strips	1 srvg	70	4	5	0.5	0	0	53	9	1	2	1 starch, 1 fat
SIDES												
Carrot & Raisin Salad	sm	260	12	4	1.5	0	5	160	39	4	2	2 veg, 2 fruit, 2 fat
Cole Slaw	sm	370	32	8	5	0	20	280	20	3	2	4 veg, 6 1/2 fat
✔Fruit Cup	med	70	0	0	0	0	0	0	17	2	1	1 fruit
Hearty Breast of Chicken Soup	sm	150	4	2	1	0	30	1040	19	2	10	1 starch, 1 lean meat, 1 fat
✔Side Salad	1 srvg	50	3	5	1.5	0	10	75	4	2	3	1 veg, 1/2 fat
Waffle Potato Fries, salted	sm	270	13	4	3	0	0	115	34	4	3	2 starch, 2 fat

✔ = Healthiest Bets

Church's Chicken
(www.churchs.com)

Light 'n Lean Choice

Crunchy Tenders *(2 individual)*
Corn on the Cob
Mashed Potatoes and Gravy *(1 serving)*
Collard Greens

Calories	475	Cholesterol (mg)	70
Fat (g)	17	Sodium (mg)	1,545
% calories from fat	32	Carbohydrate (g)	53
Saturated fat (g)	4	Fiber (g)	12
Trans fat (g)	2	Protein (g)	32

Exchanges: 3 starch, 1 veg, 2 lean meat, 1 1/2 fat

Healthy 'n Hearty Choice

Chicken Breast *(fried)*
Corn on the Cob
Cajun Rice
Cole Slaw
Apple Pie *(1/2 slice)*

Calories	750	Cholesterol (mg)	93
Fat (g)	36	Sodium (mg)	1,020
% calories from fat	43	Carbohydrate (g)	78
Saturated fat (g)	10	Fiber (g)	13
Trans fat (g)	3	Protein (g)	29

Exchanges: 3 starch, 1 veg, 2 carb, 3 lean meat, 5 fat

Church's Chicken

	Amount	Cal.	Fat (g)	% Cal. Fat	Sat. Fat (g)	Trans Fat (g)	Chol. (mg)	Sod. (mg)	Carb. (g)	Fiber (g)	Pro. (g)	Choices/Exchanges
CONDIMENTS												
✔BBQ Sauce	1 pkg	30	0	0	0	0	0	180	7	0	0	1/2 starch
✔Creamy Jalapeno Sauce	1 pkg	100	11	10	1.5	na	10	140	1	0	0	2 fat
✔Honey	1 pkg	27	0	0	0	0	0	0	7	0	0	1/2 carb
✔Honey Mustard Sauce	1 pkg	110	11	9	1.5	na	10	130	4	0	0	1/2 carb, 2 fat
✔Hot Sauce	1 pkg	18	0	0	0	0	0	120	0	0	0	Free
✔Ketchup	1 pkg	18	0	0	0	0	0	190	5	0	0	1/2 carb
✔Purple Pepper Sauce	1 pkg	45	0	0	0	0	0	26	12	0	0	1 carb
Ranch Sauce	1 pkg	130	13	9	2	na	10	320	1	0	0	2 1/2 fat

✔ = Healthiest Bets; na = not available

(Continued)

CONDIMENTS *(Continued)*	Amount	Cal.	Fat (g)	% Cal. Fat	Sat. Fat (g)	Trans Fat (g)	Chol. (mg)	Sod. (mg)	Carb. (g)	Fiber (g)	Pro. (g)	Choices/Exchanges
✔Sweet & Sour Sauce	1 pkg	30	0	0	0	0	0	120	8	0	0	1/2 carb
DESSERTS												
Apple Pie	1 srvg	260	11	4	4	2	5	250	39	1	2	2 1/2 carb, 1 1/2 fat
Edward's Double Lemon Pie	1 srvg	300	14	4	6	na	25	160	39	0	5	2 1/2 carb, 3 fat
Edward's Strawberry Cream Cheese Pie	1 srvg	280	15	5	8	na	15	130	32	2	4	2 carb, 3 fat
MAIN COURSE												
Chicken Sandwich w/ Cheese	1	510	27	5	7	2	50	1070	46	4	20	3 starch, 2 lean meat, 4 1/2 fat
Crunchy Tenders	1 pc	120	6	5	2	1	35	440	6	0	12	1/2 starch, 2 lean meat, 1/2 fat

Fried Steak Sandwich	1	490	32	6	8	2	30	880	38	2	13	2 1/2 starch, 1 lean meat, 6 fat
Fried Steak w/ Gravy	1 pc	470	28	5	7	2	65	1620	36	1	21	2 1/2 starch, 2 medium-fat meat, 3 1/2 fat
Fried Steak w/ Gravy	2 pcs	610	43	6	12	4	70	1465	31	2	24	2 starch, 3 medium-fat meat, 6 fat
✔Original Breast	1 pc	200	11	5	3	2	80	450	3	1	22	3 lean meat, 1/2 fat
✔Original Leg	1 pc	110	6	5	2	1	65	280	3	0	10	1 lean meat, 1/2 fat
Original Thigh	1 pc	330	23	6	6	3	110	680	8	1	21	1/2 starch, 3 lean meat, 3 fat
Original Wing	1 pc	300	19	6	5	3	120	540	7	3	27	1/2 starch, 4 lean meat, 1 1/2 fat
✔Spicy Breast	1 pc	320	20	6	5	4	75	760	12	2	21	1 starch, 3 lean meat, 2 1/2 fat
Spicy Crunchy Tenders	1 pc	135	7	5	2	2	25	480	7	4	11	1/2 starch, 1 lean meat, 1/2 fat

✔ = Healthiest Bets; na = not available

(*Continued*)

MAIN COURSE *(Continued)*	Amount	Cal.	Fat (g)	% Cal. Fat	Sat. Fat (g)	Trans Fat (g)	Chol. (mg)	Sod. (mg)	Carb. (g)	Fiber (g)	Pro. (g)	Choices/Exchanges
Spicy Fish Fillet	1 pc	160	9	5	2	2.5	25	350	13	1	7	1 starch, 1 lean meat, 1 1/2 fat
Spicy Fish Sandwich	1	320	20	6	4	3	25	560	25	2	10	1 1/2 starch, 1 lean meat, 3 1/2 fat
✔Spicy Leg	1 pc	180	11	6	3	2	65	470	8	1	12	1/2 starch, 1 lean meat, 1 1/2 fat
Spicy Thigh	1 pc	480	35	7	9	5	135	1035	20	2	22	1 1/2 starch, 3 lean meat, 5 1/2 fat
Spicy Wing	1 pc	430	27	6	7	4	125	1020	17	2	29	1 starch, 4 lean meat, 3 fat
SIDES												
✔Cajun Rice	reg	130	7	5	3	0	5	260	16	0	1	1 starch, 1 1/2 fat
Cole Slaw	reg	150	10	6	2	0	5	170	15	2	1	1 starch, 2 fat

✔Collard Greens	reg	25	0	0	0	0	0	170	5	2	2	1/2 starch
✔Corn on the Cob	1 ear	140	3	2	0	0	0	15	24	9	4	1 starch
French Fries	reg	290	14	4	3	3	0	320	38	4	3	2 1/2 starch, 3 fat
Honey Butter Biscuits	1	240	12	5	3	2	0	540	28	1	3	2 starch, 2 1/2 fat
Jalapeno Bombers	4	240	10	4	6	na	30	970	29	3	8	2 starch, 2 fat
Macaroni & Cheese	reg	210	11	5	4	na	15	690	23	1	8	1 1/2 starch, 2 fat
✔Mashed Potatoes & Gravy	reg	70	2	3	0	0	0	480	12	1	2	1 starch, 1/2 fat
Okra	reg	350	22	6	7	0.5	0	590	36	5	3	2 starch, 1 veg, 4 1/2 fat
Sweet Corn Nuggets	reg	600	29	4	2	na	0	1260	72	5	7	5 starch, 6 fat
✔Whole Jalapeno Peppers	2	10	0	0	0	0	0	390	2	1	0	Free

✔ = Healthiest Bets; na = not available

KFC

(www.kfc.com)

Light 'n Lean Choice

Original Drumsticks *(2)*
Corn on the Cob *(large, 5 1/2")*
Green Beans

Calories	460	Cholesterol (mg)	135
Fat (g)	21	Sodium (mg)	712
% calories from fat	41	Carbohydrate (g)	37
Saturated fat (g)	5	Fiber (g)	9
Trans fat (g)	0	Protein (g)	31

Exchanges: 2 starch, 1 veg, 3 lean meat, 2 fat

Healthy 'n Hearty Choice

Original Chicken Breast
BBQ Beans
Macaroni and Cheese

Calories	760	Cholesterol (mg)	130
Fat (g)	30	Sodium (mg)	2,550
% calories from fat	36	Carbohydrate (g)	70
Saturated fat (g)	9	Fiber (g)	7
Trans fat (g)	1	Protein (g)	51

Exchanges: 4 1/2 starch, 5 lean meat, 3 fat

KFC

	Amount	Cal.	Fat (g)	% Cal. Fat	Sat. Fat (g)	Trans Fat (g)	Chol. (mg)	Sod. (mg)	Carb. (g)	Fiber (g)	Pro. (g)	Choices/Exchanges
CHICKEN												
✔Breast	1	360	21	5	5	0	115	1020	7	0	37	1/2 starch, 5 lean meat, 1 fat
✔Breast - no skin or breading	1	140	2	1	0	0	656	520	1	0	29	3 lean meat
✔Drumstick	1	130	8	6	2	0	65	350	2	0	12	2 lean meat, 1/2 fat
Extra Crispy - Breast	1	440	27	6	6	0	105	970	15	0	34	1 starch, 4 lean meat, 2 1/2 fat
Extra Crispy - Drumstick	1	160	10	6	2	0	55	370	6	0	12	1/2 starch, 2 lean meat, 1 fat
Extra Crispy - Thigh	1	370	28	7	6	0	85	850	12	0	18	1 starch, 2 lean meat, 4 1/2 fat

✔ = Healthiest Bets

(*Continued*)

CHICKEN *(Continued)*	Amount	Cal.	Fat (g)	% Cal. Fat	Sat. Fat (g)	Trans Fat (g)	Chol. (mg)	Sod. (mg)	Carb. (g)	Fiber (g)	Pro. (g)	Choices/Exchanges
Extra Crispy - Whole Wing	1	170	11	6	2.5	0	55	350	6	1	12	1/2 starch, 2 lean meat, 1 1/2 fat
Thigh	1	330	24	7	6	0	110	870	8	0	20	1/2 starch, 3 lean meat, 3 fat
Whole Wing	1	130	8	6	2	0	50	350	4	0	11	1/2 starch, 1 lean meat, 1/2 fat
DESSERTS												
Apple Pie Mini's	3	370	20	5	6	0	0	260	44	2	2	3 carb, 3 1/2 fat
Double Chocolate Chip Cake	1 srvg	330	16	4	4	1	50	260	41	1	4	2 1/2 carb, 2 1/2 fat
Lil' Bucket Chocolate Crème	1 srvg	280	13	4	9	1	0	230	38	3	3	2 1/2 carb, 2 fat
Lil' Bucket Lemon Crème	1 srvg	410	15	3	7	1.5	0	270	61	2	7	4 carb, 2 1/2 fat

Lil' Bucket Strawberry Short Cake	1 srvg	210	7	3	5	0	10	125	33	1	2	2 carb, 1 1/2 fat
✔Sweet Life Chocolate Chip Cookie	1	160	7	4	3.5	0	10	95	23	1	2	1 1/2 carb, 1 1/2 fat
✔Sweet Life Oatmeal Raisin Cookie	1	150	5	3	2.5	0	5	135	24	1	2	1 1/2 carb, 1 fat
✔Sweet Life Sugar Cookie	1	160	6	3	2.5	0	5	120	13	0	2	1 carb, 1 1/2 fat
✔Teddy Grahams - Cinnamon	1 srvg	90	3	3	0.5	0	0	95	15	1	1	1 carb, 1/2 fat
POPCORN CHICKEN												
Popcorn Chicken	individ	400	26	6	4.5	0	60	1160	22	3	21	1 1/2 starch, 2 lean meat, 4 fat
✔Popcorn Chicken	kid's	290	19	6	3.5	0	40	850	16	2	16	1 starch, 2 lean meat, 2 1/2 fat
Popcorn Chicken	lg	550	35	6	6	0	80	1600	30	3	29	2 starch, 3 lean meat, 5 fat

✔ = Healthiest Bets

(*Continued*)

	Amount	Cal.	Fat (g)	% Cal. Fat	Sat. Fat (g)	Trans Fat (g)	Chol. (mg)	Sod. (mg)	Carb. (g)	Fiber (g)	Pro. (g)	Choices/Exchanges
POT PIE/BOWLS												
Chicken and Biscuit Bowl	1	870	44	5	11	4.5	60	2420	88	7	29	6 starch, 2 lean meat, 7 1/2 fat
Chicken Pot Pie	1	770	40	5	15	14	115	1680	70	5	33	4 1/2 starch, 3 lean meat, 6 1/2 fat
Mashed Potato w/ Gravy Bowl	1	740	35	4	9	1.5	60	2350	80	7	27	5 1/2 starch, 2 lean meat, 5 fat
Rice w/ Gravy Bowl	1	620	28	4	7	1	60	2150	67	6	26	4 1/2 starch, 2 lean meat, 4 fat
SALADS & MORE												
✔Caesar Side Salad - no dressing or croutons	1	50	3	5	2	0	10	135	2	1	4	1 veg, 1 fat
Creamy Parmesan Caesar Dressing	1 srvg	260	26	9	5	0	15	540	4	0	2	1/2 carb, 5 fat

Crispy BLT Salad - no dressing	1	330	17	5	4	0	65	1130	18	1	28	1/2 starch, 1 veg, 3 lean meat, 2 fat
Crispy Caesar Salad - no dressing or croutons	1	350	19	5	6	0	70	1080	16	3	29	1/2 starch, 1 veg, 4 lean meat, 2 fat
✔Golden Italian Dressing	1 srvg	45	3	6	0	0	0	660	6	0	0	1/2 carb, 1/2 fat
✔House Side Salad - no dressing	1	15	0	0	0	0	0	10	2	1	1	Free
Original Ranch Dressing	1 srvg	200	20	9	3	0	25	470	3	0	1	4 fat
✔Original Ranch Fat Free Dressing	1 srvg	35	0	0	0	0	0	410	8	0	1	1/2 carb
✔Parmesan Garlic Croutons	1 srvg	60	3	5	0	0	0	135	8	0	2	1 carb
✔Roasted BLT Salad - no dressing	1	200	6	3	2	0	65	880	8	4	29	1 veg, 3 lean meat, 1 fat
✔Roasted Caesar Salad - no dressing & croutons	1	220	8	3	4.5	0	70	830	6	3	30	1 veg, 4 lean meat, 2 fat

✔ = Healthiest Bets

(*Continued*)

	Amount	Cal.	Fat (g)	% Cal. Fat	Sat. Fat (g)	Trans Fat (g)	Chol. (mg)	Sod. (mg)	Carb. (g)	Fiber (g)	Pro. (g)	Choices/Exchanges
SANDWICHES AND WRAPS												
Crispy Twister	1	550	28	5	6	0	55	1500	49	3	26	3 1/2 starch, 2 lean meat, 4 fat
Double Crunch Sandwich	1	470	23	4	4.5	0	55	1190	38	2	27	2 1/2 starch, 3 lean meat, 3 fat
✔KFC Snacker	1	290	13	4	2.5	0	30	680	29	2	15	2 starch, 1 lean meat, 2 fat
KFC Snacker - Buffalo	1	260	8	3	1.5	0	25	860	31	1	15	2 starch, 1 lean meat, 1 fat
KFC Snacker - Fish	1	330	15	4	3	0	60	710	31	1	17	2 starch, 2 lean meat, 2 fat
KFC Snacker - Fish w/out sauce	1	290	12	4	2.5	0	60	610	29	1	17	2 starch, 2 lean meat, 1 1/2 fat

KFC Snacker - Honey BBQ	1	210	3	1	0.5	0	40	530	32	2	14	2 starch, 1 lean meat
KFC Snacker - Ultimate Cheese	1	280	11	4	2.5	0.5	25	780	30	1	15	2 starch, 1 lean meat, 1 1/2 fat
Oven Roasted Twister	1	420	17	4	4	0	60	1250	40	3	28	2 1/2 starch, 3 lean meat, 1 1/2 fat
Oven Roasted Twister - no sauce	1	330	7	2	2.5	0	50	2230	39	3	28	2 1/2 starch, 3 lean meat
Tender Roast Sandwich	1	380	13	3	3	0	80	1180	29	2	37	2 starch, 4 lean meat
Tender Roast Sandwich - no sauce	1	300	5	2	1.5	0	70	1060	28	2	37	2 starch, 4 lean meat
✔Toasted Wrap w/ Crispy Strip	1	350	19	5	5	0	40	880	29	1	16	2 starch, 1 lean meat, 3 fat
✔Toasted Wrap w/ Tender Roast Fillet	1	310	15	4	5	0	50	880	24	1	21	1 1/2 starch, 2 lean meat, 1 1/2 fat

✔ = Healthiest Bets

(*Continued*)

	Amount	Cal.	Fat (g)	% Cal. Fat	Sat. Fat (g)	Trans Fat (g)	Chol. (mg)	Sod. (mg)	Carb. (g)	Fiber (g)	Pro. (g)	Choices/Exchanges
SIDES (INDIVIDUAL)												
Baked Beans	1 srvg	220	1	0	0	0	0	730	45	7	8	3 starch
Biscuit	1 srvg	220	11	5	2.5	3.5	0	640	24	1	4	2 starch, 2 fat
Cole Slaw	1 srvg	180	10	5	1.5	0	5	270	22	3	1	1 starch, 1 1/2 fat
✔Corn on the Cob	3"	70	5	6	0.5	0	0	5	13	3	2	1 starch, 1/2 fat
Corn on the Cob	5.5"	150	3	2	1	0	0	10	26	7	5	2 starch, 1/2 fat
✔Green Beans	1 srvg	50	2	4	0	0	5	2	7	2	2	1 veg, 1/2 fat
Macaroni & Cheese	1 srvg	180	8	4	3.5	1	15	800	18	0	6	1 starch, 2 fat
✔Mashed Potatoes - no gravy	1 srvg	110	4	3	1	0	0	320	17	1	2	1 starch, 1 fat
✔Mashed Potatoes w/ Gravy	1 srvg	140	5	3	1	0.5	0	560	20	1	2	1 starch, 1 fat

Potato Salad	1 srvg	180	9	5	1.5	0	5	470	22	2	2	1 starch, 2 fat
Potato Wedges	1 srvg	260	13	5	2.5	0	0	740	33	3	4	2 starch, 2 fat
Seasoned Rice	1 srvg	150	4	2	0	0	0	630	32	2	4	2 starch, 1/2 fat
STRIPS												
Crispy Strips	3	350	19	5	3.5	0	70	1190	16	0	29	1 starch, 4 lean meat, 1 1/2 fat
Crispy Strips	2	240	13	5	2.5	0	50	800	11	0	20	1/2 starch, 3 lean meat, 1 fat
WINGS												
Boneless Fiery Buffalo	5	420	20	4	3.5	0	65	2260	33	3	28	2 starch, 3 lean meat, 2 fat
Boneless Honey BBQ	5	450	20	4	3.5	0	65	1880	41	4	28	2 1/2 starch, 3 lean meat, 2 1/2 fat
Boneless Sweet & Spicy	5	440	19	4	3.5	0	65	1700	38	3	27	2 1/2 starch, 3 lean meat, 2 fat

✔ = Healthiest Bets

(*Continued*)

WINGS *(Continued)*	Amount	Cal.	Fat (g)	% Cal. Fat	Sat. Fat (g)	Trans Fat (g)	Chol. (mg)	Sod. (mg)	Carb. (g)	Fiber (g)	Pro. (g)	Choices/Exchanges
Boneless Teriyaki	5	500	21	4	3.5	0	65	1730	50	3	28	3 1/2 starch, 3 lean meat, 2 1/2 fat
Fiery Buffalo	5	380	24	6	5	0	105	1480	19	2	21	1 1/2 starch, 2 lean meat, 3 1/2 fat
Honey BBQ	5	390	24	6	5	0	105	830	23	3	21	1 1/2 starch, 2 lean meat, 3 1/2 fat
Hot	5	350	24	6	5	0	105	740	14	2	20	1 starch, 2 lean meat, 3 1/2 fat
Sweet & Spicy	5	400	24	5	5	0	105	760	24	2	21	1 1/2 starch, 2 lean meat, 3 1/2 fat
Teriyaki	5	480	25	5	5	0	105	830	40	2	22	2 1/2 starch, 2 lean meat, 4 fat

✔ = Healthiest Bets

Popeyes Louisiana Kitchen
(www.popeyes.com)

Light 'n Lean Choice

Chicken Breast, mild
Cajun Rice
Green Beans

Calories	590	Cholesterol (mg)	244
Fat (g)	27	Sodium (mg)	2,060
% calories from fat	41	Carbohydrate (g)	44
Saturated fat (g)	9	Fiber (g)	4
Trans fat (g)	0.5	Protein (g)	43

Exchanges: 2 starch, 3 veg, 4 lean meat, 2 1/2 fat

Healthy 'n Hearty Choice

Chicken Breast, spicy
Corn on the Cob
Coleslaw

Calories	810	Cholesterol (mg)	185
Fat (g)	47	Sodium (mg)	1,020
% calories from fat	52	Carbohydrate (g)	59
Saturated fat (g)	12	Fiber (g)	14
Trans fat (g)	0.5	Protein (g)	37

Exchanges: 3 1/2 starch, 1 veg, 4 lean meat, 6 fat

(*Continued*)

Popeyes Louisiana Kitchen

	Amount	Cal.	Fat (g)	% Cal. Fat	Sat. Fat (g)	Trans Fat (g)	Chol. (mg)	Sod. (mg)	Carb. (g)	Fiber (g)	Pro. (g)	Choices/Exchanges
CAJUN WINGS												
Cajun Wing Segments	6 pcs	595	43	7	15	1.5	260	1274	19	0	34	1 1/2 starch, 4 lean meat, 6 fat
LOUISIANA LEGENDS												
Chicken & Sausage Jambalaya	1 srvg	660	33	5	9	3	96	2280	60	3	30	4 starch, 3 lean meat, 5 fat
Chicken Etouffee	1 srvg	480	30	6	9	0	60	2610	18	6	36	1 starch, 5 lean meat, 3 fat
Crawfish Etouffee	1 srvg	540	15	3	3	0	144	1920	75	6	12	5 starch, 3 fat
Smothered Chicken	1 srvg	630	24	3	6	0	69	2229	72	3	30	5 starch, 2 lean meat, 3 1/2 fat

MILD CHICKEN												
Breast	1	350	20	5	7	0.5	179	1130	8	0	33	1/2 starch, 4 lean meat, 1 1/2 fat
✔Leg	1	110	7	6	2.5	0	92	280	3	0	11	2 lean meat, 1/2 fat
Strips	2 pcs	250	10	4	4.5	0.5	55	1080	16	1	22	1 starch, 3 lean meat, 1/2 fat
Thigh	1	280	20	6	7	0.5	135	710	7	0	16	1/2 starch, 2 lean meat, 2 1/2 fat
Wing	1	150	10	6	3.5	0	59	690	5	0	9	1/2 starch, 1 lean meat, 1 1/2 fat
MILD CHICKEN (SKINLESS AND NO BREADING)												
✔Breast	1	120	2	2	1	0	120	540	0	0	24	2 lean meat
✔Leg	1	50	2	4	0.5	0	85	190	0	0	9	1 lean meat
✔Strips	2 pcs	130	3	2	1	0	50	620	3	0	25	3 lean meat

✔ = Healthiest Bets

(*Continued*)

MILD CHICKEN (SKINLESS & NO BREADING) *(Continued)*	Amount	Cal.	Fat (g)	% Cal. Fat	Sat. Fat (g)	Trans Fat (g)	Chol. (mg)	Sod. (mg)	Carb. (g)	Fiber (g)	Pro. (g)	Choices/Exchanges
✔Thigh	1	80	4	5	1	0	98	230	0	0	11	2 lean meat
✔Wing	1	40	2	5	0.5	0	58	400	0	0	7	1 lean meat
SANDWICHES												
Deluxe - no mayo	1	480	15	3	6	0.5	55	1290	54	3	33	3 1/2 starch, 3 lean meat, 1 fat
Deluxe w/ Mayo	1	630	31	4	8	1	71	1480	53	3	35	3 1/2 starch, 3 lean meat, 4 fat
SEAFOOD												
Popcorn Shrimp	1 srvg	280	16	5	6	1	95	1110	22	0	12	1 1/2 starch, 1 lean meat, 2 1/2 fat
SIDES												
Biscuits	1	240	13	5	7	0	0	490	36	1	4	2 starch, 2 fat
✔Cajun Rice	1 srvg	170	6	3	2	0	60	530	22	2	8	1 starch, 1 fat

Chicken Etouffee	1 srvg	160	10	6	3	0	20	870	6	2	12	1/2 starch, 2 lean meat, 1 fat
Cinnamon Apple Turnover	1	250	12	4	4	1.5	5	320	34	2	3	2 high-fat meat, 2 fat
Coleslaw	1 srvg	260	23	8	3.5	0	15	260	14	9	0	1/2 starch, 1 veg, 4 fat
✔Corn on the Cob	1 ear	190	2	1	0.5	0	0	0	37	4	6	2 starch
✔Crawfish Etouffee	1 srvg	180	5	3	1	0	48	640	25	2	7	1 1/2 starch, 1 fat
French Fries	1 srvg	310	17	5	7	1	7	660	35	3	4	2 starch, 2 fat
✔Green Beans	1 srvg	70	1	1	0	0	5	400	14	2	2	3 veg
Jambalaya	1 srvg	220	11	5	3	1	32	760	20	1	10	1 starch, 2 fat
✔Mashed Potatoes - no Gravy	1 srvg	100	3	3	1	0.5	0	380	17	0	1	1 starch, 1/2 fat
✔Mashed Potatoes w/ Gravy	1 srvg	130	4	3	2	0.5	5	580	18	2	3	1 starch, 1 fat
Red Beans & Rice	1 srvg	320	19	5	6	0	20	710	31	17	10	2 starch, 4 fat

✔ = Healthiest Bets

(*Continued*)

SIDES *(Continued)*	Amount	Cal.	Fat (g)	% Cal. Fat	Sat. Fat (g)	Trans Fat (g)	Chol. (mg)	Sod. (mg)	Carb. (g)	Fiber (g)	Pro. (g)	Choices/Exchanges
✔Smothered Chicken	1 srvg	210	8	3	2	0	23	743	24	1	10	1 1/2 starch, 1 lean meat, 1 fat
SPICY CHICKEN												
Breast	1	360	22	6	8	0.5	170	760	8	1	31	1/2 starch, 4 lean meat, 2 fat
✔Leg	1	100	5	5	2	0	71	230	3	0	9	2 lean meat
Strips	2 pcs	270	11	4	4.5	0.5	55	1430	21	0	22	1 1/2 starch, 3 lean meat, 1/2 fat
Thigh	1	300	24	7	8	0.5	131	490	7	0	15	1/2 starch, 2 lean meat, 3 1/2 fat
Wing	1	140	9	6	3.5	0	79	290	5	0	8	1/2 starch, 1 lean meat, 1 fat

SPICY CHICKEN (SKINLESS AND NO BREADING)

✔Breast	1	120	2	2	1	0	112	380	0	0	25	3 lean meat
✔Leg	1	50	2	4	0.5	0	60	135	0	0	9	1 lean meat
✔Strips	2 pcs	150	4	2	1.5	0	55	820	5	0	23	1/2 starch, 2 lean meat
✔Thigh	1	80	3	3	1	0	98	170	2	0	12	2 lean meat
✔Wing	1	40	2	5	0.5	0	66	125	0	0	6	1 lean meat

✔ = Healthiest Bets

Exclusive Web Content

Be sure to visit the following restaurants online at http://www.diabetes.org/healthyrestaurant

Carvel
Del Taco
El Pollo Loco
Frëshens
Godfather's
Jersey Mike's
Jimmy John's
Tim Hortons
Whataburger
Wienerschnitzel
Zaxby's

Seafood Catches

RESTAURANTS

Captain D's
Long John Silver's

NUTRITION PROS

- Fish and seafood are naturally low in total fat, saturated fat, and calories.
- During the years of nutrition and health consciousness, some fast-food restaurants began to bake, broil, or grill their seafood. But much of the healthier fish have headed out to sea and disappeared from the menu.
- Some healthy sides are available: baked potatoes, rice, salad, and cooked vegetables.

NUTRITION CONS

- The nutritional virtues of fish and seafood are lost in most chain seafood restaurants because their favorite preparation method is frying.
- After fish and seafood have been battered and fried, you wonder what happened to the fish. When you read the nutrition numbers, there's not much fish to speak of.
- Fried fish is often surrounded by high-fat plate fillers—hush puppies, French fries, or coleslaw drenched in a mayonnaise-based dressing. Thus, the once-healthy seafood is now part of a fat- and calorie-dense meal.

- Seafood restaurants load their starches—hush puppies, biscuits, cornbread, French fries, etc.—with fat.
- Fruit is nowhere to be found.

Healthy Tips

- ★ If you order a baked potato, have butter and sour cream held or served on the side.
- ★ Lemon is plentiful. Use it to add flavor without adding calories.
- ★ Use low-fat, low-calorie cocktail sauce to add flavor without extra calories. Substitute this for higher-calorie tartar sauce.
- ★ Not all coleslaw is created equal. Some is high in fat, and some is relatively low in fat. Check the nutrition numbers to know the score in the restaurant you choose.

Get It Your Way

- ★ Hold the tartar sauce and opt for lemon or vinegar.
- ★ Substitute a baked potato or rice for French fries or hush puppies, if available.
- ★ Substitute a cooked vegetable, such as green beans or corn, for French fries.
- ★ Substitute breadsticks or a yeast roll for biscuits or corn bread, if you have the option.

Captain D's
(www.captainds.com)

Light 'n Lean Choice

Grilled Seasoned Shrimp Salad with Fat-Free Raspberry Vinaigrette *(1.5 oz, 3 Tbsp)*

Calories	455	Cholesterol (mg)	69
Fat (g)	5	Sodium (mg)	835
% calories from fat	10	Carbohydrate (g)	74
Saturated fat (g)	2	Fiber (g)	2
Trans fat (g)	1	Protein (g)	15

Exchanges: 2 1/2 starch, 1 carb, 2 veg, 1 lean meat, 2 fat

Healthy 'n Hearty Choice

Shrimp Marinara Pasta Bowl *(1/2 serving)*
Side Salad with
Fat-Free Italian Dressing *(1 oz, 2 Tbsp)*
Breadstick *(1/2 of 1)*

Calories	560	Cholesterol (mg)	43
Fat (g)	13	Sodium (mg)	1,370
% calories from fat	21	Carbohydrate (g)	83
Saturated fat (g)	3.5	Fiber (g)	7
Trans fat (g)	1.5	Protein (g)	19

Exchanges: 5 starch, 1 veg, 1 lean meat, 2 fat

(Continued)

Captain D's

	Amount	Cal.	Fat (g)	% Cal. Fat	Sat. Fat (g)	Trans Fat (g)	Chol. (mg)	Sod. (mg)	Carb. (g)	Fiber (g)	Pro. (g)	Choices/Exchanges
ADD-A-PIECE												
Batter-Dipped Fish	1 srvg	160	10	6	4	1	25	475	10	0	8	1/2 starch, 1 lean meat, 1 1/2 fat
Chicken Tender	1 srvg	170	10	5	4	0	25	430	11	0	9	1/2 starch, 1 lean meat, 1 1/2 fat
✔Premium Shrimp	3 pc	154	6	4	3	0	45	323	0	0	8	1 lean meat, 1 fat
✔Stuffed Crab Shell	1 srvg	100	5	5	2	0	20	220	9	0	5	1/2 starch, 1/2 fat
BEVERAGES												
Iced Tea, Sweetened	23 oz.	90	0	0	0	0	0	15	23	0	0	1 1/2 carb
✔Iced Tea, Unsweetened	23 oz.	0	0	0	0	0	0	15	0	0	0	Free
Lemonade	23 oz.	180	0	0	0	0	0	80	49	0	0	3 1/2 carb

CLASSICS

Bite Size Shrimp Dinner	1 srvg	1140	61	5	24	5	150	1930	120	9	22	8 starch, 11 fat
Catfish	1 srvg	1050	63	5	24	5	120	2090	87	7	28	6 starch, 2 lean meat, 11 1/2 fat
Chicken Dinner	3 pc	1190	70	5	29	5	115	2380	102	7	33	7 starch, 2 lean meat, 12 fat
Classic Fish and Chicken Dinner	1 srvg	1250	77	6	30	5	122	2750	105	7	32	7 starch, 2 lean meat, 14 fat
Classic Fish and Shrimp Dinner	1 srvg	1285	75	5	30	5	157	2750	94	7	33	6 1/2 starch, 3 lean meat, 14 fat
Coastal Fried Flounder	1 srvg	1530	93	5	37	7	225	2980	115	8	63	7 1/2 starch, 6 lean meat, 14 fat
Country Style Fish Dinner	1 srvg	1180	68	5	28	5	130	2020	99	7	39	6 1/2 starch, 3 lean meat, 11 fat
Deluxe Seafood Platter	1 srvg	1485	85	5	34	5	197	3190	112	7	43	7 1/2 starch, 3 lean meat, 16 fat

✔ = Healthiest Bets

(*Continued*)

CLASSICS *(Continued)*	Amount	Cal.	Fat (g)	% Cal. Fat	Sat. Fat (g)	Trans Fat (g)	Chol. (mg)	Sod. (mg)	Carb. (g)	Fiber (g)	Pro. (g)	Choices/Exchanges
Fish and Fries	1 srvg	910	55	5	24	5	87	2010	81	5	22	5 1/2 starch, 1 lean meat, 10 1/2 fat
Fish Dinner	2 pc	1080	67	6	26	5	97	2320	94	7	23	6 1/2 starch, 2 lean meat, 12 fat
Fish Dinner	3 pc	1240	77	6	30	6	122	2810	104	7	30	7 starch, 1 lean meat, 14 fat
Fried Clam Platter	1 srvg	1450	87	5	23	5	75	2540	133	13	28	9 starch, 17 fat
Gulf Coast Oysters	1 srvg	1000	58	5	23	5	105	1800	100	8	16	6 1/2 starch, 11 fat
Jumbo Fish Platter	1 srvg	1500	92	6	37	6	156	3455	123	6	39	8 starch, 2 lean meat, 17 fat
Premium Shrimp Dinner	1 srvg	1090	57	5	22	4	160	1950	69	8	25	4 1/2 starch, 3 lean meat, 11 fat
Ultimate Premium Shrimp Platter	1 srvg	1290	65	5	26	5	220	2390	69	8	35	4 1/2 starch, 4 lean meat, 14 fat

Ultimate Variety Platter	1 srvg	1655	95	5	38	5	222	3620	123	7	52	8 starch, 4 lean meat, 17 fat
DESSERTS												
Cheesecake w/ Strawberries	1 pc	430	26	5	9	5	70	220	45	1	6	3 carb, 5 fat
Chocolate Cake	1 pc	300	11	3	2	1	25	270	49	2	3	3 1/2 carb, 2 fat
Pecan Pie	1 pc	470	26	5	4	4	70	270	56	2	5	3 1/2 carb, 4 fat
Pineapple Cream Cheese Pie	1 pc	320	14	4	6	2	20	300	43	0	6	3 carb, 3 fat
DRESSINGS												
Blue Cheese	1.5 oz.	230	24	9	4	0	25	440	2	0	2	5 fat
Caesar Cardini	12 oz.	365	15	4	6	1	29	605	41	2	14	3 carb, 3 fat
✔Fat-Free Italian	1 oz.	10	0	0	0	0	0	440	2	0	0	Free
✔Fat-Free Raspberry Vinaigrette	1.5 oz.	50	0	0	0	0	0	320	13	0	0	1 carb
Honey Mustard	1.5 oz.	160	16	9	2	0	15	125	5	0	0	1/2 carb, 3 fat

✔ = Healthiest Bets

(*Continued*)

DRESSINGS (Continued)	Amount	Cal.	Fat (g)	% Cal. Fat	Sat. Fat (g)	Trans Fat (g)	Chol. (mg)	Sod. (mg)	Carb. (g)	Fiber (g)	Pro. (g)	Choices/Exchanges
Ranch	1 oz.	120	12	9	2	0	10	210	1	0	0	2 1/2 fat
Thousand Island	1 oz.	120	11	8	2	0	10	320	5	0	0	1/2 carb, 2 fat
FAMILY MEALS												
Captain's Value Pack	1 srvg	1360	87	6	35	6	130	3270	114	7	30	7 1/2 starch, 1 lean meat, 15 fat
Fish or Chicken Only	10 pc	730	51	6	23	4	94	2330	47	0	23	3 starch, 2 lean meat, 9 fat
Seafood Feast	1 srvg	1350	85	6	35	6	145	3220	115	6	30	7 1/2 starch, 1 lean meat, 16 fat
KIDS MEALS												
Chicken	1 srvg	684	31	4	14	2	48	1053	86	4	13	5 1/2 starch, 5 fat
Fish	1 srvg	674	31	4	14	3	48	1098	85	4	12	5 1/2 starch, 5 fat
Shrimp	1 srvg	744	31	4	14	3	78	1043	101	5	12	6 1/2 starch, 5 fat

KITCHEN SELECTIONS												
Chicken Dinner	1 srvg	680	22	3	9	4	89	2450	84	5	30	5 1/2 starch, 2 lean meat, 3 1/2 fat
Coastal Flounder	1 srvg	720	23	3	10	2	104	1830	82	5	40	5 1/2 starch, 3 lean meat, 2 1/2 fat
Seafood Lovers Mixed Grill	1 srvg	1010	33	3	11	2	439	2100	89	5	82	6 starch, 9 lean meat, 1 fat
Seafood Scampi Platter	1 srvg	760	22	3	10	2	159	1920	82	5	43	5 1/2 starch, 4 lean meat, 2 fat
Seasoned Tilapia	1 srvg	700	22	3	10	2	94	1680	82	5	36	5 1/2 starch, 3 lean meat, 2 fat
Shrimp Skewers	1 srvg	720	17	2	6	1	319	1780	84	5	52	5 1/2 starch, 5 lean meat, 1/2 fat
Wild Alaskan Salmon	1 srvg	800	29	3	11	2	134	1800	87	5	41	6 starch, 3 lean meat, 4 fat

✔ = Healthiest Bets

(*Continued*)

	Amount	Cal.	Fat (g)	% Cal. Fat	Sat. Fat (g)	Trans Fat (g)	Chol. (mg)	Sod. (mg)	Carb. (g)	Fiber (g)	Pro. (g)	Choices/Exchanges
PASTA												
Chicken and Broccoli Alfredo Pasta Bowl	1 srvg	980	45	4	23	4	167	1991	84	3	41	5 1/2 starch, 3 lean meat, 7 fat
Shrimp Alfredo Pasta Bowl	1 srvg	870	36	4	20	1	157	1261	82	3	29	5 1/2 starch, 2 lean meat, 7 fat
Shrimp Marinara Pasta Bowl	1 srvg	670	15	2	4	1	79	1380	93	4	27	6 starch, 1 lean meat, 2 1/2 fat
Shrimp Scampi Pasta Bowl	1 srvg	810	32	4	17	3	132	1290	93	3	25	6 starch, 1 lean meat, 6 fat
SALAD												
Bite Size Shrimp	1 salad	655	26	4	11	3	114	1015	81	4	21	4 starch, 3 veg, 1 lean meat, 4 1/2 fat
Chicken Caesar	1 salad	620	41	6	10	4	129	1565	33	2	27	1 starch, 3 veg, 3 lean meat, 6 fat

✔Fried Chicken	1 salad	365	15	4	6	1	29	605	41	2	14	2 starch, 3 veg, 1 lean meat, 2 fat
✔Grilled Alaskan Salmon	1 salad	485	21	4	7	2	124	495	35	2	35	1/2 starch, 2 veg, 5 lean meat, 3 fat
✔Grilled Seasoned Shrimp	1 salad	255	5	2	2	1	69	415	30	2	12	1/2 starch, 2 veg, 1 lean meat, 2 fat
✔Side	1 salad	60	0	0	0	0	0	90	14	4	2	3 veg
SANDWICHES												
Chicken Ranch	1 sand.	770	44	5	16	1	80	2000	24	2	30	1 1/2 starch, 4 lean meat, 9 fat
Chicken Snack Smacker	1 sand.	570	30	5	11	1	90	1820	49	0	25	3 1/2 starch, 2 lean meat, 4 fat
Deluxe Classic Fish	1 sand.	690	39	5	11	2	65	1680	21	2	25	1 1/2 starch, 3 lean meat, 8 fat

✔ = Healthiest Bets

(*Continued*)

SANDWICHES ***(Continued)***	**Amount**	**Cal.**	**Fat (g)**	**% Cal. Fat**	**Sat. Fat (g)**	**Trans Fat (g)**	**Chol. (mg)**	**Sod. (mg)**	**Carb. (g)**	**Fiber (g)**	**Pro. (g)**	**Choices/Exchanges**
✔Fish Snack Smacker	1 sand.	440	26	5	8	1	40	835	41	0	12	2 1/2 starch, 1 lean meat, 5 fat
Grilled Alaskan Salmon	1 sand.	660	35	5	8	1	135	1050	6	2	38	1/2 starch, 5 lean meat, 6 fat
Grilled Tilapia	1 sand.	560	28	5	7	1	95	930	1	2	33	5 lean meat, 6 fat
SAUCES												
Ginger Teriyaki	2 oz.	60	0	0	0	0	0	1300	13	0	2	1 carb
Scampi Butter	2 oz.	120	10	8	6	1	25	360	5	0	2	1/2 carb, 2 fat
Sweet Chili	2 oz.	100	0	0	0	0	0	960	25	0	0	1 1/2 carb
SIDES												
✔Apples and Caramel	1 srvg	140	4	3	2	0	5	140	24	2	0	1 carb, 1 fruit, 1 fat

✔Baked Potato	1 potato	240	0	0	0	0	0	25	54	6	6	4 starch
Breadsticks	1 srvg	300	11	3	3	2	5	300	42	2	6	3 starch, 2 fat
✔Broccoli	1 srvg	40	1	2	0	0	0	30	5	2	2	1 veg
✔Corn-on-the-Cob	1 srvg	190	2	1	0	0	0	10	37	4	5	2 starch, 1/2 fat
Fried Okra	1 srvg	230	14	5	6	1	15	410	23	2	3	1 starch, 1 veg, 3 fat
Fries	1 srvg	310	15	4	7	2	15	450	38	4	3	3 starch, 3 fat
✔Garlic Mashed Potatoes	1 srvg	100	3	3	1	0	0	490	16	2	2	1 starch, 1/2 fat
Home-style Cole Slaw	1 srvg	170	12	6	2	0	10	310	13	2	1	1/2 carb, 1 veg, 2 fat
Hushpuppies	1 srvg	400	26	6	11	2	30	650	36	3	5	2 starch, 5 fat
✔Lemon Herb Rice	1 srvg	150	0	0	0	0	0	100	31	0	3	2 starch
Macaroni and Cheese	1 srvg	160	7	4	2	0	10	570	17	0	6	1 starch, 1 1/2 fat
Roasted Red Potatoes	1 srvg	170	7	4	4	0	10	1200	25	3	3	2 starch, 1 1/2 fat
✔Side Salad	1 salad	65	0	0	0	0	0	90	15	4	2	3 veg

✔ = Healthiest Bets

(*Continued*)

SIDES *(Continued)*	Amount	Cal.	Fat (g)	% Cal. Fat	Sat. Fat (g)	Trans Fat (g)	Chol. (mg)	Sod. (mg)	Carb. (g)	Fiber (g)	Pro. (g)	Choices/Exchanges
✔Southern-style Green Beans	1 srvg	60	2	3	0	0	5	400	10	3	1	2 veg, 1/2 fat
✔Vegetable Medley	1 srvg	35	0	0	0	0	0	30	7	3	1	1 veg
Vegetable Medley with Italian Seasoning	1 order	140	11	7	2	2	0	750	9	3	2	2 veg, 2 fat
STARTERS												
Cheesesticks	4 pc	220	12	5	6	0	20	535	16	0	10	1 starch, 1 medium-fat meat, 1 1/2 fat
Cheesesticks and Jalapeno Poppers	1 srvg	440	24	5	13	1	40	1070	32	0	21	2 starch, 2 medium-fat meat, 2 1/2 fat
Jalapeno Poppers	9 pcs	350	19	5	11	1	40	840	36	4	5	2 starch, 1 veg, 4 fat

✔ = Healthiest Bets

Long John Silver's
(www.ljsilvers.com)

Light 'n Lean Choice

Baked Cod *(1 piece)*
Corn Cobbette
Rice
Cole Slaw *(1/2 serving)*

Calories	490	Cholesterol (mg)	100
Fat (g)	20	Sodium (mg)	950
% calories from fat	37	Carbohydrate (g)	57
Saturated fat (g)	5	Fiber (g)	8
Trans fat (g)	0	Protein (g)	29

Exchanges: 2 1/2 starch, 1 veg, 3 lean meat, 2 fat

Healthy 'n Hearty Choice

Clam Chowder
Baked Cod *(1 piece)*
Corn Cobbette
Hush Puppies *(3)*

Calories	560	Cholesterol (mg)	105
Fat (g)	25	Sodium (mg)	2,060
% calories from fat	40	Carbohydrate (g)	61
Saturated fat (g)	7	Fiber (g)	6
Trans fat (g)	4	Protein (g)	32

Exchanges: 2 starch, 1 veg, 1 milk, 3 lean meat, 3 fat

(Continued)

Long John Silver's

	Amount	Cal.	Fat (g)	% Cal. Fat	Sat. Fat (g)	Trans Fat (g)	Chol. (mg)	Sod. (mg)	Carb. (g)	Fiber (g)	Pro. (g)	Choices/Exchanges
CHICKEN												
✔Chicken Plank	1 pc	140	8	5	2	2.5	20	480	9	0	8	1/2 starch, 1 lean meat, 1 fat
DESSERTS												
Chocolate Cream Pie	1 pc	310	22	6	14	1.5	15	170	24	1	5	1 1/2 carb, 4 1/2 fat
Pecan Pie	1 pc	370	15	4	2.5	2	4	190	55	2	4	3 1/2 carb, 2 1/2 fat
Pineapple Cream Pie	1 pc	290	13	4	7	1.5	15	210	39	1	4	2 1/2 carb, 2 fat
DIPPING SAUCES												
✔Cocktail Sauce	1 oz	25	0	0	0	0	0	250	6	0	0	Free
Tartar Sauce	1 oz	100	9	8	1.5	0	15	250	4	0	0	1/2 carb, 2 fat

FISH AND SEAFOOD												
Alaskan Flounder	1 pc	250	11	4	2.5	3	35	910	36	2	12	2 starch, 1 lean meat, 1 1/2 fat
✔Baked Cod	1 pc	120	5	4	1	0	90	240	1	0	22	3 lean meat
Battered Fish	1 pc	260	16	6	4	4.5	35	790	17	0	12	1 starch, 1 lean meat, 2 1/2 fat
Battered Shrimp	1 pc	45	3	6	1	1	15	160	3	0	2	1 fat
Breaded Clams	1 snack box	320	19	5	4.5	7	353	1190	29	2	9	2 starch, 4 fat
Buttered Lobster Bites	1 snack box	250	9	3	3	3.5	65	560	27	2	14	2 starch, 1 lean meat, 1 fat
Popcorn Shrimp	1 snack box	270	16	5	4	4.5	75	570	23	1	9	1 1/2 starch, 1 lean meat, 3 fat
SALADS & DRESSINGS												
Crispy Chicken Club Salad	1	510	30	5	9	6.5	65	1550	35	5	28	1 starch, 3 veg, 4 lean meat, 4 fat

✔ = Healthiest Bets

(*Continued*)

SALADS & DRESSINGS *(Continued)*	Amount	Cal.	Fat (g)	% Cal. Fat	Sat. Fat (g)	Trans Fat (g)	Chol. (mg)	Sod. (mg)	Carb. (g)	Fiber (g)	Pro. (g)	Choices/Exchanges
Garden Ranch Dressing	1 pouch	230	24	9	4	0	10	400	2	0	1	5 fat
✔Lite Italian Dressing	1 pouch	20	1	5	0	0	0	780	3	0	0	Free
✔Shrimp & Seafood Salad	1	260	12	4	4.5	2	85	820	22	4	18	1/2 starch, 3 veg, 2 lean meat, 1 fat
Thousand Island Dressing	1 pouch	220	21	9	3.5	0	25	350	7	0	0	1/2 carb, 4 fat
SANDWICHES												
✔Chicken Sandwich	1	360	15	4	3.5	2.5	25	90	40	3	14	2 1/2 starch, 1 lean meat, 2 1/2 fat
Fish Sandwich	1	470	23	4	5	4.5	45	1210	48	3	18	3 starch, 1 lean meat, 3 1/2 fat
Ultimate Fish Sandwich	1	530	28	5	8	5	60	1400	49	3	21	3 1/2 starch, 2 lean meat, 4 fat

SIDES AND STARTERS

✔Cheesesticks	3	140	8	5	2	1.5	10	320	12	1	4	1 starch, 1 1/2 fat
Clam Chowder	1 bowl	170	8	4	3.5	0.5	15	1220	19	0	4	1 milk, 1 fat
Cole Slaw	1 srvg	200	15	7	2.5	0	20	340	15	3	1	1 veg, 1/2 carb, 3 fat
✔Corn Cobbette	1	90	3	3	0.5	0	0	0	14	3	3	1/2 starch, 1 veg, 1 fat
Crumblies	1 srvg	170	12	6	2.5	4	0	420	14	1	1	1 starch, 2 1/2 fat
Hushpuppies	1	60	3	5	0.5	1	0	200	9	1	1	1 starch, 1/2 fat
Large Fries	1 srvg	390	17	4	4	5	0	580	56	5	4	4 starch, 3 fat
✔Lobster Stuffed Crab Cake	1	170	9	5	2	0	30	390	16	1	6	1 starch, 1 1/2 fat
✔Regular Fries	1 srvg	230	10	4	2.5	3	0	350	34	3	3	2 starch, 1 1/2 fat
✔Rice	1 srvg	180	4	2	2	0	0	540	34	3	3	2 starch, 1 fat

✔ = Healthiest Bets

Family Fare

RESTAURANTS

Bob Evans Restaurants

Boston Market

Denny's

Romano's Macaroni Grill

EXCLUSIVE WEB CONTENT

Zaxby's (http://www.diabetes.org/healthyrestaurant)

Note: You might not find several large chains you expect to see in this chapter. That's because they don't provide nutrition information for their menu aside from the information for several healthier items.

NUTRITION PROS

- Some restaurants serving family fare have added healthier options to their menus.
- You can pick and choose among the appetizers, salads, soups, and side dishes to put together healthy, portion-controlled meals.
- Healthier preparation methods are available—stir-frying, grilling, and blackening.
- Time and the desire to please are on your side. This makes special requests easier for you and for the kitchen.
- Portions are large, but take-home containers are at the ready.
- Some of these restaurants serve their breakfast-to-dinner menu 24 hours a day. This puts variety on your side.

- These restaurants hardly limit their menu to American specialties. They globe trot to bring you Mexican fajitas or salads, Italian pastas or pizzas, and Chinese potstickers or stir-fry dishes. This helps widen the variety of healthier choices.
- Raw and cooked vegetables can be found, but just be careful they aren't drenched in fat or fried.
- Condiments to help you add taste without adding fat might be found in the kitchen—teriyaki or soy sauce, lemons, limes, a variety of vinegars, ketchup, barbecue sauce, and low-calorie salad dressings. Ask, and maybe you'll receive.

NUTRITION CONS

- Bread, rolls, crackers, or breadsticks and butter might greet you at the table.
- These restaurants love to fry—from fried mozzarella sticks to fried shrimp, chicken fingers, French fries, and onion rings.
- Sandwiches and other entrees may be accompanied by French fries, onion rings, potato chips, or creamy coleslaw.
- Some foods get a healthy start—vegetables, potatoes, or pasta. But then they are drenched in salad dressing or cheese sauce or dropped a foot deep in oil and fried.
- Salads can start off healthy but end up with high-fat toppers—avocado, cheese, bacon, or croutons.
- Portions are frequently too big…many are way too big.
- Plain fruit is often not available. The apples buried between a double crust are not the healthiest way to eat your fruits.

- Cheese is in, on, and around a startling number of menu items—melted cheese on a sandwich or cheese sauce on vegetables or pasta. This makes the calories, saturated fat, and cholesterol counts rise.

Healthy Tiops

★ Combine a soup, salad, and side dish or combine one or two appetizers and a salad for a healthy, portion-controlled meal.

★ Share two complementary entrees—pasta topped with a tomato-based sauce or vegetables and a Mexican salad, for example.

★ Split everything with your dining partner, from appetizer to dessert.

★ Request a take-home container when you order your meal. Pack up the portion to take home when your food arrives.

Get It Your Way

★ Ask for your salad dressing on the side—all of the time.

★ Ask that high-fat salad toppers be used lightly or left in the kitchen.

★ Request to substitute high-fat, high-calorie sides with lower-fat, lower-calorie items. Substitute a baked potato for French fries or onion rings, request a sandwich on

(*Continued*)

whole-wheat bread rather than on a croissant, or opt for mustard rather than mayonnaise. Each and every change improves the healthiness of your meals.

- ★ Ask the kitchen to hold the butter or cheese sauce on vegetables.
- ★ Skip the fried tortilla shell in which big salads may be served.
- ★ Request some lemon or lime slices, vinegar, or soy or teriyaki sauce on the side to flavor menu items with fewer calories.

Exclusive Web Content

Be sure to visit the following restaurants online at http://www.diabetes.org/healthyrestaurant

Carvel
Del Taco
El Pollo Loco
Frëshens
Godfather's
Jersey Mike's
Jimmy John's
Tim Hortons
Whataburger
Wienerschnitzel
Zaxby's

Bob Evans Restaurants

(www.bobevans.com)

Light 'n Lean Choice

Fruit Cup *(1/2 serving)*
Egg Beaters Omelet
Lite Sausage Link *(2)*
Grits *(1 serving)*

Calories	602	Cholesterol (mg)	23
Fat (g)	26	Sodium (mg)	724
% calories from fat	39	Carbohydrate (g)	68
Saturated fat (g)	6	Fiber (g)	6
Trans fat (g)	1	Protein (g)	27

Exchanges: 3 1/2 starch, 1 fruit, 3 medium-fat meat, 2 fat

Healthy 'n Hearty Choice

Salmon with Wildfire Barbecue Sauce
Buttered Corn
Glazed Carrots
Applesauce

Calories	715	Cholesterol (mg)	115
Fat (g)	24	Sodium (mg)	543
% calories from fat	30	Carbohydrate (g)	82
Saturated fat (g)	7	Fiber (g)	11
Trans fat (g)	1	Protein (g)	45

Exchanges: 3 starch, 2 veg, 1 1/2 fruit, 5 lean meat, 1 1/2 fat

(*Continued*)

Bob Evans Restaurants

	Amount	Cal.	Fat (g)	% Cal. Fat	Sat. Fat (g)	Trans Fat (g)	Chol. (mg)	Sod. (mg)	Carb. (g)	Fiber (g)	Pro. (g)	Choices/Exchanges
BREAKFAST												
Eggs Benedict	1	826	52	6	19	5	564	3137	44	0	44	3 starch, 5 medium-fat meat, 5 fat
Fruit and Yogurt Plate	1	403	2	0	1	0	5	109	93	9	9	3 carb, 2 fruit, 1 milk
Spinach, Bacon, and Tomato Country Benedict	1	729	48	6	16	5	494	1885	42	1	30	3 starch, 3 medium-fat meat, 6 1/2 fat
✔Strawberry Banana Mini Fruit & Yogurt Parfait	1 srvg	157	1	1	0	0	3	58	34	3	5	2 starch
✔Strawberry Blueberry Mini Fruit Parfait	1 srvg	166	1	1	0	0	3	65	35	3	5	1 fruit, 1 milk
Sunshine Skillet	1	728	52	6	16	3	522	1387	35	4	29	2 1/2 starch, 3 medium-fat meat, 7 1/2 fat

BREAKFAST SANDWICHES

Border Scramble Burrito	1	1103	64	5	21	1	561	1999	80	12	51	5 1/2 starch, 5 medium-fat meat, 7 fat
Country Breakfast Biscuit	1	659	45	6	16	6	269	1703	40	1	24	2 1/2 starch, 3 high-fat meat, 2 1/2 fat
Sausage Country Benedict	1	936	66	6	24	5	536	2098	40	0	44	2 1/2 starch, 6 high-fat meat, 3 fat

BREAKFAST SIDES

Bacon	1 slice	36	4	10	2	0	5	54	0	0	1	1 fat
✔Eggs	1	101	8	7	2	0	229	68	1	0	7	1 medium-fat meat
✔French Toast	1 slice	131	2	1	0	0	25	175	13	1	3	1 starch, 1 fat
Grits	1 srvg	178	7	4	2	1	9	172	28	2	3	2 starch, 1 fat
✔Hard cooked Egg	1	60	4	6	2	0	190	55	1	0	6	1 medium-fat meat
✔Mush	1 srvg	79	3	3	1	0	0	466	11	2	1	1 starch, 1/2 fat

✔ = Healthiest Bets

(*Continued*)

BREAKFAST SIDES *(Continued)*	**Amount**	**Cal.**	**Fat (g)**	**% Cal. Fat**	**Sat. Fat (g)**	**Trans Fat (g)**	**Chol. (mg)**	**Sod. (mg)**	**Carb. (g)**	**Fiber (g)**	**Pro. (g)**	**Choices/Exchanges**
✔Oatmeal	cup	64	1	1	0	0	0	146	12	2	2	1 starch
✔Oatmeal	bowl	172	3	2	0	0	0	394	32	4	6	2 starch, 1/2 fat
Pot Roast Hash	1 srvg	652	39	5	14	1	533	1081	34	34	38	2 1/2 starch, 4 medium-fat meat, 3 1/2 fat
Sausage Gravy	cup	134	9	6	5	0	8	619	10	0	4	1 starch, 2 fat
Sausage Gravy	bowl	268	17	6	11	0	17	1238	21	0	7	1 starch, 3 1/2 fat
Sausage Link	1	125	11	8	3	0	14	184	0	0	5	1 high-fat meat, 1 fat
Sausage Patty	1	141	11	7	4	0	24	315	0	0	8	1 high-fat meat, 1/2 fat
Scrambled Eggs	3	255	17	6	5	0	723	213	2	0	20	3 medium-fat meat, 1/2 fat
Scrambled Eggs	2	170	11	6	3	0	482	142	1	0	14	2 medium-fat meat, 1/2 fat
✔Scrambled Eggs w/ Egg Lites	1 srvg	120	7	5	1	0	0	238	1	0	11	2 medium-fat meat

Smoked Ham	1 slice	87	2	2	1	0	52	1131	2	0	14	2 lean meat
Turkey Sausage	1 order	346	12	3	2	0	31	815	34	3	24	2 1/2 starch, 2 lean meat, 1 fat
CONDIMENTS												
✔Apple Butter	.5 oz	33	0	0	0	0	0	2	8	0	0	1/2 carb
Butter Cups	1	37	4	10	3	0	11	30	0	0	0	1 fat
✔Diet Blackberry Jam	5	0	0	0	0	0	0	5	0	0	1	Free
Half and Half Cups	.5 oz	40	3	7	0	0	15	15	1	0	1	1 fat
✔Margarine Cup	1	102	3	3	1	4	0	34	0	0	0	2 fat
Pancake Syrup	3 oz	213	0	0	0	0	0	101	55	0	0	3 carb
✔Strawberry Jam	.5 oz	36	0	0	0	0	0	1	9	0	0	1/2 carb
✔Sugar Free Strawberry Jam	3 oz	39	0	0	0	0	0	79	10	0	0	Free

✔ = Healthiest Bets

(*Continued*)

	Amount	Cal.	Fat (g)	% Cal. Fat	Sat. Fat (g)	Trans Fat (g)	Chol. (mg)	Sod. (mg)	Carb. (g)	Fiber (g)	Pro. (g)	Choices/Exchanges
DESSERTS												
Chocolate Fudge Sundae	1	624	29	4	20	0	75	213	85	1	9	5 1/2 carb, 5 fat
Coconut Cream Pie	1 slice	534	27	5	19	0	16	422	65	2	8	4 1/2 carb, 5 fat
Hershey's Hot Fudge Cake	1 pc	845	40	4	25	1	35	633	115	5	7	7 1/2 carb, 6 fat
Hershey's Hot Fudge Cake a la mode	1 pc	968	46	4	29	1	60	676	130	5	9	8 1/2 carb, 7 fat
Lemon Meringue Pie	1 slice	504	17	3	5	1	19	387	87	0	4	6 carb, 4 1/2 fat
NSA Apple Pie	1 slice	491	30	5	5	13	0	419	55	4	4	3 1/2 carb, 4 1/2 fat
NSA Apple Pie a la mode	1 slice	650	38	5	11	13	34	470	74	4	7	5 carb, 6 fat
Peanut Butter Cup Sundae	1	816	40	4	24	0	77	328	103	2	13	7 carb, 6 fat
Strawberry Short Cake	1	671	31	4	15	4	25	981	91	5	9	6 carb, 4 1/2 fat
Strawberry Sundae	1	496	24	4	19	0	75	121	64	2	8	4 1/2 carb, 4 1/2 fat

Strawberry Supreme Pie	1 slice	574	36	6	19	1	56	343	58	3	6	4 carb, 6 1/2 fat
✔Vanilla Ice Cream	1 srvg	116	6	5	4	0	25	37	14	0	2	1 fat
DINNER												
Bob-B-Q Chicken	1 srvg	545	14	2	4	0	95	1498	66	5	35	4 1/2 starch, 3 lean meat, 1 fat
Bob-B-Q Ribs	1 srvg	787	25	3	10	0	154	1931	84	5	52	5 1/2 starch, 5 medium-fat meat
Bob-B-Q Ribs Combo	1 srvg	534	13	2	5	0	77	1189	75	5	26	5 starch, 2 medium-fat meat, 1 fat
Chicken Parmesan	1 srvg	798	29	3	9	0	115	3014	85	6	39	5 1/2 starch, 3 lean meat, 4 fat
Chicken Salad Plate	1 srvg	763	46	5	7	0	88	1132	72	11	22	5 starch, 1 lean meat, 7 1/2 fat
Chicken Stir Fry	1 srvg	636	20	3	4	0	75	2681	77	6	38	5 starch, 3 lean meat, 2 fat

✔ = Healthiest Bets

(*Continued*)

DINNER *(Continued)*	Amount	Cal.	Fat (g)	% Cal. Fat	Sat. Fat (g)	Trans Fat (g)	Chol. (mg)	Sod. (mg)	Carb. (g)	Fiber (g)	Pro. (g)	Choices/Exchanges
Chicken-N-Noodles Deep Dish	1 srvg	845	43	5	14	4	114	2554	67	2	32	4 1/2 starch, 3 lean meat, 7 fat
Country Fried Steak - no Gravy	1 srvg	496	33	6	11	2	51	1217	31	0	18	2 starch, 2 medium-fat meat, 5 fat
Country Fried Steak w/ Gravy	1 srvg	552	38	6	12	3	51	1520	37	0	19	2 1/2 starch, 2 medium-fat meat, 6 fat
✔Fried Chicken Breast	1 srvg	285	13	4	3	0	89	758	13	1	29	1 starch, 4 lean meat, 1/2 fat
Fried Chicken Strips	1 strip	137	8	5	1	0	8	302	10	0	7	1/2 starch, 1 lean meat, 1 fat
✔Fried Haddock	1 srvg	363	18	4	4	0	41	608	27	0	24	2 starch, 3 lean meat, 2 fat
Garden Vegetable Alfredo	1 srvg	899	45	5	18	3	45	2590	99	12	21	6 starch, 1 veg, 8 1/2 fat
Garden Vegetable and Chicken Alfredo	1 srvg	951	44	4	17	1	111	3073	85	7	46	5 starch, 1 veg, 4 lean meat, 6 fat

Garden Vegetable and Salmon Alfredo	1 srvg	1074	52	4	18	2	137	2492	86	8	58	5 starch, 1 veg, 6 lean meat, 7 1/2 fat
✔Garlic Butter Grilled Chicken Breast	1 srvg	271	16	5	4	1	87	911	3	0	30	4 lean meat, 1/2 fat
✔Garlic Butter Salmon	1 srvg	326	16	4	4	1	103	377	2	0	40	6 lean meat
Green Pepper and Onion Pasta	1 srvg	558	19	3	4	0	3	2537	83	7	8	5 starch, 1 veg, 3 fat
✔Grilled Chicken Breast	1 srvg	232	13	5	3	0	85	635	0	0	29	4 lean meat
✔Grilled Chicken Tenders	1 tender	93	6	6	1	0	29	257	0	0	10	1 lean meat, 1/2 fat
Italian Sausage and Pepper Pasta	1 srvg	822	40	4	12	0	40	3041	76	5	27	4 starch, 1 veg, 2 medium-fat meat, 6 fat
✔Meatloaf	1 srvg	283	20	6	8	1	101	948	9	1	19	1/2 starch, 2 medium-fat meat, 1 1/2 fat
Open Faced Roast Beef	1 srvg	510	25	4	8	0	103	1038	24	1	33	1 1/2 starch, 4 medium-fat meat, 1 fat

✔ = Healthiest Bets

(*Continued*)

DINNER *(Continued)*	Amount	Cal.	Fat (g)	% Cal. Fat	Sat. Fat (g)	Trans Fat (g)	Chol. (mg)	Sod. (mg)	Carb. (g)	Fiber (g)	Pro. (g)	Choices/Exchanges
Pot Roast Beef Stew Deep Dish	1 srvg	763	39	5	15	4	79	2851	65	2	26	4 1/2 starch, 2 medium-fat meat, 6 fat
✔Potato Crusted Flounder	1 srvg	254	17	6	4	0	25	552	8	0	17	1/2 starch, 2 lean meat, 2 fat
✔Salmon	1 srvg	287	13	4	3	0	101	101	0	0	40	6 lean meat
Salmon Stir Fry	1 srvg	750	27	3	5	0	101	2086	77	6	50	5 starch, 5 lean meat, 2 1/2 fat
Sirloin Steak	1 srvg	403	27	6	8	0	77	638	3	0	33	5 medium-fat meat, 1/2 fat
Slow-Roasted Chicken Pot Pie	1 srvg	908	60	6	16	13	129	2847	64	5	33	4 1/2 starch, 3 lean meat, 10 fat
✔Slow-Roasted Chicken-N-Noodles	1 srvg	296	16	5	3	0	72	846	23	1	13	1 1/2 starch, 1 lean meat, 2 1/2 fat
✔Slow-Roasted Turkey	1 srvg	144	4	3	1	0	47	674	1	0	16	2 lean meat

✔Steak Tips	1 srvg	279	16	5	4	0	85	828	3	0	29	4 medium-fat meat
Steak Tips and Noodles	1 srvg	1024	46	4	12	1	270	4137	81	4	76	5 1/2 starch, 9 medium-fat meat, 1/2 fat
Steak Tips Stir Fry	1 srvg	1022	47	4	11	0	170	3641	84	6	69	5 1/2 starch, 7 medium-fat meat, 2 fat
Turkey and Dressing	1 srvg	551	28	5	9	3	113	2357	33	1	37	2 starch, 4 lean meat, 3 fat
Vegetable Stir Fry	1 srvg	505	15	3	2	0	0	2011	86	9	13	4 1/2 starch, 1 veg, 3 fat
✔Wildfire Grilled Chicken Breast	1 srvg	325	13	4	3	0	85	784	22	2	29	1 1/2 starch, 4 lean meat, 1/2 fat
✔Wildfire Salmon	1 srvg	380	13	3	3	0	101	250	22	2	40	1 1/2 starch, 5 lean meat
FIT FROM THE FARM												
✔Breakfast w/ a Parfait	1	359	12	3	3	0	34	707	38	3	25	2 1/2 starch, 2 medium-fat meat

✔ = Healthiest Bets

(*Continued*)

FIT FROM THE FARM *(Continued)*	Amount	Cal.	Fat (g)	% Cal. Fat	Sat. Fat (g)	Trans Fat (g)	Chol. (mg)	Sod. (mg)	Carb. (g)	Fiber (g)	Pro. (g)	Choices/Exchanges
Breakfast w/ a Yogurt Crepe	1	557	24	4	7	2	110	975	54	8	30	3 1/2 starch, 3 medium-fat meat, 2 fat
✔Breakfast w/ Oatmeal	1	364	13	3	3	0	35	815	37	2	25	2 1/2 starch, 3 medium-fat meat
HOTCAKES AND CREPES												
Blueberry Crepes	2	1046	75	6	25	5	178	718	79	4	12	5 starch, 14 fat
✔Blueberry Hotcakes	1	328	9	2	2	3	0	749	55	2	6	4 starch, 1 1/2 fat
✔Buttermilk Hotcake	1	318	9	3	2	3	0	748	53	2	6	4 starch, 2 fat
Cinnamon Hotcake	1	417	15	3	4	5	0	749	66	2	6	4 starch, 2 fat
✔Multigrain Hotcake	1	322	10	3	3	1	0	733	52	3	7	3 starch, 2 fat
Plain Crepe	1	459	36	7	12	2	89	352	27	1	6	2 starch, 7 fat

Stacked and Stuffed Caramel Banana Pecan Hotcakes	1 srvg	1543	77	4	26	9	55	2259	198	8	21	13 starch, 12 fat
Stacked and Stuffed Cinnamon Cream Hotcakes	1 srvg	1032	49	4	23	9	52	1552	136	4	14	9 starch, 7 1/2 fat
Stacked and Stuffed Cream Hotcakes	1 srvg	1099	42	3	21	6	50	1835	164	6	18	11 starch, 6 fat
Stacked and Stuffed Strawberry Banana Cream Hotcakes	1 srvg	1204	42	3	21	6	50	1820	193	12	20	13 starch, 5 fat
Strawberry Banana Crepes	2	1059	75	6	25	5	178	705	84	6	13	6 starch, 13 fat
Strawberry Banana Fruit & Yogurt Crepe	2	734	26	3	10	4	159	656	107	9	18	7 starch, 4 fat
Strawberry Blueberry Fruit and Yogurt Crepe	2	695	27	3	10	4	159	663	96	8	18	6 starch, 5 1/2 fat

✔ = Healthiest Bets

(*Continued*)

HOTCAKES & CREPES *(Continued)*	Amount	Cal.	Fat (g)	% Cal. Fat	Sat. Fat (g)	Trans Fat (g)	Chol. (mg)	Sod. (mg)	Carb. (g)	Fiber (g)	Pro. (g)	Choices/Exchanges
Stuffed French Toast - no topping	1 srvg	599	20	3	12	0	99	689	53	3	11	4 starch, 6 fat
Sweet Cream Waffles - no topping	1 srvg	598	12	2	7	3	149	1288	100	3	15	7 starch, 2 fat
KID'S MEAL												
✔Fresh Garden Salad	1	60	4	6	2	0	12	82	3	2	4	1 veg, 1 fat
Fried Chicken Strips	1	137	8	5	1	0	8	302	10	0	7	1/2 starch, 1 lean meat, 1 fat
Fruit & Yogurt Dippers	1 srvg	275	2	1	1	0	5	95	61	5	7	3 carb, 1 milk
Fudge Blast Sundae	1	248	11	4	8	0	25	86	34	0	3	2 1/2 carb, 1 1/2 fat
✔Grilled Cheese Triangles	1 srvg	290	16	5	7	1	30	796	26	1	9	1 1/2 starch, 1 medium-fat meat, 2 1/2 fat
Grilled Chicken Tenders	1	93	6	6	1	0	29	257	0	0	10	1 lean meat, 1/2 fat

✔Kid's Pasta	1 srvg	206	5	2	1	0	0	858	35	2	3	2 carb, 1 veg
Kid's Strawberry Sundae	1	242	13	5	10	0	25	47	30	1	3	2 carb, 1 1/2 fat
✔Macaroni & Cheese	1 srvg	320	11	3	3	0	23	778	45	2	11	3 starch, 2 fat
✔Mini Cheeseburgers	2	306	19	6	7	0	40	525	21	1	12	1 1/2 starch, 1 medium-fat meat, 2 1/2 fat
Plenty-O-Pancakes	1 srvg	501	17	3	6	4	0	1071	79	2	9	5 starch, 2 1/2 fat
Reese I'm Smiling Sundae	1	332	16	4	10	0	25	134	42	1	5	3 carb, 2 fat
Smiley Face Potatoes	1 srvg	524	31	5	6	0	2	646	57	3	5	4 starch, 5 fat
✔Turkey Lurkey	1 srvg	141	6	4	2	0	49	802	2	0	16	2 lean meat
OMELETS												
Border Scramble Omelet	1	726	56	7	19	0	791	1042	14	3	41	1 starch, 5 medium-fat meat, 5 1/2 fat
Border Scramble Omelet w/ Egg Lites	1	493	31	6	13	0	68	1187	14	3	37	1 starch, 5 lean meat, 3 1/2 fat

✔ = Healthiest Bets

(*Continued*)

OMELETS ***(Continued)***	Amount	Cal.	Fat (g)	% Cal. Fat	Sat. Fat (g)	Trans Fat (g)	Chol. (mg)	Sod. (mg)	Carb. (g)	Fiber (g)	Pro. (g)	Choices/Exchanges
✔Egg Lites Omelet Shell	1 srvg	149	7	4	1	0	0	357	2	0	17	2 medium-fat meat
Farmer's Market Omelet	1	778	60	7	24	1	810	1739	13	2	42	1 starch, 6 medium-fat meat, 6 1/2 fat
Farmer's Market Omelet w/ Egg Lites	1	544	35	6	18	1	87	1883	13	2	38	1 starch, 5 medium-fat meat, 2 fat
Garden Harvest Omelet	1	654	50	7	20	1	782	1241	13	2	33	1 starch, 4 medium-fat meat, 5 1/2 fat
Garden Harvest Omelet w/ Egg Lites	1	420	26	6	13	2	59	1385	13	2	29	1 starch, 4 medium-fat meat, 1 1/2 fat
Ham & Cheese	1	634	48	7	17	0	798	1419	3	1	44	6 lean meat, 6 fat
Ham & Cheese w/ Egg Lites	1	402	24	5	11	0	75	1564	4	1	40	1/2 starch, 6 lean meat, 1 1/2 fat
Omelet Shell	6 oz	383	31	7	7	0	723	213	2	0	20	3 medium-fat meat, 3 1/2 fat

Omelet Shell	4 oz	298	26	8	6	0	482	142	1	0	14	2 medium-fat meat, 3 fat
Sausage & Cheddar	1	741	61	7	21	0	847	942	3	1	42	6 medium-fat meat, 6 fat
Sausage & Cheddar w/ Egg Lites	1	478	34	6	14	0	57	1071	3	1	37	5 medium-fat meat, 1 1/2 fat
Three Cheese Omelet w/ Egg Lites	1	411	28	6	15	0	73	1170	4	1	32	1/2 starch, 4 medium-fat meat, 1 fat
Turkey & Spinach Omelet	1	736	54	7	20	0	883	1702	6	1	49	1/2 starch, 7 medium-fat meat, 4 fat
Turkey & Spinach Omelet w/ Egg Lites	1	472	27	5	14	0	105	1830	6	1	44	1/2 starch, 6 medium-fat meat
Western	1	654	48	7	17	0	798	1420	8	2	44	1/2 starch, 6 medium-fat meat, 3 1/2 fat
Western w/ Egg Lites	1	423	24	5	11	0	75	1566	9	2	41	1/2 starch, 6 medium-fat meat

✔ = Healthiest Bets

(*Continued*)

	Amount	Cal.	Fat (g)	% Cal. Fat	Sat. Fat (g)	Trans Fat (g)	Chol. (mg)	Sod. (mg)	Carb. (g)	Fiber (g)	Pro. (g)	Choices/Exchanges
SALAD DRESSING												
Avocado Ranch, side portion	1	205	22	10	3	0	13	359	2	0	1	4 1/2 fat
Avocado Ranch, dinner portion	1	411	43	9	7	0	25	718	3	0	1	8 1/2 fat
Bleu Cheese, side portion	1	220	23	9	4	0	22	337	3	0	1	4 1/2 fat
Bleu Cheese, dinner portion	1	440	47	10	9	0	44	675	6	0	3	1/2 carb, 9 1/2 fat
Buttermilk Ranch, side portion	1	156	16	9	3	0	14	312	1	0	1	3 fat
Buttermilk Ranch, dinner ptn	1	312	31	9	6	0	28	624	3	0	3	6 1/2 fat
Colonial, side portion	1	232	21	8	3	0	0	193	12	0	0	1 carb, 4 fat
Colonial, dinner portion	1	464	41	8	6	0	0	387	23	0	0	1 1/2 carb, 8 fat
French, side portion	1	219	21	9	3	0	14	247	10	0	0	1/2 carb, 4 fat
French, dinner portion	1	439	41	8	7	0	27	494	19	0	0	1 1/2 carb, 7 1/2 fat
Honey Mustard, side portion	1	192	18	8	3	0	21	247	8	0	0	1/2 carb, 3 1/2 fat

Honey Mustard, dinner portion	1	384	36	8	5	0	41	494	16	0	0	1 carb, 7 fat
Hot Bacon, side portion	1	106	3	3	1	0	4	189	18	0	0	1 carb, 1/2 fat
Hot Bacon, dinner portion	1	213	6	3	2	0	7	378	35	0	0	2 1/2 carb, 1 fat
Lite Ranch, side portion	1	103	10	9	2	0	11	377	2	0	1	2 fat
Lite Ranch, dinner portion	1	206	20	9	3	0	22	754	5	1	2	1/2 carb, 4 fat
Sweet Italian, side portion	1	173	10	5	3	0	0	505	8	0	0	1/2 carb, 3 fat
Sweet Italian, dinner portion	1	346	21	5	5	0	0	1010	16	0	0	1 carb, 5 fat
Swiss Bacon, side portion	1	227	26	10	4	0	21	397	1	0	1	5 fat
Swiss Bacon, dinner portion	1	454	51	10	9	0	43	794	3	0	3	10 fat
Thousand Island, side portion	1	213	20	8	3	0	14	354	7	0	0	1/2 carb, 4 fat
Thousand Island, dinner portion	1	425	40	8	6	0	28	709	14	0	0	1 carb, 8 fat
✔Vinegar & Oil, side portion	1	27	3	10	0	0	0	0	0	0	0	1/2 fat
Vinegar & Oil, dinner portion	1	54	6	10	1	0	0	0	0	0	0	1 fat

✔ = Healthiest Bets

(Continued)

SALAD DRESSING (Continued)	Amount	Cal.	Fat (g)	% Cal. Fat	Sat. Fat (g)	Trans Fat (g)	Chol. (mg)	Sod. (mg)	Carb. (g)	Fiber (g)	Pro. (g)	Choices/Exchanges
Wildfire Ranch, side portion	1	121	1	1	1	0	8	307	9	0	1	1/2 carb, 1/2 fat
Wildfire Ranch, dinner portion	1	241	3	1	3	0	15	614	18	0	1	1 carb, 1 fat
SALADS												
Chili and Cheese Taco Salad	1	928	62	6	18	0	91	1724	73	16	30	3 1/2 starch, 3 veg, 3 medium-fat meat, 9 1/2 fat
Chili and Cheese Taco Salad	savor size	715	46	6	14	0	70	1305	62	11	23	2 1/2 starch, 3 veg, 2 medium-fat meat, 7 fat
Cobb Salad	1	698	46	6	19	0	350	1819	14	5	60	3 veg, 8 medium-fat meat, 1 fat
Cobb Salad	savor size	469	30	6	12	0	293	1180	10	3	41	2 veg, 6 medium-fat meat
Country Spinach Salad	1	605	41	6	10	0	304	1464	13	5	52	3 veg, 7 medium-fat meat

Country Spinach Salad	savor size	505	35	6	9	0	274	1183	12	4	40	3 veg, 6 medium-fat meat
Cranberry Pecan Chicken Salad	1	836	46	5	15	0	123	2112	49	7	46	2 1/2 starch, 3 veg, 6 lean meat, 6 fat
Cranberry Pecan Chicken Salad	savor size	647	38	5	13	0	85	1502	42	5	31	2 starch, 3 veg, 4 lean meat, 5 fat
✓Garden Salad	1	137	4	3	0	0	0	347	22	3	4	4 veg, 1 fat
Heritage Chef Salad	1	456	26	5	12	0	286	1582	14	5	41	3 veg, 6 lean meat, 1 1/2 fat
✓Heritage Chef Salad	savor size	259	15	5	7	0	237	793	9	3	23	2 veg, 3 lean meat, 1 fat
✓Specialty Garden Salad	1	171	9	5	4	0	23	432	14	2	9	3 veg, 2 fat
Wildfire Fried Chicken Salad	1	789	21	2	10	0	49	1442	81	10	34	4 starch, 4 veg, 3 lean meat, 4 fat
Wildfire Fried Chicken Salad	savor size	631	30	4	9	0	41	1131	68	8	26	3 1/2 starch, 3 veg, 2 lean meat, 4 fat

✓ = Healthiest Bets

(*Continued*)

SALADS *(Continued)*	Amount	Cal.	Fat (g)	% Cal. Fat	Sat. Fat (g)	Trans Fat (g)	Chol. (mg)	Sod. (mg)	Carb. (g)	Fiber (g)	Pro. (g)	Choices/Exchanges
Wildfire Grilled Chicken Salad	1	654	21	3	9	0	112	1308	53	9	43	2 1/2 starch, 3 veg, 5 lean meat, 3 fat
Wildfire Grilled Chicken Salad	savor size	541	26	4	8	0	82	1041	49	7	31	1 starch, 3 veg, 4 lean meat, 3 1/2 fat
SANDWICHES												
Bacon Cheeseburger	1	716	48	6	20	2	135	1335	32	3	38	2 starch, 5 medium-fat meat, 5 fat
Bob-B-Q Pulled Pork Sandwich	1	655	30	4	5	1	98	788	68	4	37	4 1/2 starch, 3 medium-fat meat, 2 fat
Bob's BLT&E	1	645	38	5	15	1	278	1065	27	2	19	2 starch, 3 high-fat meat, 4 1/2 fat
Cheeseburger	1	645	41	6	17	2	125	1226	32	3	37	2 starch, 4 medium-fat meat, 4 fat

Chicken Salad Sandwich	1	649	38	5	6	0	62	1282	43	6	22	3 starch, 2 lean meat, 6 1/2 fat
Fried Chicken Club Sandwich	1	660	35	5	12	0	123	1609	44	3	40	3 starch, 4 lean meat, 4 1/2 fat
Fried Chicken Sandwich	1	503	21	4	4	0	89	1125	43	2	34	3 starch, 4 lean meat, 2 fat
Fried Haddock Sandwich	1	786	34	4	10	1	70	1650	78	2	40	5 starch, 3 lean meat, 4 fat
✔Grilled Cheese Sandwich	1	396	16	4	6	1	29	777	25	2	9	Free
Grilled Chicken Club Sandwich	1	606	35	5	12	1	118	1485	31	2	41	2 starch, 5 lean meat, 4 fat
✔Grilled Chicken Sandwich	1	399	15	3	3	1	85	945	30	1	38	2 starch, 5 lean meat, 1/2 fat
✔Half Chicken Salad Sandwich	1	331	19	5	3	0	34	644	28	3	12	2 starch, 1 lean meat, 3 1/2 fat

✔ = Healthiest Bets

(*Continued*)

SANDWICHES *(Continued)*	Amount	Cal.	Fat (g)	% Cal. Fat	Sat. Fat (g)	Trans Fat (g)	Chol. (mg)	Sod. (mg)	Carb. (g)	Fiber (g)	Pro. (g)	Choices/Exchanges
✔Half Pot Roast Sandwich	1	390	19	4	7	0	66	808	31	2	23	2 starch, 2 medium-fat meat, 1 1/2 fat
✔Half Turkey Bacon Melt	1	306	14	4	6	0	43	905	26	1	16	1 1/2 starch, 2 medium-fat meat, 1 1/2 fat
Hamburger	1	539	32	5	11	2	96	756	31	3	31	2 starch, 4 medium-fat meat, 3 fat
✔Hamburger Patty	1	321	24	7	10	1	96	389	1	1	26	4 medium-fat meat, 1 fat
Knife and Fork Bob-B-Q Chicken Sandwich	1	748	20	2	9	0	108	1619	75	6	36	5 starch, 3 lean meat, 3 1/2 fat
Knife and Fork Bob-B-Q Pulled Pork Sandwich	1	817	36	4	10	0	127	1080	67	5	37	4 1/2 starch, 3 medium-fat meat, 4 fat
Knife and Fork Meatloaf Sandwich	1	720	38	5	17	1	145	2591	41	3	28	2 1/2 starch, 3 medium-fat meat, 6 fat
Knife and Fork Turkey Sandwich	1	696	36	5	12	1	80	2439	46	2	24	3 starch, 2 lean meat, 7 fat

Pot Roast Sandwich	1	610	28	4	11	1	80	1361	58	3	31	4 starch, 3 medium-fat meat, 3 fat
Ranch Steak Burger	1	937	68	7	27	2	165	2007	35	3	42	2 1/2 starch, 5 medium-fat meat, 8 1/2 fat
Turkey Bacon Melt	1	617	29	4	11	1	87	1818	53	3	33	3 1/2 starch, 3 lean meat, 4 fat
SAUCES AND TOPPINGS												
✔American Cheese	1 slice	53	4	7	3	0	15	235	1	0	3	1/2 fat
✔Beef Gravy	2 oz	22	1	4	0	0	1	372	3	0	1	Free
Blue Cheese	1 oz	97	8	7	5	0	22	381	0	0	6	1 medium-fat meat, 1/2 fat
Blueberry Topping	3 oz	103	0	0	0	0	0	14	25	2	1	1 1/2 carb
Caramel Topping	1 oz	74	0	0	0	0	1	79	18	0	1	1 carb
✔Chicken-Roasted Gravy	2 oz	53	4	7	1	0	4	256	3	0	1	1 fat

✔ = Healthiest Bets

(*Continued*)

SAUCES AND TOPPINGS *(Continued)*	Amount	Cal.	Fat (g)	% Cal. Fat	Sat. Fat (g)	Trans Fat (g)	Chol. (mg)	Sod. (mg)	Carb. (g)	Fiber (g)	Pro. (g)	Choices/Exchanges
Chocolate Fudge Topping	1 oz	86	2	2	1	0	0	46	16	0	1	1 carb, 1/2 fat
Citrus Stir Fry Sauce	2 oz	51	0	0	0	0	0	335	12	0	1	1 carb
✔Cocktail Sauce	1 oz	31	0	0	0	0	0	414	7	0	1	1/2 carb
Country Gravy	3 oz	56	4	6	1	2	0	303	6	0	0	1/2 carb, 1 fat
Cranberries	.7 oz	68	0	0	0	0	0	0	17	1	0	1 carb
✔Garlic Butter	1 oz	40	3	7	1	1	2	276	2	0	0	1 fat
✔Hollandaise Sauce	2 oz	50	3	5	1	1	2	211	5	0	1	1 fat
Honey Roasted Pecans	.7 oz	142	14	9	1	0	0	72	6	2	2	1/2 carb, 3 fat
✔Marinara Sauce	3 oz	35	1	3	0	0	0	374	5	1	1	1/2 carb
✔Monterey Jack Cheese	1 slice	76	6	7	5	0	23	364	0	0	4	1 fat
✔Pork-Roasted Gravy	2 oz	63	5	7	3	0	12	297	3	0	1	1 1/2 fat
✔Raisins	1 oz	70	0	0	0	0	0	2	17	1	1	1 fruit

✔Ranchero Picante	1 oz	28	0	0	0	0	0	71	0	0	7	1 veg
Sour Cream	1 oz	57	5	8	3	0	19	24	2	0	1	1 fat
Strawberry Topping	3.6 oz	66	0	0	0	0	0	1	17	2	1	1 carb
Tartar Sauce	1 oz	166	18	10	3	0	20	176	1	0	0	3 fat
Whipped Topping	1 oz	90	7	7	6	0	0	5	7	0	2	1 1/2 fat
✔Wildfire BBQ Sauce	1.5 oz	94	0	0	0	0	0	149	22	2	0	1 1/2 carb
SENIORS												
Chicken Parmesan	1 srvg	615	26	4	9	0	115	2405	53	4	37	3 1/2 starch, 4 lean meat, 3 fat
Chicken Stir Fry	1 srvg	368	13	3	2	0	37	1385	44	5	21	3 starch, 2 lean meat, 1 1/2 fat
Country Fried Steak - no Gravy	1 srvg	496	33	6	11	2	51	1217	31	0	18	2 starch, 2 medium-fat meat, 5 fat
Country Fried Steak w/ Gravy	1 srvg	552	38	6	12	3	51	1520	37	0	19	2 1/2 starch, 2 medium-fat meat, 6 fat

✔ = Healthiest Bets

(Continued)

SENIORS *(Continued)*	Amount	Cal.	Fat (g)	% Cal. Fat	Sat. Fat (g)	Trans Fat (g)	Chol. (mg)	Sod. (mg)	Carb. (g)	Fiber (g)	Pro. (g)	Choices/Exchanges
✔Fried Chicken Breast	1 srvg	285	13	4	3	0	89	758	13	1	29	1 starch, 4 lean meat, 1/2 fat
✔Fried Haddock	1 srvg	363	18	4	4	0	41	608	27	0	24	2 starch, 3 lean meat, 2 fat
Garden Vegetable Alfredo	1 srvg	457	23	5	9	1	24	1322	49	6	11	3 starch, 1 veg, 4 fat
Garden Vegetable and Chicken Alfredo	1 srvg	545	26	4	10	1	62	1678	49	6	25	3 1/2 starch, 2 lean meat, 4 fat
Green Pepper and Onion Pasta	1 srvg	352	14	4	3	0	3	1679	48	5	6	2 1/2 starch, 1 veg, 3 fat
✔Grilled Chicken Breast	1 srvg	232	13	5	3	0	85	635	0	0	29	4 lean meat
Italian Sausage and Pepper Pasta	1 srvg	616	36	5	12	0	40	2183	41	3	24	2 1/2 starch, 2 medium-fat meat, 5 fat

✔Meatloaf	1 srvg	283	20	6	8	1	101	948	9	1	19	1/2 starch, 2 medium-fat meat, 1 1/2 fat
Opened-Faced Roast Beef	1 srvg	510	25	4	80	0	103	1038	24	1	33	1 1/2 starch, 4 medium-fat meat, 1 1/2 fat
Sausage Gravy	cup	134	9	6	5	0	8	619	10	0	4	1 starch, 2 fat
Slow-Roasted Chicken Pot Pie	1 srvg	908	60	6	16	13	129	2847	64	5	33	4 1/2 starch, 3 lean meat, 10 fat
Steak Tip Stir Fry	1 srvg	560	26	4	6	0	85	1865	48	5	37	3 starch, 4 medium-fat meat, 1 fat
Steak Tips and Noodles	1 srvg	523	24	4	6	0	136	2255	42	2	37	3 starch, 4 medium-fat meat, 1/2 fat
Turkey and Dressing	1 srvg	438	23	5	7	3	66	1699	33	1	21	2 starch, 2 lean meat, 3 1/2 fat
Turkey Sausage	1 srvg	346	12	3	2	0	31	815	34	2	24	2 1/2 starch, 2 medium-fat meat

✔ = Healthiest Bets

(*Continued*)

SENIORS *(Continued)*	Amount	Cal.	Fat (g)	% Cal. Fat	Sat. Fat (g)	Trans Fat (g)	Chol. (mg)	Sod. (mg)	Carb. (g)	Fiber (g)	Pro. (g)	Choices/Exchanges
Vegetable Stir Fry	1 srvg	281	10	3	1	0	0	1037	44	5	7	2 starch, 1 veg, 2 fat
SIDES												
Applesauce	1 srvg	83	0	0	0	0	0	14	21	2	0	1 1/2 fruit
✔Baked Potato	1 srvg	207	0	0	0	0	0	16	54	6	8	3 1/2 starch
Bread & Celery Dressing	1 srvg	272	15	5	5	3	15	786	29	1	5	2 starch, 3 fat
✔Broccoli Florets	1 srvg	32	0	0	0	0	0	29	6	3	3	1 veg
✔Caramelized Onions	1 srvg	38	2	5	0	0	0	208	6	1	1	1/2 veg, 1/2 fat
Coleslaw	1 srvg	203	14	6	2	0	12	235	19	2	1	1/2 starch, 1 veg, 2 fat
✔Corn	1 srvg	169	8	4	3	1	10	184	25	3	4	2 starch, 1 fat
✔Cottage Cheese	1 srvg	115	5	4	3	0	34	410	4	0	14	1/2 milk, 1 fat
✔Cranberry Relish	1 srvg	57	0	0	0	0	0	6	13	1	0	1 carb
✔Dill Pickle Slices	1 srvg	1	0	0	0	0	0	159	0	0	0	Free

French Fries	1 srvg	354	15	4	3	0	1	102	51	1	5	3 starch, 2 fat
✔Fruit Cup	1 srvg	150	1	1	0	0	0	11	38	4	2	2 fruit
✔Fruit Dish	1 srvg	71	0	0	0	0	0	10	18	1	1	1 1/2 fruit
Garden Vegetables	1 srvg	121	7	5	3	1	9	212	14	5	3	3 veg, 1 fat
✔Glazed Carrots	1 srvg	83	3	3	1	0	4	95	14	4	1	2 veg, 1/2 fat
✔Green Beans	1 srvg	79	3	3	1	0	8	885	9	3	5	2 veg
Grilled Mushrooms	1 srvg	152	12	7	2	0	0	1005	10	5	4	2 veg, 2 fat
Home Fries	1 srvg	186	7	3	1	1	0	547	27	3	3	2 starch, 1 1/2 fat
✔Lettuce & Tomato	1 srvg	4	0	0	0	0	0	2	1	0	0	Free
✔Lettuce, Tomato and Pickle	1 srvg	6	0	0	0	0	0	161	1	0	0	Free
Loaded Baked Potato	1 srvg	373	13	3	7	0	40	437	56	7	19	4 starch, 2 fat
✔Mashed Potatoes	1 srvg	205	7	3	5	0	22	458	17	1	3	1 starch, 1 fat
Onions Petals	1 srvg	302	18	5	2	2	0	466	35	2	3	2 starch, 3 fat

✔ = Healthiest Bets

(*Continued*)

SIDES *(Continued)*	Amount	Cal.	Fat (g)	% Cal. Fat	Sat. Fat (g)	Trans Fat (g)	Chol. (mg)	Sod. (mg)	Carb. (g)	Fiber (g)	Pro. (g)	Choices/Exchanges
Rice Pilaf	1 srvg	129	4	3	1	0	0	600	20	1	2	1 starch, 1 fat
✔Strawberry Yogurt	1 srvg	145	1	1	1	0	5	85	28	1	6	1 carb, 1 milk
Sweet Corn Griddle Cakes	1 srvg	400	18	4	6	1	131	310	54	3	7	4 starch, 3 fat
✔Tomato Slices	1 srvg	4	0	0	0	0	0	2	1	0	0	Free
SOUP												
✔Bean Soup	cup	144	3	2	1	0	8	776	19	5	10	1 starch, 1/2 fat
Bean Soup	bowl	205	5	2	2	0	12	1111	27	7	14	2 starch, 1 fat
Cheddar Baked Potato Soup	bowl	371	25	6	10	4	42	1474	24	2	13	2 starch, 5 fat
Cheddar Baked Potato Soup	cup	294	20	6	8	3	34	1168	19	1	10	1 starch, 4 fat
Sausage Chili	bowl	376	24	6	9	0	59	962	26	10	22	1 1/2 starch, 2 medium-fat meat, 2 fat

✔Sausage Chili	cup	268	17	6	6	0	42	687	18	7	16	1 starch, 2 medium-fat meat, 1 fat
✔Vegetable Beef Soup	cup	135	5	3	2	0	14	370	17	3	6	1 starch, 1 fat
✔Vegetable Beef Soup	bowl	193	7	3	2	0	20	528	25	4	9	2 starch, 1 1/2 fat

✔ = Healthiest Bets

Exclusive Web Content

Be sure to visit the following restaurants online at http://www.diabetes.org/healthyrestaurant

Carvel **Frëshens** **Jimmy John's** **Wienerschnitzel**
Del Taco **Godfather's** **Tim Hortons** **Zaxby's**
El Pollo Loco **Jersey Mike's** **Whataburger**

Boston Market
(www.bostonmarket.com)

Light 'n Lean Choice

Macaroni and Cheese
Butternut Squash
Steamed Broccoli with Garlic Butter
Seasonal Fresh Fruit Salad

Calories	580	Cholesterol (mg)	40
Fat (g)	22	Sodium (mg)	1,385
% calories from fat	34	Carbohydrate (g)	81
Saturated fat (g)	12	Fiber (g)	8
Trans fat (g)	0	Protein (g)	17

Exchanges: 4 starch, 1 veg, 1 fruit, 3 1/2 fat

Healthy 'n Hearty Choice

1/4 White Meat Chicken *(no skin or wing)*
Sweet Corn
Green Bean Casserole
Cinnamon Apples

Calories	650	Cholesterol (mg)	140
Fat (g)	11	Sodium (mg)	1,370
% calories from fat	15	Carbohydrate (g)	99
Saturated fat (g)	2.5	Fiber (g)	7
Trans fat (g)	0	Protein (g)	50

Exchanges: 4 starch, 2 veg, 2 fruit, 4 lean meat

Boston Market

	Amount	Cal.	Fat (g)	% Cal. Fat	Sat. Fat (g)	Trans Fat (g)	Chol. (mg)	Sod. (mg)	Carb. (g)	Fiber (g)	Pro. (g)	Choices/Exchanges
DESSERTS												
Cherry Cobbler	1 srvg	430	6	1	3.5	0	15	190	113	3	3	7 1/2 carb
Chocolate Cake	1 srvg	580	34	5	11	0	45	360	57	3	5	4 carb, 6 1/2 fat
Chocolate Chip Cookie	1	370	19	5	9	0	20	340	49	2	4	3 1/2 carb, 3 1/2 fat
Chocolate Chip Fudge Brownie	1	580	23	4	5	0	90	390	81	3	9	5 1/2 carb, 4 fat
✔Cornbread	1 pc	180	5	3	1.5	1.5	10	320	31	0	2	2 starch, 1/2 fat
FAMILY MEALS												
✔Award Winning Roasted Sirloin	5 oz	290	15	5	6	1	125	440	0	0	39	6 lean meat

✔ = Healthiest Bets

(Continued)

FAMILY MEALS *(Continued)*	Amount	Cal.	Fat (g)	% Cal. Fat	Sat. Fat (g)	Trans Fat (g)	Chol. (mg)	Sod. (mg)	Carb. (g)	Fiber (g)	Pro. (g)	Choices/Exchanges
Meatloaf	7.7 oz	480	36	7	16	1.5	145	1030	21	0	29	1 1/2 starch, 4 medium-fat meat, 3 fat
✔Roasted Turkey	5 oz	180	3	2	1	0	72	635	0	0	38	4 lean meat
✔Rotisserie Chicken	6 oz	290	14	4	4	0	175	710	4	0	39	6 lean meat
INDIVIDUAL MEALS												
✔1 Thigh & 1 Drumstick	5.5 oz	300	17	5	5	0	180	630	6	0	32	1/2 starch, 4 lean meat, 1 fat
3 Piece Dark	2 Thighs & Drumstick	510	30	5	9	0	295	1020	8	0	52	1/2 starch, 7 lean meat, 1 1/2 fat
✔3 Piece Dark Skinless	2 Thighs & Drumstick	310	13	4	4	0	240	690	6	0	42	1/2 starch, 5 lean meat
✔3 Piece Skinless	Thigh & 2 Drumsticks	240	8	3	2.5	0	205	650	7	0	37	1/2 starch, 4 lean meat

✔Award Winning Roasted Sirloin	5 oz	290	15	5	6	1	125	440	0	0	39	5 lean meat
✔Dark Individual Meal	7 oz	380	19	5	6	0	250	880	7	0	45	1/2 starch, 6 lean meat
✔Dark Tuscan Herb Roasted Chicken	1/4 chicken	310	17	5	5	0	180	810	6	1	33	1/2 starch, 5 lean meat, 1/2 fat
Meatloaf	7.6 oz	520	36	6	16	1.5	145	1030	21	0	29	1 1/2 starch, 4 medium-fat meat, 3 fat
Pastry Top Chicken Pot Pie	15 oz	780	47	5	17	7	125	930	60	4	29	4 starch, 2 lean meat, 7 1/2 fat
✔Roasted Turkey	5 oz	180	3	2	1	0	72	635	0	0	38	4 lean meat
Tuscan Herb Roasted Chicken	Thigh & 2 Drumsticks	390	20	5	6	0	250	1050	8	1	45	1/2 starch, 6 lean meat, 1/2 fat
Tuscan Herb Roasted Chicken	2 Thighs & Drumstick	520	31	5	9	0	295	1190	9	1	53	1/2 starch, 7 lean meat, 2 fat
Tuscan Herb Roasted Chicken	1/2 Chicken	610	28	4	9	0	350	1760	11	2	78	1/2 starch, 10 lean meat

✔ = Healthiest Bets

(*Continued*)

INDIVIDUAL MEALS *(Continued)*	Amount	Cal.	Fat (g)	% Cal. Fat	Sat. Fat (g)	Trans Fat (g)	Chol. (mg)	Sod. (mg)	Carb. (g)	Fiber (g)	Pro. (g)	Choices/Exchanges
✔White Rotisserie Chicken	1/4 chicken	290	11	3	3.5	0	170	780	4	0	45	1/2 starch, 5 lean meat
✔White Rotisserie Chicken - no skin	1/4 chicken	210	2	1	0.5	0	135	640	6	0	42	1/2 starch, 4 lean meat
✔White Tuscan Herb Roasted Chicken	1/4 chicken	300	11	3	305	0	170	960	5	1	45	1/2 starch, 5 lean meat
SALADS												
Caesar Salad Dressing	2.5 oz	360	38	10	6	0.5	30	910	4	1	2	1/2 carb, 7 1/2 fat
Caesar Salad Entrée	1	500	45	8	11	0	45	1190	12	3	13	3 veg, 2 lean meat, 7 fat
✔Caesar Salad Entrée - no dressing	1	140	8	5	5	0	15	280	8	2	11	2 veg, 2 fat
✔Lite Ranch Dressing	1.5 oz	70	4	5	0.5	0	0	310	8	0	1	1/2 carb, 1 fat
Roasted Sirloin	3 oz	160	6	3	2	0	75	170	0	0	26	3 lean meat

✔Roasted Turkey	3 oz	140	6	4	1	0	25	370	1	0	19	3 lean meat
✔Rotisserie Chicken	5 oz	160	1	1	0	0	105	520	3	0	35	3 lean meat
Tuscan Chicken Mixed Green Salad	1	530	24	4	5	0	125	1990	37	7	43	1 starch, 3 veg, 6 lean meat, 1 1/2 fat
Tuscan Herb Chicken Salad	1	420	32	7	7	0.5	105	970	12	2	22	1 starch, 3 veg, 3 lean meat, 2 fat
SANDWICHES												
✔Beef Au Jus	1 srvg	20	0	0	0	0	0	760	4	0	1	Free
Boston Chicken Carver	1	700	29	4	7	0	90	1560	68	3	44	4 1/2 starch, 4 lean meat, 2 1/2 fat
Boston Meatloaf Carver	1	980	46	4	20	2	165	2200	96	4	48	6 1/2 starch, 4 medium-fat meat, 4 fat
Boston Sirloin Dip Carver	1	1000	51	5	15	2	200	1690	70	3	67	4 1/2 starch, 8 lean meat, 5 1/2 fat

✔ = Healthiest Bets

(*Continued*)

SANDWICHES *(Continued)*	Amount	Cal.	Fat (g)	% Cal. Fat	Sat. Fat (g)	Trans Fat (g)	Chol. (mg)	Sod. (mg)	Carb. (g)	Fiber (g)	Pro. (g)	Choices/Exchanges
Boston Turkey Carver	1	770	27	3	8	0	125	1810	68	3	66	4 1/2 starch, 7 lean meat
Boston Turkey Dip Carver	1	770	27	3	8	0	125	1890	67	3	66	4 1/2 starch, 8 lean meat, 1/2 fat
✔Half Boston Chicken Carver	1	340	15	4	4	0	65	710	29	1	24	2 starch, 3 lean meat, 1 1/2 fat
Half Boston Sirloin Carver	1	500	25	5	8	1	100	850	35	1	33	2 1/2 starch, 4 medium-fat meat, 1 1/2 fat
✔Half Boston Turkey Carver	1	390	14	3	4	0	60	910	34	2	33	2 1/2 starch, 4 lean meat, 1/2 fat
✔Half Boston Turkey Dip	1	380	14	3	4	0	60	950	33	1	33	2 starch, 4 lean meat, 1/2 fat
Meatloaf Open-faced Sandwich	1	670	38	5	17	1.5	145	1760	48	1	34	3 starch, 3 medium-fat meat, 3 1/2 fat

✔Poultry Au Jus	1 srvg	15	1	6	0	0	0	570	4	0	1	Free
Roasted Sirloin Open-faced Sandwich	1	410	15	3	6	1	100	1640	32	1	35	2 starch, 4 lean meat, 1/2 fat
Roasted Turkey Open-faced Sandwich	1	350	7	2	1.5	0	40	1540	45	2	27	3 starch, 2 lean meat
Rotisserie Chicken Open-faced Sandwich	1	330	9	2	2	0	70	1540	38	1	25	2 1/2 starch, 2 lean meat, 1/2 fat
Tuscan Chicken Carver	1	770	34	4	9	1	95	1600	70	3	49	4 1/2 starch, 5 lean meat, 3 fat
Tuscan Herb Chicken Salad Sandwich	1	1190	77	6	18	1.5	160	2110	79	4	46	5 1/2 starch, 4 lean meat, 12 fat
SOUPS & SIDES												
✔4-Cheese Cavatappi	1 srvg	300	15	5	9	0	30	520	30	1	11	2 starch, 1 medium-fat meat, 2 1/2 fat
✔Beef Gravy	3 oz	35	2	5	0.5	0	0	500	4	0	1	1/2 fat

✔ = Healthiest Bets

(*Continued*)

SOUPS & SIDES *(Continued)*	Amount	Cal.	Fat (g)	% Cal. Fat	Sat. Fat (g)	Trans Fat (g)	Chol. (mg)	Sod. (mg)	Carb. (g)	Fiber (g)	Pro. (g)	Choices/Exchanges
✔Broccoli w/ Garlic Butter	1 srvg	80	6	7	2	0	0	230	6	3	3	1 veg, 1 fat
✔Butternut Squash	1 srvg	140	5	3	3	0	10	35	25	2	2	2 starch, 1/2 fat
Caesar Salad Dressing	2.5 oz	360	38	10	6	0.5	30	910	4	1	2	1/2 carb, 7 1/2 fat
Caesar Side Salad	1 srvg	400	40	9	8	0.5	30	980	7	2	5	1 veg, 8 fat
✔Caesar Side Salad - no dressing	1 srvg	40	2	5	1.5	0	5	75	3	1	3	1 veg, 1/2 fat
✔Chicken Noodle Soup	6 oz	170	5	3	1.5	0	60	930	17	1	13	1 starch, 1 lean meat
✔Chicken Tortilla Soup - no toppings	6 oz	90	5	5	1	0	15	900	7	1	5	1/2 starch, 1 lean meat, 1/2 fat
Chicken Tortilla Soup w/ toppings	6 oz	340	22	6	7	0	45	1310	24	1	12	1 1/2 starch, 1 lean meat, 4 fat
Cinnamon Apples	1 srvg	210	3	1	0	0	0	15	47	3	0	3 fruit

✔Cranberry Walnut Relish	1 srvg	140	2	1	0	0	0	0	30	2	1	2 carb
Creamed Spinach	1 srvg	280	23	7	15	0	70	580	12	4	9	1 veg, 4 1/2 fat
✔Fresh Steamed Vegetables	1 srvg	60	2	3	0	0	0	40	8	3	2	2 veg
Fresh Vegetable Stuffing	1 srvg	190	8	4	1	0	0	580	25	2	3	2 starch, 1 1/2 fat
Garden Fresh Coleslaw	1 srvg	170	9	5	2	0	10	270	21	2	2	1 starch, 1 veg, 1 1/2 fat
✔Garlic Dill New Potatoes	1 srvg	140	3	2	1	0	0	120	24	3	3	2 starch, 1/2 fat
Garlic Spinach	1 srvg	130	9	6	6	0	20	200	9	5	5	2 veg, 2 fat
✔Green Bean Casserole	1 srvg	60	2	3	1	0	5	620	9	2	2	2 veg
✔Green Beans	1 srvg	60	4	6	1.5	0	0	180	7	3	2	1 veg, 1/2 fat
Macaroni & Cheese	1 srvg	300	11	3	7	0	30	1100	35	2	11	2 starch, 2 fat
Mashed Potatoes	1 srvg	270	11	4	7	0	30	810	36	4	5	2 starch, 2 fat
✔Poultry Gravy	4 oz	15	1	6	0	0	0	570	4	0	1	Free
✔Seasonal Fresh Fruit Salad	1 srvg	60	0	0	0	0	0	20	15	1	1	1 fruit

✔ = Healthiest Bets

(*Continued*)

SOUPS & SIDES ***(Continued)***	Amount	Cal.	Fat (g)	% Cal. Fat	Sat. Fat (g)	Trans Fat (g)	Chol. (mg)	Sod. (mg)	Carb. (g)	Fiber (g)	Pro. (g)	Choices/Exchanges
Spinach Artichoke Dip	1 srvg	100	8	7	3.5	0	15	220	3	1	3	1 veg, 1 1/2 fat
Squash Casserole	1 srvg	320	24	7	11	0.5	50	1380	21	3	9	1 starch, 5 fat
Sweet Corn	1 srvg	170	4	2	1	0	0	95	37	2	6	2 starch
Sweet Potato Casserole	1 srvg	460	17	3	6	0	20	210	77	3	4	5 starch, 1 1/2 fat

✔ = Healthiest Bets

Exclusive Web Content

Be sure to visit the following restaurants online at http://www.diabetes.org/healthyrestaurant

Carvel
Del Taco
El Pollo Loco
Frëshens
Godfather's
Jersey Mike's
Jimmy John's
Tim Hortons
Whataburger
Wienerschnitzel
Zaxby's

Denny's
(www.dennys.com)

Light 'n Lean Choice

Grapefruit *(1/2)*
Veggie-Cheese Omelette with Egg Beaters
English Muffin, dry
Cream Cheese *(1 Tbsp)*

Calories	606	Cholesterol (mg)	39
Fat (g)	29	Sodium (mg)	1,134
% calories from fat	43	Carbohydrate (g)	55
Saturated fat (g)	10	Fiber (g)	11
Trans fat (g)	0	Protein (g)	32

Exchanges: 2 starch, 1 veg, 1 fruit, 3 1/2 lean meat, 3 fat

Healthy 'n Hearty Choice

Vegetable Beef Soup
Vegetable Beef Entrée
Vegetable Beef Entrée sides and toppings

Calories	630	Cholesterol (mg)	85
Fat (g)	27	Sodium (mg)	2,470
% calories from fat	39	Carbohydrate (g)	46
Saturated fat (g)	6.6	Fiber (g)	6
Trans fat (g)	0.5	Protein (g)	52

Exchanges: 2 starch, 2 veg, 4 medium-fat meat, 1 fat

(Continued)

Denny's

	Amount	Cal.	Fat (g)	% Cal. Fat	Sat. Fat (g)	Trans Fat (g)	Chol. (mg)	Sod. (mg)	Carb. (g)	Fiber (g)	Pro. (g)	Choices/Exchanges
APPETIZERS												
Buffalo Chicken Strips	5 pcs	734	42	5	4	0	96	1673	43	0	48	3 starch, 6 lean meat, 5 fat
Buffalo Wings	9 pcs	974	72	7	18	0	267	4049	11	2	67	1/2 starch, 9 lean meat, 9 fat
Chicken Strips	5 pcs	720	33	4	4	0	95	1666	56	0	47	3 1/2 starch, 5 lean meat, 3 1/2 fat
Mozzarella Sticks	8 pcs	710	41	5	24	0	48	5220	49	6	36	3 1/2 starch, 4 medium-fat meat, 4 1/2 fat
Nachos	1 srvg	1278	64	5	31	0	181	1654	117	11	54	8 starch, 4 medium-fat meat, 8 fat
Sampler	1	1405	80	5	24	1	75	5305	124	4	47	8 1/2 starch, 3 medium-fat meat, 12 fat

Smothered Cheese Fries	1 srvg	767	48	6	17	3	78	875	69	0	27	4 1/2 starch, 2 medium-fat meat, 6 1/2 fat
BEVERAGES												
✔Cappuccino French Vanilla	8 oz.	100	3	3	0	3	0	220	28	1	3	2 carb
Cherry Limeade	15 oz.	240	0	0	0	0	0	45	62	0	0	4 carb, fat
✔Hot Chocolate	8 oz.	100	2	2	0	2	0	219	28	1	3	2 carb
Island Fizz	15 oz.	250	0	0	0	0	0	35	64	0	0	4 1/2 carb, fat
Lemonade w/ Ice	16 oz.	150	0	0	0	0	0	38	35	0	0	2 carb
OJ Mango	14 oz.	240	0	0	0	0	0	5	60	0	0	4 carb, fat
Pineapple Dream	15 oz.	180	0	0	0	0	0	35	64	1	0	4 1/2 carb
✔Raspberry Iced Tea w/ Ice	16 oz.	78	0	0	0	0	0	0	21	0	0	1 1/2 carb
Razzdango	15 oz.	220	0	0	0	0	0	40	59	1	0	4 carb, fat
Strawberry Mango Pucker	15 oz.	200	0	0	0	0	0	10	51	1	0	3 1/2 carb
Very Double Berry	14 oz.	280	0	0	0	0	0	10	69	0	0	4 1/2 carb, fat

✔ = Healthiest Bets

(*Continued*)

	Amount	Cal.	Fat (g)	% Cal. Fat	Sat. Fat (g)	Trans Fat (g)	Chol. (mg)	Sod. (mg)	Carb. (g)	Fiber (g)	Pro. (g)	Choices/Exchanges
BREAKFAST												
All American Slam w/ Hash Browns	1 srvg	950	75	7	25	1	775	2230	21	2	48	1 1/2 starch, 6 medium-fat meat, 8 1/2 fat
Belgian Waffle Platter	1 waffle	619	45	7	22	0	274	1683	28	0	22	2 starch, 2 medium-fat meat, 6 1/2 fat
Buttermilk Pancake	3 pancakes	410	5	1	1	0	0	1350	82	3	9	5 starch
Center Cut Sirloin & Eggs	1 srvg	370	15	4	5	0	520	870	1	0	54	7 medium-fat meat
✔Cereal	1 srvg	100	0	0	0	0	0	276	23	1	2	1 1/2 starch
Country Fried Potatoes	1 srvg	394	20	5	6	3	9	938	23	10	3	2 starch, 6 fat
Country Fried Steak & Eggs w/ Hash Browns	1 srvg	740	46	6	14	0	510	2340	49	2	32	3 1/2 starch, 3 medium-fat meat, 6 fat

French Toast Platter	3 slices	1261	79	6	30	0	422	2495	110	3	44	7 1/2 starch, 3 medium-fat meat, 11 fat
French Toast Slam	2 slices	1180	75	6	27	0	760	2520	74	2	49	5 starch, 5 medium-fat meat, 9 1/2 fat
✔Grits	1 srvg	80	0	0	0	0	0	520	18	0	2	1 starch
Ham & Cheddar Omelette	1 srvg	595	47	7	16	0.5	783	1200	5	0	41	1/2 starch, 6 medium-fat meat, 3 1/2 fat
Ham & Cheddar Omelette w/ Egg Beaters	1 srvg	468	32	6	11	0	58	1351	5	0	37	1/2 starch, 5 lean meat, 3 1/2 fat
Hash Browns	1 srvg	197	12	5	2	0	0	446	20	2	2	1 starch, 2 1/2 fat
Hash Browns w/ Onions, Cheese, Gravy	1 srvg	493	25	5	9	0	29	3534	54	3	14	4 starch, 5 fat
Hash Browns w/ Cheddar Cheese	1 srvg	280	19	6	6	0	23	583	21	2	7	1 starch, 4 fat

✔ = Healthiest Bets

(Continued)

BREAKFAST *(Continued)*	Amount	Cal.	Fat (g)	% Cal. Fat	Sat. Fat (g)	Trans Fat (g)	Chol. (mg)	Sod. (mg)	Carb. (g)	Fiber (g)	Pro. (g)	Choices/Exchanges
Heartland Scramble	1 srvg	1080	63	5	22	0.5	545	2710	93	6	35	6 starch, 2 medium-fat meat, 10 fat
Lumberjack Slam w/ Hash Browns	1 srvg	1040	53	5	20	0	555	3380	84	4	47	5 1/2 starch, 4 medium-fat meat, 6 1/2 fat
Meat Lover's Scramble	1 srvg	1180	74	6	26	0.5	560	3360	78	4	47	5 starch, 4 medium-fat meat, 10 fat
Moons Over My Hammy	1 srvg	760	40	5	15	0.5	540	2490	52	2	46	3 1/2 starch, 5 lean meat, 5 fat
Original Grand Slam	1 srvg	740	43	5	12	0	505	2320	56	2	33	3 1/2 starch, 3 medium-fat meat, 5 fat
T-bone Steak & Eggs	1 srvg	991	77	7	31	0	657	1003	1	1	73	10 medium-fat meat, 5 fat
Ultimate Omelette w/ Hash Browns	1 srvg	830	62	7	19	0.5	745	1910	26	3	40	1 1/2 starch, 5 medium-fat meat, 7 1/2 fat

Veggie-Cheese Omelette w/ Egg Beaters	1 srvg	346	22	6	7	0	23	849	11	3	25	1 veg, 4 lean meat, 2 1/2 fat
Veggie-Cheese Omelette w/ Hash Browns	1 srvg	670	48	6	15	0	705	1280	28	4	30	2 starch, 3 medium-fat meat, 6 fat
BREAKFAST: A LA CARTE												
✔Applesauce	1 srvg	60	0	0	0	0	0	13	15	1	0	1 fruit
Bacon	4 strips	162	18	10	5	0	36	640	1	0	12	2 high-fat meat
Bagel, dry	1	310	1	0	0	0	0	640	65	2	11	4 starch
✔Banana	1	110	0	0	0	0	0	0	29	4	1	2 fruit
✔Biscuit	1 srvg	192	10	5	2	4	<1	519	22	0	3	1 1/2 starch, 2 fat
✔Egg Beaters Egg Substitute	1 srvg	56	0	0	0	0	0	186	2	0	11	1 lean meat
✔English Muffin, dry	1	150	2	1	0	0	0	230	27	2	5	2 starch
✔Fruit Medley	1 srvg	80	0	0	0	0	0	1	20	2	1	1 fruit

✔ = Healthiest Bets

(Continued)

BREAKFAST: A LA CARTE *(Continued)*	Amount	Cal.	Fat (g)	% Cal. Fat	Sat. Fat (g)	Trans Fat (g)	Chol. (mg)	Sod. (mg)	Carb. (g)	Fiber (g)	Pro. (g)	Choices/Exchanges
✔Grapefruit	1/2	60	0	0	0	0	0	0	16	6	1	1 fruit
✔Grapes	1 srvg	55	1	2	0	0	0	0	15	1	1	1 fruit
Ham, grilled slice, Honey Smoked	1 srvg	85	3	3	2	0	49	1700	6	0	15	2 lean meat
One Egg	1 egg	120	10	8	3	0	210	120	>1	0	6	1 medium-fat meat, 2 fat
✔Quaker Oatmeal	1 srvg	100	2	2	0	0	0	175	18	3	5	1 starch
Sausage	4 links	354	32	8	12	0	64	944	0	0	16	2 high-fat meat, 2 fat
✔Toast, dry	1 slice	90	1	1	0	0	0	166	17	1	3	1 starch
Two Eggs and More Breakfast	1 srvg	630	47	7	13	0	515	1760	21	2	31	1 1/2 starch, 4 medium-fat meat, 5 1/2 fat
BREAKFAST TOPPINGS												
Cream Cheese	1 oz.	100	10	9	6	0	31	90	1	0	2	2 fat

Maple-Flavored Syrup	3 Tbsp.	143	0	0	0	0	0	26	36	0	0	2 fruit
✔Sugar-Free Maple-Flavored Syrup	3 Tbsp.	23	0	0	0	0	0	71	9	0	0	1/2 fruit
DESSERT TOPPINGS												
✔Cherry Topping	2 oz.	57	0	0	0	0	0	3	14	0	0	1 carb
Chocolate Topping	2 oz.	133	1	1	0	0	0	109	34	1	2	2 carb
Cinnamon Apple Filling	3 oz.	90	2	2	0	0	0	70	19	1	0	1 veg
Fudge Topping	2 oz.	201	10	4	7	0	3	96	30	1	1	2 carb, 1 fat
✔Strawberry Topping	2 oz.	77	1	1	0	0	0	8	17	1	1	1 carb
✔Whipped Cream	2 Tb	23	2	8	0	0	7	3	2	0	0	1/2 fat
DESSERTS												
Apple Crisp a la mode	1 srvg	723	21	3	8	0	32	394	133	6	6	9 carb, 2 fat
Apple Pie	1 srvg	470	21	4	5	2	0	650	68	3	4	4 1/2 carb, 3 1/2 fat

✔ = Healthiest Bets

(*Continued*)

DESSERTS *(Continued)*	Amount	Cal.	Fat (g)	% Cal. Fat	Sat. Fat (g)	Trans Fat (g)	Chol. (mg)	Sod. (mg)	Carb. (g)	Fiber (g)	Pro. (g)	Choices/Exchanges
Banana Split	1 srvg	894	43	4	19	0	78	177	121	6	15	8 carb, 7 fat
Carrot Cake	1 srvg	799	45	5	13	3	125	630	99	2	9	6 1/2 carb, 7 fat
Cheesecake	1 srvg	580	38	6	24	2	174	380	51	0	8	3 1/2 carb, 7 fat
Coconut Cream Pie	1 srvg	701	32	4	20	1	1	963	100	4	4	6 1/2 carb, 5 fat
Double Scoop/ Sundae w/o Toppings	1 srvg	375	27	6	12	0	74	86	29	0	6	2 carb, 5 1/2 fat
Floats (Root Beer or Cola)	12 oz.	280	10	3	6	0	39	109	47	0	3	3 carb, 2 fat
French Silk Pie	1 srvg	737	56	7	31	0	96	353	58	2	5	4 carb, 10 fat
Hershey's Chocolate Cake	1 srvg	631	33	5	13	2	40	420	79	2	5	5 1/2 carb, 5 fat
Hot Fudge Brownie a la mode	1 srvg	997	42	4	6	3.5	14	82	147	6	12	10 carb, 6 fat
Malted Milkshake (Vanilla/ Chocolate)	12 oz.	583	26	4	16	0	100	278	82	< 1	12	5 1/2 carb, 5 fat

Milkshake (Vanilla/ Chocolate)	12 oz.	560	26	4	16	0	100	272	76	< 1	11	5 carb, 5 fat
Oreo Blender Blast Off (Kids)	10 oz.	580	29	5	15	0	87	194	72	1	11	5 carb, 2 fruit, 5 fat
Oreo Blender Blaster	15 oz.	895	46	5	23	0	135	280	112	2	16	7 1/2 carb, 9 fat
Single Scoop/ Sundae w/o Toppings	1 srvg	290	16	5	11	0	35	95	35	0	4	2 1/2 carb, 3 fat
DINNER ENTREES												
Chicken Strips	1 srvg	635	25	4	1	0	95	1510	55	0	47	3 1/2 starch, 5 lean meat, 2 fat
Country Fried Steak	1 srvg	644	46	6	10	0	89	2149	30	11	28	2 starch, 3 medium-fat meat, 6 fat
Fish & Chips	1 srvg	958	54	5	30	0	88	1390	83	6	34	5 1/2 starch, 2 lean meat, 9 fat
Grilled Chicken Dinner	1 srvg	280	5	2	4	0	135	1190	4	0	55	1/2 starch, 8 lean meat, 3 1/2 fat

✔ = Healthiest Bets

(*Continued*)

DINNER ENTREES *(Continued)*	Amount	Cal.	Fat (g)	% Cal. Fat	Sat. Fat (g)	Trans Fat (g)	Chol. (mg)	Sod. (mg)	Carb. (g)	Fiber (g)	Pro. (g)	Choices/Exchanges
Grilled Shrimp Skewers/ Pilaf/Garlic Bread	1 srvg	570	24	4	5	3	135	1750	58	3	26	4 starch, 2 lean meat, 3 1/2 fat
Grilled Tilapia Dinner	1 srvg	530	18	3	5	0	110	1720	33	1	53	2 starch, 7 lean meat
Lemon Pepper Tilapia	1 srvg	810	48	5	11	0	130	3290	38	3	55	2 1/2 starch, 7 lean meat, 5 1/2 fat
Meat Loaf Dinner	1 srvg	930	60	6	25	0	145	4400	51	2	42	3 1/2 starch, 5 medium-fat meat, 7 1/2 fat
Mushroom Swiss Chopped Steak	1 srvg	930	76	7	29	0	175	1540	13	1	46	1 starch, 6 medium-fat meat, 9 fat
Sirloin Steak & Breaded Shrimp Dinner	1 srvg	440	15	3	4	0	145	1470	23	2	52	1 1/2 starch, 5 medium-fat meat
✔Sirloin Steak Dinner	1 srvg	220	6	2	2	0	65	600	1	0	41	4 medium-fat meat
T-bone Steak Dinner	1 srvg	630	29	4	11	0	165	1110	0	0	88	9 medium-fat meat

DINNER SIDES												
✔Applesauce	1 srvg	60	0	0	0	0	0	13	15	1	0	1 fruit
✔Corn	1 srvg	110	2	2	0	0	0	180	23	3	3	2 starch, 1/2 fat
✔Cottage Cheese	1 srvg	72	3	4	2	0	10	281	2	0	9	1 milk
Mashed Potatoes, plain	1 srvg	170	7	4	3	0	10	500	23	2	3	2 starch, 1 1/2 fat
✔Sliced Tomatoes	1 srvg	13	0	0	0	0	0	6	3	1	1	1 veg
✔Vegetable Blend	1 srvg	60	4	6	0.5	0	0	50	5	1	1	1/2 fat
Vegetable Rice Pilaf	1 srvg	173	3	2	1	0	0	1033	33	1	4	2 starch, 1/2 fat
FIT FARE: DINNER												
Grilled Chicken Breast Dinner w/ Vegetables	1 srvg	390	11	3	2	0	135	1270	12	2	57	2 veg, 7 lean meat
Tilapia/ Rice/ Vegetable Blend/Tomato Slices	1 srvg	420	13	3	3	0	50	1190	40	5	34	2 1/2 starch, 4 lean meat, 1/2 fat

✔ = Healthiest Bets

(Continued)

	Amount	Cal.	Fat (g)	% Cal. Fat	Sat. Fat (g)	Trans Fat (g)	Chol. (mg)	Sod. (mg)	Carb. (g)	Fiber (g)	Pro. (g)	Choices/Exchanges
KID'S MENU												
✔Applesauce	1 srvg	84	0	0	0	0	0	38	19	1	0	1 fruit
Brownie	1 srvg	344	16	4	4	1.5	25	245	49	2	4	3 1/2 carb, 2 1/2 fat
✔Cheeseburger	1 srvg	341	20	5	6	1	40	580	24	1	15	1 1/2 starch, 1 medium-fat meat, 2 1/2 fat
✔Chicken Nuggets	1 srvg	190	13	6	4	0	30	340	9	0	9	1/2 starch, 1 lean meat, 2 fat
Deep-Sea Salad w/ Ranch	1 srvg	240	20	8	3	0	16	359	13	1	3	2 veg, 4 fat
French Toastix	1 srvg	627	71	10	13	0	190	1068	71	1	18	5 starch, 14 fat
✔Goldfish Galaxy	1 srvg	284	3	1	9	0	473	36	0	0	0	Free
✔Grapes	1 srvg	60	0	0	0	0	0	2	15	1	0	1 fruit
✔Grilled Cheese	1 srvg	334	20	5	2	0.5	24	828	28	2	9	2 starch, 4 fat

Hotcakes w/ meat	1 srvg	340	12	3	5	0	45	1060	49	1	9	3 1/2 starch, 2 1/2 fat
✔Hotcakes w/o meat	1 srvg	230	3	1	0.5	0	0	710	47	1	5	3 starch, 1/2 fat
Junior Grand Slam	1 srvg	400	21	5	7	0	240	900	38	1	16	2 1/2 starch, 1 medium-fat meat, 3 fat
Little Dippers w/ Apple-sauce & Marinara	1 srvg	566	27	4	13	0	22	1504	50	5	27	3 starch, 1 fruit, 5 1/2 fat
Little Dippers w/ Marinara & Fries	1 srvg	860	43	5	17	1.5	22	1679	80	8	32	5 1/2 starch, 2 medium-fat meat, 6 1/2 fat
Macaroni & Cheese	1 srvg	353	13	3	4	0	19	651	48	2	12	3 starch, 2 1/2 fat
✔Moon Crater Mashed w/ Brown Gravy	1 srvg	145	6	4	2	0.5	6	557	20	2	3	1 1/2 starch, 1 fat
✔Pizza	1 srvg	331	14	4	5	0	16	514	38	2	13	2 1/2 starch, 1 medium-fat meat, 2 fat
Sundae	1 srvg	413	19	4	9	0	44	111	59	2	6	4 carb, 3 fat

✔ = Healthiest Bets

(*Continued*)

	Amount	Cal.	Fat (g)	% Cal. Fat	Sat. Fat (g)	Trans Fat (g)	Chol. (mg)	Sod. (mg)	Carb. (g)	Fiber (g)	Pro. (g)	Choices/Exchanges
LUNCH SIDES												
Coleslaw	1 srvg	260	22	8	3.5	0	35	520	15	3	2	1/2 starch, 1 veg, 4 fat
French Fries, unsalted	1 srvg	423	20	4	5	3	0	221	57	5	6	4 starch, 3 1/2 fat
Onion Rings	1 srvg	381	23	5	6	0	6	1003	38	1	5	3 starch, 4 fat
Seasoned Fries	1 srvg	460	28	5	6	8	0	880	46	4	4	3 starch, 5 fat
OTHER SIDES												
✔BBQ Sauce	1.5 oz.	47	1	2	0	0	0	595	11	0	0	1/2 carb
Butter Roll	2 pcs	260	9	3	0.5	5	10	330	38	1	5	3 starch, 2 fat
Croutons (for salad)	1 srvg	112	6	5	0	1	0	195	12	1	2	1 starch, 1/2 fat
Garlic Dinner Bread	2 pcs	170	11	6	1	2	0	325	15	1	2	1 starch, 2 fat
✔Pico de Gallo	1 srvg	21	0	0	0	0	0	125	5	1	1	1 veg
Sour Cream	1.5 oz.	91	9	9	0	6	19	23	2	0	1	2 fat

✔Whipped Margarine	1 Tbsp.	40	5	11	1	0.5	0	30	0	0	0	1 fat
SALAD DRESSING												
Blue Cheese Dressing	1 oz.	163	18	10	0	3	20	205	1	0	1	3 1/2 fat
Caesar Dressing	1 oz.	133	14	9	0	2	2	380	1	0	1	3 fat
✔Fat-Free Italian	1 oz.	15	0.5	3	0	0	0	390	3	0	0	Free
✔Fat-Free Ranch Dressing	1 oz.	25	0.2	1	0	0	0	300	6	0	0.1	1/2 carb
✔French Dressing	1 oz.	106	10	8	0	2	7	274	3	0	0	2 fat
Honey Mustard Dressing	1 oz.	160	15	8	0	8	20	123	20	0	0	1 1/2 carb, 2 fat
Ranch Dressing	1 oz.	129	14	10	0	2	8	189	1	0	0	3 fat
Thousand Island Dressing	1 oz.	118	11	8	0	2	15	170	5	0	0	1/2 carb, 2 fat
SALADS												
Fried Chicken Strip Salad	1 srvg	438	26	5	6	0	78	1030	26	4	33	1 starch, 2 veg, 4 lean meat, 2 fat

✔ = Healthiest Bets

(Continued)

SALADS *(Continued)*	Amount	Cal.	Fat (g)	% Cal. Fat	Sat. Fat (g)	Trans Fat (g)	Chol. (mg)	Sod. (mg)	Carb. (g)	Fiber (g)	Pro. (g)	Choices/Exchanges
✔Grilled Chicken Breast Salad	1 srvg	259	11	4	5	0	90	724	10	4	32	2 veg, 4 lean meat
Side Garden Salad w/o Dressing	1 srvg	113	7	6	5	0	0	144	6	2	7	1 veg
✔Turkey Breast Salad w/o Dressing	1 srvg	248	8	3	4	0	86	798	12	4	31	2 veg, 3 lean meat
SANDWICHES												
Bacon Cheddar Burger	1 srvg	970	70	6	31	3.5	225	2250	33	4	56	2 starch, 7 medium-fat meat, 6 fat
Bacon, Lettuce, & Tomato	1 srvg	570	37	6	9	0.5	55	850	36	5	20	2 1/2 starch, 3 high-fat meat, 2 1/2 fat
Boca Burger	1 srvg	510	16	3	3.5	0	15	1220	64	9	31	4 1/2 starch, 3 lean meat, 1 fat

Boca Burger w/ Small Fruit Bowl	1 srvg	570	11	2	3.5	0	10	1070	83	23	34	4 starch, 1 fruit, 3 lean meat
Chicken Ranch Melt	1 srvg	920	42	4	11	0	115	2800	79	4	53	5 1/2 starch, 5 lean meat, 5 fat
Classic Burger	1 srvg	780	45	5	17	2.5	125	1550	56	5	39	3 1/2 starch, 4 medium-fat meat, 4 fat
Classic Burger w/ Cheese	1 srvg	940	59	6	26	2.5	165	2180	56	5	49	3 1/2 starch, 5 medium-fat meat, 5 1/2 fat
Club Sandwich	1 srvg	658	34	5	7	0.5	60	1640	55	4	29	3 1/2 starch, 3 medium-fat meat, 4 fat
Grilled Chicken Sandwich w/o Dressing	1 srvg	490	13	2	2.5	0	80	1510	57	4	39	4 starch, 4 lean meat
Mushroom Swiss Burger	1 srvg	900	55	6	22	3.5	150	1990	62	5	46	4 starch, 5 medium-fat meat, 5 1/2 fat
Philly Melt	1 srvg	740	43	5	13	0	95	1650	51	3	40	3 1/2 starch, 4 medium-fat meat, 4 fat

✔ = Healthiest Bets

(*Continued*)

SANDWICHES *(Continued)*	Amount	Cal.	Fat (g)	% Cal. Fat	Sat. Fat (g)	Trans Fat (g)	Chol. (mg)	Sod. (mg)	Carb. (g)	Fiber (g)	Pro. (g)	Choices/Exchanges
Spicy Buffalo Chicken Melt	1 srvg	930	46	4	12	4	100	3700	79	4	46	5 1/2 starch, 4 lean meat, 6 1/2 fat
Super Bird Sandwich	1 srvg	570	27	4	9	0	55	1800	43	2	38	3 starch, 4 medium-fat meat, 1 fat
Western Burger w/ Fries	1 srvg	1580	95	5	33	6	190	2780	122	10	61	8 starch, 5 medium-fat meat, 12 fat
SENIORS' MENU												
Bacon Cheddar Burger w/ Fries	1 srvg	433	25	5	8	3	57	608	27	2	24	2 starch, 3 medium-fat meat, 2 1/2 fat
Belgian Waffle Slam	1 srvg	580	41	6	20	0	485	1170	29	1	23	2 starch, 2 medium-fat meat, 5 1/2 fat
Country Fried Steak	1 srvg	341	23	6	5	0	44	1464	18	6	14	1 starch, 1 medium-fat meat, 3 fat

Fish & Chips w/ Coleslaw	1 srvg	756	47	6	35	0	67	1116	64	6	20	4 1/2 starch, 1 lean meat, 9 fat
French Toast Slam	1 srvg	591	43	7	15	0	378	690	37	1	22	2 1/2 starch, 2 medium-fat meat, 6 fat
Grilled Cheese Sandwich	1 srvg	540	30	5	12	0.5	45	1540	50	2	17	3 1/2 starch, 1 medium-fat meat, 5 fat
✔Grilled Chicken Breast	1 srvg	200	5	2	1	0	67	824	15	1	25	1 starch, 2 lean meat
✔Grilled Tilapia	1 srvg	248	10	4	3	0	201	180	0	0	39	5 lean meat
Homestyle Meatloaf	1 srvg	570	42	7	14	2	170	2450	18	0	27	1 starch, 3 medium-fat meat, 5 fat
Lemon Pepper Tilapia	1 srvg	509	41	7	9	0	104	1821	6	1	33	1/2 starch, 5 lean meat, 5 1/2 fat
Omelette w/ Hash Browns/Toast	1 srvg	760	55	7	19	0.5	515	755	36	4	32	2 1/2 starch, 4 medium-fat meat, 7 1/2 fat

✔ = Healthiest Bets

(*Continued*)

SENIORS' MENU *(Continued)*	Amount	Cal.	Fat (g)	% Cal. Fat	Sat. Fat (g)	Trans Fat (g)	Chol. (mg)	Sod. (mg)	Carb. (g)	Fiber (g)	Pro. (g)	Choices/Exchanges
Scrambled Eggs & Cheddar	1 srvg	790	46	5	16	0	575	2290	56	2	39	3 1/2 starch, 4 medium-fat meat, 4 1/2 fat
Senior Club	1 srvg	570	33	5	5	0.5	60	1660	40	3	27	2 1/2 starch, 3 medium-fat meat, 4 fat
Senior Starter w/ Hash Browns/Biscuit	1 srvg	410	42	9	11	0	245	631	23	2	16	1 1/2 starch, 2 medium-fat meat, 4 1/2 fat
SOUPS												
✔Chicken Noodle	1 srvg	170	9	5	2	1	70	340	14	0	10	1 starch, 2 fat
Clam Chowder	1 srvg	170	11	6	3	3	15	290	13	0	4	1 starch, 1 milk, 1 fat
Tomato Basil	1 srvg	240	15	6	10	0	40	1610	21	3	4	1/2 starch, 2 veg, 3 fat
✔Vegetable Beef	1 srvg	140	5	3	0	0	10	1290	17	3	7	1 starch, 1 fat

✔ = Healthiest Bets

Romano's Macaroni Grill

(www.macaronigrill.com)

Light 'n Lean Choice

Pollo Magro "Skinny Chicken"
Garden della Casa *(House)*
with Low-Fat Caesar *(1 oz, 2 Tbsp)*

Calories	490	Cholesterol (mg)	na
Fat (g)	12	Sodium (mg)	1,570
% calories from fat	22	Carbohydrate (g)	48
Saturated fat (g)	3	Fiber (g)	8
Trans fat (g)	na	Protein (g)	49

Exchanges: 2 starch, 3 veg, 4 lean meat, 1 1/2 fat

Healthy 'n Hearty Choice

Mama's Trio *(1/2 serving)*
Caesar della Casa *(House)*
with Low-Fat Caesar *(1 oz, 2 Tbsp)*

Calories	785	Cholesterol (mg)	na
Fat (g)	41	Sodium (mg)	2,360
% calories from fat	47	Carbohydrate (g)	53
Saturated fat (g)	21	Fiber (g)	4
Trans fat (g)	na	Protein (g)	50

Exchanges: 2 1/2 starch, 3 veg, 5 medium-fat meat, 2 1/2 fat

(Continued)

Romano's Macaroni Grill

	Amount	Cal.	Fat (g)	% Cal. Fat	Sat. Fat (g)	Trans Fat (g)	Chol. (mg)	Sod. (mg)	Carb. (g)	Fiber (g)	Pro. (g)	Choices/Exchanges
AMORE DE LA GRILL - LISTED W/ SIDES												
Boursin Filet	1 srvg	930	63	6	26	na	na	2920	39	5	52	2 1/2 starch, 6 medium-fat meat, 6 fat
Chicken Portobello	1 srvg	1020	66	6	11	na	na	2760	61	5	46	3 starch, 2 veg, 5 lean meat, 11 fat
Chicken Sorrentino	1 srvg	1050	46	4	10	na	na	1660	85	6	72	5 1/2 starch, 8 lean meat, 4 fat
Grilled Halibut	1 srvg	830	43	5	12	na	na	1440	56	2	52	3 1/2 starch, 6 lean meat, 5 fat
Grilled Pork Chops	1 srvg	1940	111	5	44	na	na	4980	93	8	114	6 starch, 14 medium-fat meat, 9 fat
Grilled Salmon (Teriyaki)	1 srvg	1230	74	5	9	na	na	6590	79	5	56	5 1/2 starch, 6 lean meat, 11 fat

Honey Balsamic Chicken	1 srvg	1190	59	4	10	na	na	1580	94	10	68	6 1/2 starch, 7 lean meat, 7 fat
✔Pollo Magro Skinny Chicken	1 srvg	330	5	1	1	na	na	770	29	5	42	2 starch, 4 lean meat
Simple Salmon	1 srvg	600	42	6	7	na	na	2340	18	8	51	1 starch, 7 lean meat, 4 fat
Tuscan Ribeye	1 srvg	1000	66	6	23	na	na	5180	40	6	58	2 1/2 starch, 7 medium-fat meat, 6 fat
ANTIPASTI												
Calamari Fritti	1 srvg	1210	78	6	13	na	na	4170	66	4	62	4 1/2 starch, 7 lean meat, 11 fat
Crab Stuffed Mushrooms	1 srvg	750	38	5	10	na	na	1000	71	12	32	4 1/2 starch, 3 lean meat, 5 fat
Mozzarella Fritta	1 srvg	880	63	6	18	na	na	1770	54	3	24	3 1/2 starch, 2 medium-fat meat, 10 fat

✔ = Healthiest Bets; na = not available

(*Continued*)

ANTIPASTI *(Continued)*	Amount	Cal.	Fat (g)	% Cal. Fat	Sat. Fat (g)	Trans Fat (g)	Chol. (mg)	Sod. (mg)	Carb. (g)	Fiber (g)	Pro. (g)	Choices/Exchanges
Parmesan Crusted Artichokes	1 srvg	820	62	7	18	na	na	1570	40	6	27	2 1/2 starch, 3 medium-fat meat, 9 fat
Peasant Bread	1 loaf	520	11	2	0	na	na	2140	89	4	14	6 starch, 2 fat
Romano's Sampler - Fried Calamari Only	1 srvg	670	29	4	5	na	na	2060	59	3	39	4 starch, 4 lean meat, 3 fat
Romano's Sampler - Fried Mozzarella Only	1 srvg	480	32	6	10	na	na	770	32	1	15	2 starch, 1 medium-fat meat, 5 fat
Romano's Sampler - Garnish Only	1 srvg	60	4	6	1	na	na	370	4	1	1	1/2 starch, 1 fat
Romano's Sampler - Tomato Bruschetta Only	1 srvg	450	33	7	5	na	na	820	31	2	8	2 starch, 6 1/2 fat
Romano's Sampler (All 3)	1 srvg	1640	98	5	22	na	na	4000	126	7	62	8 1/2 starch, 5 medium-fat meat, 14 fat
Shrimp & Artichoke Dip w/ Romano Croutons	1 srvg	980	52	5	24	na	na	3350	88	7	43	6 starch, 4 lean meat, 7 fat

Tomato Bruschetta	1 srvg	1000	70	6	11	na	na	1810	75	6	17	5 starch, 14 fat
BRICK-OVEN PIZZA												
BBQ Chicken Pizza	whole pizza	970	24	2	14	na	na	2700	135	6	48	9 starch, 3 lean meat, 2 fat
Pesto Chicken Pizza	whole pizza	1940	101	5	34	na	na	3000	163	18	97	11 starch, 9 medium-fat meat, 9 fat
Pizza Margherita	whole pizza	1010	34	3	18	na	na	2070	123	7	49	8 starch, 3 medium-fat meat, 3 fat
Sicilian Pizza	whole pizza	1450	70	4	36	na	na	3520	124	7	75	8 1/2 starch, 7 medium-fat meat, 6 fat
CLASICO ITALIAN												
Chicken & Shrimp Scaloppine, Dinner	1 srvg	1380	97	6	36	na	na	3410	68	6	45	4 1/2 starch, 4 lean meat, 17 fat
Chicken & Shrimp Scaloppine, Lunch	1 srvg	1260	89	6	34	na	na	3150	66	6	38	4 1/2 starch, 4 lean meat, 15 1/2 fat

✔ = Healthiest Bets; na = not available

(*Continued*)

CLASICO ITALIAN *(Continued)*	Amount	Cal.	Fat (g)	% Cal. Fat	Sat. Fat (g)	Trans Fat (g)	Chol. (mg)	Sod. (mg)	Carb. (g)	Fiber (g)	Pro. (g)	Choices/Exchanges
Chicken Marsala, Dinner	1 srvg	1090	66	5	23	na	na	2060	76	4	33	5 starch, 3 lean meat, 12 fat
Chicken Marsala, Lunch	1 srvg	980	59	5	22	na	na	1820	73	4	26	5 starch, 2 lean meat, 11 fat
Chicken Scaloppini, Dinner	1 srvg	1110	71	6	30	na	na	2870	68	6	42	4 1/2 starch, 4 lean meat, 12 fat
Chicken Scaloppini, Lunch	1 srvg	1010	64	6	28	na	na	2650	65	6	35	4 1/2 starch, 3 lean meat, 11 fat
Eggplant Parmesan, Dinner	1 srvg	1240	64	5	36	na	na	2560	118	23	45	8 starch, 3 medium-fat meat, 9 fat
Eggplant Parmesan, Lunch	1 srvg	1080	57	5	33	na	na	2170	102	17	40	7 starch, 3 medium-fat meat, 9 fat
Fettuccine Alfredo	1 srvg	1130	81	6	53	na	na	1120	68	4	28	4 1/2 starch, 2 medium-fat meat, 14 fat

Fettuccine Alfredo w/ Chicken	1 srvg	1370	97	6	57	na	na	1260	68	4	51	4 1/2 starch, 5 lean meat, 16 fat
Fettuccine Alfredo w/ Shrimp	1 srvg	1320	95	6	56	na	na	1300	70	4	43	4 1/2 starch, 4 lean meat, 16 fat
Layers & Layers of Lasagna, Dinner	1 srvg	1680	87	5	41	na	na	4290	120	9	100	8 starch, 11 medium-fat meat, 6 fat
Layers & Layers of Lasagna, Lunch	1 srvg	890	47	5	23	na	na	2250	61	4	53	4 starch, 6 medium-fat meat, 3 fat
Mama's Trio	1 srvg	1290	69	5	38	na	na	3260	81	4	86	5 1/2 starch, 10 medium-fat meat, 3 fat
Parmesan Crusted Sole, Dinner	1 srvg	2170	135	6	54	na	na	3530	148	9	83	10 starch, 8 lean meat, 22 fat
Parmesan Crusted Sole, Lunch	1 srvg	1800	129	6	52	na	na	3220	106	7	47	7 starch, 4 lean meat, 23 fat
Primo Chicken Parmesan, Dinner	1 srvg	2220	148	6	52	na	na	4440	126	5	90	8 1/2 starch, 9 lean meat, 23 fat

✔ = Healthiest Bets; na = not available

(*Continued*)

CLASICO ITALIAN *(Continued)*	Amount	Cal.	Fat (g)	% Cal. Fat	Sat. Fat (g)	Trans Fat (g)	Chol. (mg)	Sod. (mg)	Carb. (g)	Fiber (g)	Pro. (g)	Choices/Exchanges
Primo Chicken Parmesan, Lunch	1 srvg	1380	86	6	29	na	na	2710	89	4	51	6 starch, 5 lean meat, 14 fat
Spaghetti & Meat Sauce, Dinner	1 srvg	1110	63	5	35	na	na	2380	87	8	44	6 starch, 4 medium-fat meat, 9 fat
Spaghetti & Meat Sauce, Lunch	1 srvg	830	46	5	25	na	na	1830	66	6	35	4 1/2 starch, 3 medium-fat meat, 6 fat
Spaghetti & Meatballs w/ Meat Sauce, Dinner	1 srvg	2430	128	5	57	na	na	5290	207	14	96	14 starch, 8 medium-fat meat, 17 fat
Spaghetti & Meatballs w/ Meat Sauce, Lunch	1 srvg	1290	79	6	39	na	na	3590	84	8	59	5 1/2 starch, 6 medium-fat meat, 9 fat
Spaghetti & Meatballs w/ Tomato Sauce, Dinner	1 srvg	1430	81	5	41	na	na	4540	119	11	56	8 starch, 5 medium-fat meat, 11 fat
Spaghetti & Meatballs w/ Tomato Sauce, Lunch	1 srvg	1080	63	5	34	na	na	3350	89	8	40	6 starch, 3 medium-fat meat, 9 fat

Spaghetti & Stuffed Meatballs, w/ Meat Sauce, Dinner	1 srvg	2080	102	4	47	na	na	3770	191	13	83	12 1/2 starch, 6 medium-fat meat, 13 fat
Spaghetti & Stuffed Meatballs, w/ Meat Sauce, Lunch	1 srvg	1060	61	5	32	na	na	2570	73	7	51	5 starch, 5 medium-fat meat, 7 fat
Spaghetti & Stuffed Meatballs, w/ Red Sauce, Dinner	1 srvg	1760	74	4	34	na	na	3420	196	12	63	13 starch, 3 medium-fat meat, 11 fat
Spaghetti & Stuffed Meatballs, w/ Red Sauce, Lunch	1 srvg	900	49	5	29	na	na	2460	79	7	36	5 1/2 starch, 3 medium-fat meat, 6 fat
Veal Marsala	1 srvg	1320	66	5	36	na	na	3160	132	4	39	9 starch, 2 medium-fat meat, 11 fat
Veal Parmesan	1 srvg	1270	64	5	44	na	na	2660	116	6	56	7 1/2 starch, 5 medium-fat meat, 7 fat

✔ = Healthiest Bets; na = not available

(*Continued*)

	Amount	Cal.	Fat (g)	% Cal. Fat	Sat. Fat (g)	Trans Fat (g)	Chol. (mg)	Sod. (mg)	Carb. (g)	Fiber (g)	Pro. (g)	Choices/Exchanges
DESSERTS												
Amaretto Apple Crispetti	1 srvg	1300	45	3	28	na	na	570	218	3	10	14 1/2 carb, 7 fat
Dessert Ravioli	1 srvg	1630	74	4	33	na	na	1150	223	3	19	15 carb, 13 fat
Italian Sorbetto w/ Biscotti	1 srvg	330	4	1	2	na	na	80	71	0	2	4 1/2 carb, 1 fat
Lemon Passion	1 srvg	1150	56	4	29	na	na	910	149	0	17	10 carb, 10 fat
New York Cheesecake	1 srvg	980	69	6	41	na	na	620	75	0	16	5 carb, 14 fat
New York Cheesecake w/ Caramel Fudge Sauce	1 srvg	1610	96	5	54	na	na	960	169	1	21	11 1/2 carb, 18 fat
Smothered Chocolate Cake	1 srvg	1180	68	5	30	na	na	930	140	6	15	9 1/2 carb, 12 fat
Three Berry Tiramisu	1 srvg	930	70	7	38	na	na	260	65	2	12	4 carb, 1 fruit, 13 fat
Tiramisu	1 srvg	1000	64	6	36	na	na	160	89	1	12	6 carb, 12 fat

Vanilla Ice Cream w/ Chocolate Sauce (Kid's)	1 scoop	400	23	5	14	na	na	100	43	0	3	3 carb, 4 fat
DRESSINGS												
✔Balsamic Vinaigrette	1 oz.	100	9	8	1	na	na	320	2	0	0	2 1/2 fat
Caesar	1 oz.	160	16	9	3	na	na	260	1	0	1	3 1/2 fat
Cider Vinaigrette	1 oz.	140	11	7	2	na	na	30	9	0	0	1/2 carb, 2 fat
Creamy Italian	1 oz.	110	10	8	2	na	na	450	5	0	0	1/2 carb, 2 fat
✔Fat-Free Creamy Italian	1 oz.	30	0	0	0	na	na	440	5	1	0	1/2 carb
Honey Mustard	1 oz.	130	12	8	2	na	na	170	6	0	0	1/2 carb, 2 1/2 fat
✔Italian	1 oz.	90	8	8	1	na	na	470	2	0	0	2 fat
✔Low-Fat Caesar	1 oz.	30	2	6	0	na	na	340	4	0	1	1/2 fat
✔Parmesan Peppercorn Ranch	1 oz.	90	9	9	2	na	na	150	1	0	2	2 fat

✔ = Healthiest Bets; na = not available

(*Continued*)

DRESSINGS *(Continued)*	Amount	Cal.	Fat (g)	% Cal. Fat	Sat. Fat (g)	Trans Fat (g)	Chol. (mg)	Sod. (mg)	Carb. (g)	Fiber (g)	Pro. (g)	Choices/Exchanges
Roasted Garlic Lemon Vinaigrette	1 oz.	170	17	9	3	na	na	120	4	0	0	1/2 carb, 3 1/2 fat
Toscana	1 oz.	160	17	10	3	na	na	380	1	0	0	3 1/2 fat
INSALATA (SALADS)												
Caesar della Casa (House)	1	260	21	7	4	na	na	650	13	2	6	3 veg, 4 fat
✔Caesar della Casa (House) w/o Dressing	1	110	5	4	2	na	na	390	12	2	6	3 veg, 1 fat
Chicken Caesar	1	920	69	7	16	na	na	1660	24	6	54	1 starch, 3 veg, 7 lean meat, 9 fat
✔Chicken Caesar w/o Dressing	1	464	20	4	8	na	na	890	20	6	51	1/2 starch, 3 veg, 7 lean meat
Chicken Florentine	1	840	53	6	8	na	na	5460	62	7	33	3 starch, 3 veg, 3 lean meat, 8 fat
Chicken Florentine w/o Dressing	1	490	19	3	3	na	na	4940	50	7	33	2 starch, 3 veg, 4 lean meat, 1 1/2 fat

Garden della Casa (House)	1	240	15	6	3	na	na	900	20	3	6	1/2 starch, 3 veg, 3 fat
✔Garden della Casa (House) w/o Dressing	1	130	5	3	2	na	na	460	15	3	6	3 veg, 1 fat
Insalata Blu	1	640	53	7	14	na	na	1590	13	5	18	1/2 starch, 2 veg, 2 medium-fat meat, 8 fat
Insalata Blu w/ Chicken	1	760	56	7	15	na	na	1650	13	5	41	1/2 starch, 2 veg, 6 lean meat, 8 fat
Insalata Blu w/ Chicken, w/o Dressing	1	570	38	6	12	na	na	1020	9	5	41	2 veg, 6 lean meat, 4 1/2 fat
Insalata Blu w/ Steak	1	830	62	7	18	na	na	1950	13	5	48	1/2 starch, 2 veg, 7 medium-fat meat, 6 fat
Insalata Blu w/ Steak, w/o Dressing	1	640	44	6	15	na	na	1320	9	5	48	2 veg, 7 medium-fat meat, 2 fat
Insalata Blu w/o Dressing	1	440	36	7	12	na	na	970	9	5	18	2 veg, 3 medium-fat meat, 4 1/2 fat

✔ = Healthiest Bets; na = not available

(*Continued*)

INSALATA (SALADS) *(Continued)*	Amount	Cal.	Fat (g)	% Cal. Fat	Sat. Fat (g)	Trans Fat (g)	Chol. (mg)	Sod. (mg)	Carb. (g)	Fiber (g)	Pro. (g)	Choices/Exchanges
Mozzarella Alla Caprese, full order	5 each	450	36	7	12	na	na	760	9	2	19	2 veg, 3 lean meat, 5 1/2 fat
Mozzarella Alla Caprese, half order	3 each	260	21	7	7	na	na	410	5	1	11	1 veg, 2 lean meat, 3 1/2 fat
Parmesan-Crusted Chicken	1	1190	63	5	17	na	na	3230	60	5	91	3 starch, 3 veg, 12 lean meat, 5 fat
Parmesan-Crusted Chicken w/o Dressing	1	1060	49	4	15	na	na	2880	59	5	88	3 starch, 3 veg, 11 lean meat, 3 fat
Seared Sea Scallops	1	1320	91	6	25	na	na	2860	40	6	80	2 starch, 3 veg, 11 lean meat, 12 fat
Seared Sea Scallops w/o Dressing	1	1050	68	6	22	na	na	2810	22	6	81	1/2 starch, 3 veg, 11 lean meat, 7 fat
KID'S												
Chicken Fingerias only	1 srvg	650	45	6	7	na	na	1790	39	1	23	2 1/2 starch, 2 lean meat, 7 fat

Fettuccine Alfredo	1 srvg	580	30	5	17	na	na	1430	53	3	23	3 1/2 starch, 2 medium-fat meat, 4 fat
✔Grilled Chicken & Broccoli	1 srvg	390	5	1	2	na	na	560	51	6	33	3 starch, 1 veg, 2 lean meat
Macaroni 'n' Cheese	1 srvg	600	31	5	20	na	na	1720	54	3	34	3 1/2 starch, 3 medium-fat meat, 2 fat
Mona Lisa's Cheese Masterpizza	1 srvg	840	20	2	13	na	na	1870	120	6	41	8 starch, 2 medium-fat meat, 1 fat
Mona Lisa's Pepperoni Masterpizza	1 srvg	920	27	3	16	na	na	2140	120	6	44	8 starch, 3 medium-fat meat, 2 fat
Spaghetti & Meatballs w/ Meat Sauce	1 srvg	550	24	4	10	na	na	1550	56	4	27	3 1/2 starch, 2 medium-fat meat, 2 fat
Spaghetti & Meatballs w/ Tomato Sauce	1 srvg	500	20	4	8	na	na	1520	58	4	22	4 starch, 1 medium-fat meat, 2 fat

✔ = Healthiest Bets; na = not available

(*Continued*)

	Amount	Cal.	Fat (g)	% Cal. Fat	Sat. Fat (g)	Trans Fat (g)	Chol. (mg)	Sod. (mg)	Carb. (g)	Fiber (g)	Pro. (g)	Choices/Exchanges
KID'S SIDES												
Caesar della Casa w/ Caesar Dressing	1 side	170	12	6	3	na	na	460	11	2	4	2 veg, 3 fat
Garden della Casa w/ Creamy Italian Dressing	1 side	120	8	6	2	na	na	390	9	1	3	2 veg, 1 1/2 fat
✔Grilled Asparagus	1 side	40	2	5	0	na	na	590	4	2	2	1 veg, 1/2 fat
✔Grilled Broccoli	1 side	80	3	3	0	na	na	320	11	5	3	2 veg, 1/2 fat
Shoestring Fries	1 side	250	15	5	3	na	na	690	27	2	3	2 starch, 3 fat
OVER STUFFED PASTA												
Chicken Cannelloni - Dinner	1 srvg	1080	58	5	36	na	na	3050	62	4	73	4 starch, 9 lean meat, 6 fat
Chicken Cannelloni - Lunch	1 srvg	720	39	5	24	na	na	2050	42	3	49	3 starch, 6 lean meat, 4 fat

Lobster Ravioli	1 srvg	1090	78	6	54	na	na	1910	55	4	36	3 1/2 starch, 4 medium-fat meat, 12 fat
Marsala Chicken Ravioli	1 srvg	1300	85	6	35	na	na	2100	55	3	64	3 1/2 starch, 8 lean meat, 13 fat
Mushroom Ravioli	1 srvg	990	67	6	28	na	na	1510	57	4	27	3 starch, 2 veg, 3 lean meat, 12 1/2 fat
PASTA DI PRIMA												
Carmela's Chicken Rigatoni - Dinner	1 srvg	1320	85	6	35	na	na	1540	84	6	36	5 1/2 starch, 3 lean meat, 16 fat
Carmela's Chicken Rigatoni - Lunch	1 srvg	1030	64	6	27	na	na	1270	64	5	32	4 1/2 starch, 3 lean meat, 11 fat
Pasta Milano - Dinner	1 srvg	1120	57	5	22	na	na	2110	108	13	46	7 starch, 3 medium-fat meat, 7 fat
Pasta Milano - Lunch	1 srvg	920	48	5	17	na	na	1630	83	10	40	5 1/2 starch, 3 medium-fat meat, 5 fat

✔ = Healthiest Bets; na = not available

(*Continued*)

PASTA DI PRIMA *(Continued)*	Amount	Cal.	Fat (g)	% Cal. Fat	Sat. Fat (g)	Trans Fat (g)	Chol. (mg)	Sod. (mg)	Carb. (g)	Fiber (g)	Pro. (g)	Choices/Exchanges
Penne Rustica - Dinner	1 srvg	1540	80	5	39	na	na	3360	101	9	92	6 1/2 starch, 10 medium-fat meat, 5 fat
Penne Rustica - Lunch	1 srvg	1300	71	5	33	na	na	2900	76	6	79	5 starch, 9 medium-fat meat, 5 fat
Penne w/ Oven Roasted Chicken	1 srvg	1330	80	5	21	na	na	2690	83	8	60	5 1/2 starch, 6 lean meat, 12 1/2 fat
Seafood Linguine	1 srvg	1130	71	6	23	na	na	1940	79	6	38	5 1/2 starch, 3 lean meat, 12 fat
Shrimp Portofino - Dinner	1 srvg	1110	78	6	29	na	na	1940	66	5	35	4 1/2 starch, 3 lean meat, 13 fat
Shrimp Portofino - Lunch	1 srvg	1070	78	7	29	na	na	1890	66	5	29	4 1/2 starch, 2 lean meat, 13 fat
Sizzling Shrimp Scampi	1 srvg	1380	97	6	44	na	na	2510	94	7	20	6 1/2 starch, 19 1/2 fat

Vodka Rustica	1 srvg	1160	58	5	24	na	na	2650	77	6	59	5 starch, 6 medium-fat meat, 6 fat
SANDWICHES												
Brick-Oven Meatball Sandwich	1	1890	115	5	38	na	na	4660	149	10	62	10 starch, 5 medium-fat meat, 18 fat
Chicken Caesar Calzonetto	1	1540	88	5	23	na	na	3740	124	8	65	8 1/2 starch, 6 lean meat, 13 fat
Roasted Chicken & Cheese Sandwich	1	1630	91	5	23	na	na	2520	128	8	68	8 1/2 starch, 6 lean meat, 14 fat
SAUCES												
Basil Aioli	1 oz.	130	14	10	2	na	na	200	1	0	2	3 fat
✔Pizzaiola	1 oz.	30	2	6	0	na	na	190	2	0	0	1/2 fat
SIGNATURE SIDES												
Garlic Mashed Potatoes	1 srvg	280	14	5	3	na	na	640	35	3	3	2 1/2 starch, 3 fat
✔Grilled Asparagus	1 srvg	30	1	3	0	na	na	590	4	2	2	1 veg

✔ = Healthiest Bets; na = not available

(*Continued*)

SIGNATURE SIDES *(Continued)*	Amount	Cal.	Fat (g)	% Cal. Fat	Sat. Fat (g)	Trans Fat (g)	Chol. (mg)	Sod. (mg)	Carb. (g)	Fiber (g)	Pro. (g)	Choices/Exchanges
Pasta Salad	1 srvg	460	16	3	2	na	na	380	69	4	12	4 1/2 starch, 3 fat
Romano's Parmesan Chips	1 srvg	660	51	7	11	na	na	390	39	3	8	2 1/2 starch, 10 fat
Sautéed Broccoli	1 srvg	260	22	8	4	na	na	350	12	5	4	2 veg, 4 1/2 fat
SIGNATURE SOUPS												
Chicken Toscana Soup	1 cup	260	16	6	8	na	na	1640	18	1	11	1 starch, 1 lean meat, 2 1/2 fat
Chicken Toscana Soup	1 bowl	510	32	6	15	na	na	3240	36	2	21	2 1/2 starch, 2 lean meat, 5 fat
Italian Wedding Soup	1 bowl	370	21	5	8	na	na	3120	26	3	20	1 1/2 starch, 2 lean meat, 3 fat
Italian Wedding Soup	1 cup	190	11	5	4.5	na	na	1570	13	2	10	1 starch, 1 lean meat, 1 1/2 fat

✓ = Healthiest Bets; na = not available

Soups, Sandwiches, Salads, and Subs

RESTAURANTS

Arby's
Au Bon Pain
Blimpie Subs and Salads
Panera Bread
Schlotzsky's
Steak 'n' Shake
Subway

EXCLUSIVE WEB CONTENT

Jersey Mike's (http://www.diabetes.org/healthyrestaurant)
Jimmy John's (http://www.diabetes.org/healthyrestaurant)
Wienerschnitzel
(http://www.diabetes.org/healthyrestaurant)

NUTRITION PROS

- Healthier condiments, such as all types of mustards and vinegars, are available. They keep your sandwich or sub moist without adding a lot of calories and fat.
- Subs and sandwiches are often made to order. That's good because you can specify what you want and don't want.
- Healthier breads, even whole wheat with extra fiber, are becoming easier to order.
- Healthy sub and sandwich fillers are available—turkey, smoked turkey, ham, chicken breast (grilled, plain), and roast beef.
- Healthy broth-based vegetable, grain, and/or bean-based soups are warm and ready in some sandwich

shops. Gazpacho, a healthy cold tomato-based soup with a kick, is often available in the warm weather months or warmer climates.

- Sub shops offer smaller-sized sandwiches. In some, it's the 6" size, and in others, it's half a large sandwich (or the "regular" size).
- Salads with light or fat-free salad dressings are an option in most sub and sandwich shops.

Healthy Tips

- ★ To keep your sodium meter on low, go light with or hold the pickles and olives.
- ★ Complement a sub or sandwich with something healthier than a fried snack food (potato chips, tortilla chips, and the like). For some crunch, try a side salad, popcorn, baked chips, or pretzels.
- ★ Ask to have large subs cut into two. Pack up half for another day.
- ★ In sandwich shops, order a cup of broth-based vegetable or bean soup. They'll fill you up and not out.
- ★ A Greek salad and piece of pita bread make a moderate-carbohydrate and light-on-protein meal. Ask for dressing on the side.
- ★ Pack a piece of fruit from home to bring to the sub or sandwich shop.

NUTRITION CONS

- Large sandwiches and long subs can be stuffed with enough protein to meet your entire daily requirement.
- Common sub and sandwich condiments, such as mayonnaise and oil, are high in fat.
- Tuna fish, chicken, and seafood salads sound healthy, but they are chock full of fat and calories.
- Cheese is a frequent sub or sandwich addition. Some restaurants give their nutrition information minus the cheese. Make sure you read the numbers for the way you eat your sandwich.
- Fruit and cooked vegetables are rarely available.
- Common sides are chips and French fries.

Get It Your Way

★ Hold the mayonnaise and oil. Substitute mustard or vinegar (any type).

★ Ask the sandwich maker to go light on the meat and heavy on the lettuce, onions, tomatoes, peppers, and any other vegetables they have on hand.

★ Hold the cheese.

★ Ask for the salad dressing on the side.

Arby's

(www.arbys.com)

Light 'n Lean Choice

Jr. Roast Beef Sandwich
Curly Fries *(1/2 small)*

Calories	441	Cholesterol (mg)	29
Fat (g)	20	Sodium (mg)	1,136
% calories from fat	41	Carbohydrate (g)	54
Saturated fat (g)	6	Fiber (g)	4
Trans fat (g)	0	Protein (g)	18

Exchanges: 3 1/2 starch, 1 1/2 medium-fat meat, 2 1/2 fat

Healthy 'n Hearty Choice

Martha's Vineyard Salad with
Raspberry Vinaigrette *(1/2 packet, 2 T)*
Ham and Swiss Melt Sandwich

Calories	638	Cholesterol (mg)	86
Fat (g)	21	Sodium (mg)	1,845
% calories from fat	30	Carbohydrate (g)	69
Saturated fat (g)	7	Fiber (g)	5
Trans fat (g)	0	Protein (g)	39

Exchanges: 3 starch, 1/2 carb, 3 veg, 4 1/2 lean meat, 1 1/2 fat

Arby's

	Amount	Cal.	Fat (g)	% Cal. Fat	Sat. Fat (g)	Trans Fat (g)	Chol. (mg)	Sod. (mg)	Carb. (g)	Fiber (g)	Pro. (g)	Choices/Exchanges
ARBY'S CHICKEN												
Chicken Cordon Bleu Sandwich - Crispy	1	590	26	4	5	0	76	1987	48	2	38	3 starch, 4 lean meat, 3 fat
Chicken Cordon Bleu Sandwich - Grilled	1	476	19	4	4	0	85	1725	37	1	43	2 1/2 starch, 5 lean meat, 1/2 fat
Chicken Fillet Sandwich - Crispy	1	510	24	4	4	0	52	1265	49	3	27	3 1/2 starch, 2 lean meat, 3 1/2 fat
✔Chicken Fillet Sandwich - Grilled	1	395	17	4	3	0	60	1002	38	2	32	2 1/2 starch, 3 lean meat, 1 fat
Chicken, Bacon & Swiss - Crispy	1	557	24	4	5	0	68	1684	51	2	33	3 1/2 starch, 3 lean meat, 3 fat

✔ = Healthiest Bets

(*Continued*)

ARBY'S CHICKEN *(Continued)*	Amount	Cal.	Fat (g)	% Cal. Fat	Sat. Fat (g)	Trans Fat (g)	Chol. (mg)	Sod. (mg)	Carb. (g)	Fiber (g)	Pro. (g)	Choices/Exchanges
Chicken, Bacon & Swiss - Grilled	1	443	17	3	4	0	77	1421	40	2	38	2 1/2 starch, 4 lean meat, 1 fat
✔Popcorn Chicken	reg	363	16	4	3	0	54	930	27	2	24	2 starch, 3 lean meat, 1 1/2 fat
Popcorn Chicken	lg	529	24	4	4	0	79	1354	39	3	35	2 1/2 starch, 4 lean meat, 2 1/2 fat
Popcorn Chicken Shakers	1 srvg	582	24	4	4	0	79	2483	51	3	36	3 1/2 starch, 4 lean meat, 2 1/2 fat
BREAKFAST												
Bacon & Egg Croissant	1	337	22	6	10	0	187	651	23	1	11	1 1/2 starch, 1 high-fat meat, 2 fat
Bacon Biscuit	1	340	21	6	6	0	13	1028	29	1	9	2 starch, 3 1/2 fat
Bacon, Egg & Cheese Biscuit	1	461	28	5	8	0	169	1446	30	1	17	2 starch, 2 medium-fat meat, 4 fat

Bacon, Egg & Cheese Croissant	1	378	22	5	10	0	198	850	23	1	14	1 1/2 starch, 1 medium-fat meat, 3 fat
Bacon, Egg & Cheese Sourdough	1	437	16	3	5	0	174	1220	40	2	20	2 1/2 starch, 2 medium-fat meat, 1 1/2 fat
Bacon, Egg & Cheese Wrap	1	515	29	5	8	0.5	165	1367	50	2	16	3 1/2 starch, 1 medium-fat meat, 5 fat
Blueberry Muffin	1	320	12	3	2	0	20	190	49	1	4	3 1/2 starch, 2 1/2 fat
✔Breakfast Syrup	1 oz	78	0	0	0	0	0	25	20	0	0	1 carb
Chicken Biscuit	1	417	23	5	5	0	17	1240	39	1	15	2 1/2 starch, 1 lean meat, 4 fat
✔Croissant	1	190	10	5	6	0	30	190	21	1	3	1 starch, 2 fat
Egg & Cheese Sourdough	1	392	12	3	3	0	166	1058	40	2	17	2 1/2 starch, 1 medium-fat meat, 1 fat
✔French Toastix	1 order	312	13	4	2	0	0	492	44	1	6	3 starch, 3 fat

✔ = Healthiest Bets

(Continued)

BREAKFAST *(Continued)*	Amount	Cal.	Fat (g)	% Cal. Fat	Sat. Fat (g)	Trans Fat (g)	Chol. (mg)	Sod. (mg)	Carb. (g)	Fiber (g)	Pro. (g)	Choices/Exchanges
✔Ham & Swiss Croissant	1	281	12	4	7	0	55	918	22	1	14	1 1/2 starch, 1 medium-fat meat, 1 fat
Ham Biscuit	1	323	17	5	4	0	15	1315	29	1	14	2 starch, 1 lean meat, 2 1/2 fat
Ham, Egg & Cheese Biscuit	1	444	24	5	6	0	171	1734	31	1	21	2 starch, 2 medium-fat meat, 2 1/2 fat
Ham, Egg & Cheese Croissant	1	361	18	4	9	0	200	1138	23	1	19	1 1/2 starch, 2 medium-fat meat, 1 1/2 fat
Ham, Egg, & Cheese Sourdough	1	442	14	3	4	0	180	1586	41	2	26	2 1/2 starch, 3 medium-fat meat, 1/2 fat
Ham, Egg, & Cheese Wrap	1	575	31	5	10	1	185	2005	51	2	25	3 1/2 starch, 2 medium-fat meat, 4 fat
Sausage & Egg Wrap	1	433	32	7	13	0	206	781	23	1	12	1 1/2 starch, 1 medium-fat meat, 5 1/2 fat

Sausage Biscuit	1	436	31	6	9	0	32	1160	28	1	10	2 starch, 1 medium-fat meat, 5 1/2 fat
Sausage Gravy Biscuit	1	961	68	6	14	0	12	3755	107	1	7	7 starch, 1 high-fat meat, 7 fat
Sausage Patty	1	210	20	9	7	0	40	480	0	0	6	1 high-fat meat, 2 1/2 fat
Sausage, Egg & Cheese Biscuit	1	557	38	6	11	0	187	1579	30	1	18	2 starch, 2 medium-fat meat, 6 fat
Sausage, Egg & Cheese Croissant	1	475	32	6	13	0	216	982	23	1	15	1 1/2 starch, 1 medium-fat meat, 5 fat
Sausage, Egg & Cheese Sourdough	1	556	28	5	9	0	197	1431	40	2	22	2 1/2 starch, 2 medium-fat meat, 3 1/2 fat
Sausage, Egg & Cheese Wrap	1	689	45	6	15	1	202	1849	50	2	21	3 1/2 starch, 2 medium-fat meat, 7 fat

✔ = Healthiest Bets

(Continued)

	Amount	Cal.	Fat (g)	% Cal. Fat	Sat. Fat (g)	Trans Fat (g)	Chol. (mg)	Sod. (mg)	Carb. (g)	Fiber (g)	Pro. (g)	Choices/Exchanges
CHICKEN DIPPING SAUCES												
✔BBQ	1 oz	44	0	0	0	0	0	343	11	0	0	1/2 carb
✔Buffalo	1 oz	10	1	9	0	0	0	790	2	0	0	Free
Honey Mustard	1 oz	129	12	8	2	0.25	9	151	6	0	0	1/2 carb, 2 1/2 fat
KID'S MENU												
✔Fruit Cup	1	35	0	0	0	0	0	0	9	1	0	1 fruit
✔Junior Roast Beef Sandwich	1	272	10	3	4	0	29	740	34	2	16	2 1/2 starch, 1 medium-fat meat, 1/2 fat
✔Kid's Meal - Popcorn Chicken	1 srvg	272	12	4	2	0	41	698	20	1	18	1 1/2 starch, 2 lean meat, 1 fat
✔Mini Ham & Cheese Sandwich	1	235	5	2	2	0	26	992	28	2	15	2 starch, 1 lean meat
✔Mini Turkey & Cheese Sandwich	1	244	5	2	1	0	37	854	28	2	19	2 starch, 2 lean meat

MARKET FRESH SALADS												
Chicken Club Salad	1	425	22	5	7	0	180	894	26	4	28	1 starch, 3 veg, 4 lean meat, 2 1/2 fat
✔Martha's Vineyard	1	273	9	3	4	0	61	609	25	4	22	1/2 starch, 3 veg, 3 lean meat
✔Santa Fe Salad	1	415	17	4	5	0	55	806	37	6	25	1 1/2 starch, 3 veg, 3 lean meat, 1 1/2 fat
✔Santa Fe Salad w/ Grilled Chicken	1	279	9	3	1	0	61	679	21	6	18	1/2 starch, 3 veg, 2 lean meat, 1/2 fat
MARKET FRESH SANDWICHES & WRAPS												
Corned Beef Reuben Sandwich	1	590	32	5	9	0.5	77	1685	55	3	32	3 1/2 starch, 3 medium-fat meat, 2 1/2 fat
Corned Reuben Wrap	1	560	29	5	8	0.5	77	1556	42	11	36	3 starch, 4 medium-fat meat, 1 fat
Pecan Chicken Salad Sandwich	1	769	39	5	10	0	74	1240	79	9	30	5 1/2 starch, 2 lean meat, 5 1/2 fat

✔ = Healthiest Bets

(*Continued*)

MARKET FRESH SANDWICHES & WRAPS *(Continued)*	Amount	Cal.	Fat (g)	% Cal. Fat	Sat. Fat (g)	Trans Fat (g)	Chol. (mg)	Sod. (mg)	Carb. (g)	Fiber (g)	Pro. (g)	Choices/Exchanges
Pecan Chicken Salad Wrap	1	638	38	5	10	1	74	1199	48	8	30	3 starch, 3 medium-fat meat, 4 fat
Roast Ham & Swiss Sandwich	1	691	31	4	8	0.5	59	1952	75	5	33	5 starch, 3 lean meat, 4 fat
Roast Turkey & Bacon Sandwich	1	818	38	4	11	0.5	102	2146	75	5	46	5 starch, 4 lean meat, 4 1/2 fat
Roast Turkey & Swiss Sandwich	1	708	30	4	8	0.5	83	1677	74	5	41	5 starch, 4 lean meat, 3 fat
Roast Turkey Ranch & Bacon Wrap	1	683	37	5	11	1	102	2103	44	4	45	3 starch, 5 lean meat, 4 1/2 fat
Roast Turkey Reuben Sandwich	1	594	30	5	8	0.5	86	1318	56	3	40	3 1/2 starch, 4 lean meat, 2 1/2 fat
Roast Turkey Wrap	1	564	27	4	7	0	86	1189	43	11	44	3 starch, 5 lean meat, 2 fat

Southwest Chicken Wrap	1	563	30	5	9	1	77	1609	42	4	32	3 starch, 3 lean meat, 4 fat
Ultimate BLT Sandwich	1	779	45	5	11	0.5	51	1571	75	6	23	5 starch, 1 medium-fat meat, 7 1/2 fat
Ultimate BLT Wrap	1	648	44	6	11	1	51	1530	45	6	23	3 starch, 2 medium-fat meat, 6 1/2 fat
MARKET SALAD DRESSINGS & TOPPINGS												
Buttermilk Ranch Dressing	2 oz	325	34	9	5	0.5	28	657	4	0	1	1/2 carb, 7 fat
✔Garlic & Cheese Croutons	1 srvg	77	5	6	1	0	1	116	7	0	2	1/2 starch, 1 fat
Light Buttermilk Ranch Dressing	2 oz	112	6	5	1	0	1	472	12	1	1	1 carb, 1 fat
Raspberry Vinaigrette	2 oz	194	14	6	2	0	0	387	18	0	0	1 carb, 3 fat
Santa Fe Ranch Dressing	2 oz	296	31	9	5	0	21	692	4	0	1	1/2 carb, 6 fat
✔Seasoned Crouton Strips	1 srvg	71	3	4	0	0	0	25	9	1	1	1/2 starch, 1/2 fat
Sliced Almonds	1 srvg	81	8	9	1	0	0	0	2	1	4	2 fat

✔ = Healthiest Bets

(*Continued*)

	Amount	Cal.	Fat (g)	% Cal. Fat	Sat. Fat (g)	Trans Fat (g)	Chol. (mg)	Sod. (mg)	Carb. (g)	Fiber (g)	Pro. (g)	Choices/Exchanges
ROAST BEEF SANDWICHES & MELTS												
✔Arby's Melt	1	302	12	4	4	1	30	921	36	2	16	2 1/2 starch, 1 medium-fat meat, 1 fat
✔Arby's Sauce	.5 oz	15	0	0	0	0	0	177	4	0	0	Free
Bacon Beef 'n Cheddar Sandwich	1	521	27	5	9	1.5	64	1573	45	2	27	3 starch, 3 medium-fat meat, 3 fat
BBQ Beef 'n Jack	1	360	16	4	5	0.5	37	1175	42	2	19	3 starch, 2 medium-fat meat, 1 fat
Beef 'n Cheddar Sandwich	1	445	21	4	6	1.5	51	1274	44	2	22	3 starch, 2 medium-fat meat, 2 1/2 fat
Ham & Swiss Melt Sandwich	1	268	5	2	2	0	25	1042	35	1	17	2 1/2 starch, 1 lean meat
Horsey Sauce	.5 oz	62	5	7	1	0	5	173	3	0	0	1 fat

✔Junior Roast Beef Sandwich	1	272	10	3	4	0	29	740	34	2	16	2 1/2 starch, 1 medium-fat meat, 1/2 fat
Roast Beef Sandwich	med	415	21	5	9	1	73	1379	34	2	31	2 1/2 starch, 3 medium-fat meat, 1/2 fat
Roast Beef Sandwich	super	398	19	4	6	0.5	44	1060	40	2	21	2 1/2 starch, 2 medium-fat meat, 2 fat
✔Roast Beef Sandwich	reg	320	14	4	5	0.5	44	953	34	2	21	2 1/2 starch, 2 medium-fat meat, 1 fat
Roast Beef Sandwich	lg	547	28	5	12	1.5	102	1869	41	3	42	2 1/2 starch, 5 medium-fat meat, 1/2 fat
Sourdough Ham Melt	1	380	13	3	3	0	31	1280	39	2	19	2 1/2 starch, 2 lean meat, 1 1/2 fat
Sourdough Roast Beef Melt	1	355	14	4	5	1	30	1047	40	2	18	2 1/2 starch, 1 medium-fat meat, 1 1/2 fat
✔Spicy Three Pepper Sauce	.5 oz	22	1	4	0	0	0	140	3	0	0	1/2 fat

✔ = Healthiest Bets

(*Continued*)

ROAST BEEF SANDWICHES & MELTS *(Continued)*	Amount	Cal.	Fat (g)	% Cal. Fat	Sat. Fat (g)	Trans Fat (g)	Chol. (mg)	Sod. (mg)	Carb. (g)	Fiber (g)	Pro. (g)	Choices/Exchanges
✔Swiss Melt	1	303	12	4	4	1	29	919	37	2	16	2 1/2 starch, 1 medium-fat meat, 1 fat

SHAKES & DESSERTS

Apple Turnover	1	337	16	4	5	6.5	0	201	65	2	4	4 starch, 1 1/2 fat
Berry Delight Swirl Shake	1	651	16	2	9	0.5	39	439	112	0	15	7 starch, 2 fat
Cherry Turnover	1	337	15	4	5	6	0	201	65	2	4	4 starch, 2 fat
✔Chocolate Chip Cookie	1	202	10	4	4	2	15	213	26	1	2	2 starch, 2 fat
Chocolate Shake	reg	507	13	2	8	0	34	357	83	0	13	6 starch, 2 1/2 fat
Chocolate Shake	lg	660	17	2	10	0.5	43	455	110	1	17	7 starch, 2 fat
Chocolate Turnover	1	400	25	6	7	7	0	190	37	4	6	2 starch, 5 fat
Jamocha Shake	reg	498	13	2	8	0	34	393	81	0	13	5 starch, 2 fat
Jamocha Shake	lg	647	17	2	10	0.5	43	509	107	1	17	7 starch, 2 1/2 fat

Strawberry Shake	reg	498	13	2	8	0	34	363	81	0	13	5 starch, 1 1/2 fat
Strawberry Shake	lg	646	17	2	10	0.5	43	464	107	1	16	7 starch, 2 1/2 fat
Vanilla Shake	reg	437	13	3	8	0	34	350	66	0	13	4 starch, 2 1/2 fat
Vanilla Shake	lg	555	17	3	10	0.5	43	445	83	0	16	6 starch, 3 1/2 fat
SIDES & SIDEKICKERS												
Bronco Berry Dipping Sauce	2 oz	122	0	0	0	0	0	36	30	0	0	2 carb
✔Cheddar Cheese Sauce	side portion	30	2	6	1	0.5	1	181	2	0	0	1 fat
Cheddar Fries	med	465	28	5	6	2	2	1311	51	5	6	3 starch, 5 fat
Cool Ranch Sour Cream Dipping Sauce	1.5 oz	158	16	9	4	0	0	277	2	0	1	3 fat
Curly Fries	sm	338	20	5	4	0	0	791	39	4	4	3 starch, 3 1/2 fat
Curly Fries	med	397	24	5	4	0	0	928	45	4	5	3 starch, 4 fat

✔ = Healthiest Bets

(*Continued*)

SIDES & SIDEKICKERS *(Continued)*	Amount	Cal.	Fat (g)	% Cal. Fat	Sat. Fat (g)	Trans Fat (g)	Chol. (mg)	Sod. (mg)	Carb. (g)	Fiber (g)	Pro. (g)	Choices/Exchanges
Curly Fries	lg	631	37	5	7	1	0	1476	73	7	8	5 starch, 6 fat
Jalapeño Bites, med	5	305	21	6	9	1	28	526	29	2	5	2 starch, 4 fat
Jalapeño Bites, lg	10	611	43	6	18	1.5	56	1052	58	4	11	4 starch, 7 1/2 fat
Loaded Potato Bites, med	5	353	22	6	7	0.5	13	800	27	2	11	2 starch, 4 1/2 fat
Loaded Potato Bites, lg	10	707	44	6	14	1.5	27	1601	54	5	23	4 starch, 9 fat
✔Marinara Sauce	1.5 oz	30	2	6	0	0	0	0	4	1	1	Free
Mozzarella Sticks, med	4	426	28	6	13	1	45	1370	38	2	18	2 1/2 starch, 1 medium-fat meat, 3 fat
Mozzarella Sticks, lg	8	849	56	6	26	2	90	2730	75	4	36	5 starch, 11 fat
Onion Petals	reg	331	23	6	4	0	1	332	35	2	4	2 starch, 4 fat
Onion Petals	lg	828	57	6	9	1	2	831	88	5	10	6 starch, 8 fat
Potato Cakes	2	246	18	7	4	1	0	391	26	2	2	2 starch, 3 fat

Potato Cakes	3	369	28	7	5	1.5	0	587	39	3	3	3 starch, 4 fat
Tangy Southwest Sauce	2 oz	333	35	9	5	0.5	29	371	5	0	1	7 fat
T.J. CINNAMONS												
Chocolate Twist	1	250	12	4	4	0	5	110	34	2	4	2 1/2 carb, 2 1/2 fat
Cinnamon Twist	1	260	14	5	5	4	5	190	33	1	3	2 carb, 3 fat
Original Gourmet Cinnamon Roll	1	507	10	2	4	0	7	373	73	4	10	5 carb, 2 fat
Pecan Sticky Bun	1	688	22	3	5	0	7	420	91	5	12	6 carb, 4 1/2 fat
T.J. Cinnamon Mocha Chill	1	306	7	2	4	0	29	214	48	1	11	3 carb, 1 1/2 fat
T.J. Icing	1 oz	117	5	4	2	1	8	50	18	0	1	1 carb, 1 fat
TOASTED SUBS												
Classic Italian	1	787	39	4	9	0.5	81	1642	67	3	33	4 1/2 starch, 3 medium-fat meat, 5 fat

✓ = Healthiest Bets

(*Continued*)

TOASTED SUBS *(Continued)*	Amount	Cal.	Fat (g)	% Cal. Fat	Sat. Fat (g)	Trans Fat (g)	Chol. (mg)	Sod. (mg)	Carb. (g)	Fiber (g)	Pro. (g)	Choices/Exchanges
French Dip & Swiss	1	622	20	3	7	1.5	79	3397	68	3	37	4 1/2 starch, 3 medium-fat meat, 1/2 fat
Philly Beef	1	739	37	5	9	1	85	1881	64	3	32	4 1/2 starch, 3 medium-fat meat, 4 1/2 fat
Turkey Bacon	1	619	18	3	4	0	82	2052	65	3	42	4 1/2 starch, 4 medium-fat meat

✔ = Healthiest Bets

Au Bon Pain

(www.aubonpain.com)

Light 'n Lean Choice

Southern Black-Eyed Pea Soup
Artisan Baguette *(salad size)*
Garden Salad with Light
Olive Oil Vinaigrette *(1/2 packet/2 Tbsp)*

Calories.......................535	Cholesterol (mg) 5
Fat (g) 11	Sodium (mg) 1,885
% calories from fat..19	Carbohydrate (g).........91
Saturated fat (g) 1	Fiber (g)....................16
Trans fat (g)...............0	Protein (g) 22

Exchanges: 5 starch, 1/2 carb, 2 veg, 1 lean meat, 1 1/2 fat

Healthy 'n Hearty Choice

Wild Mushroom Bisque *(medium, 12 oz)*
Maya Chicken Hot Wrap

Calories.......................780	Cholesterol (mg) 45
Fat (g) 22	Sodium (mg) 2,400
% calories from fat..25	Carbohydrate (g).......115
Saturated fat (g) 5	Fiber (g).....................8
Trans fat (g)...............0	Protein (g) 29

Exchanges: 4 starch, 3 carb, 2 veg, 2 lean meat, 3 fat

(Continued)

Au Bon Pain

	Amount	Cal.	Fat (g)	% Cal. Fat	Sat. Fat (g)	Trans Fat (g)	Chol. (mg)	Sod. (mg)	Carb. (g)	Fiber (g)	Pro. (g)	Choices/Exchanges
BAGELS												
Asiago Cheese	1	340	6	2	4	0	15	600	55	0	15	4 starch, 1 fat
Cinnamon Crisp	1	410	7	2	3	0	0	190	76	2	10	5 starch, 1 fat
Cinnamon Raisin	1	310	1	0	0	0	0	440	66	1	11	4 starch
Everything	1	340	5	1	0	0	0	980	62	1	13	4 starch, 1 fat
Honey 9 Grain	1	360	4	1	0	0	0	510	71	4	13	5 starch, 1/2 fat
Jalapeño Double Cheddar	1	340	10	3	5	0	30	630	52	0	17	3 starch, 2 fat
Onion Dill	1	290	1	0	0	0	0	440	58	1	11	4 starch
Plain	1	280	1	0	0	0	0	430	57	0	11	4 starch
Poppy	1	320	4	1	0	0	0	430	58	1	12	4 starch, 1 fat

Sesame Seed	1	320	5	1	1	0	0	430	58	1	12	4 starch, 1 fat
BLASTS & SMOOTHIES												
Banana Wildberry Smoothie	med	340	7	2	5	0	25	15	72	5	1	5 carb, 1 fat
Banana Wildberry Smoothie	lg	530	8	1	5	0	25	20	119	11	3	8 carb
Caramel Blast	med	540	17	3	12	0	60	105	104	0	6	7 carb, 3 fat
Caramel Blast	lg	760	21	2	15	0	75	130	151	0	8	10 carb, 3 fat
Coffee Blast	med	440	21	4	15	0	75	115	71	0	8	4 1/2 carb, 3 fat
Coffee Blast	lg	690	29	4	21	0	105	170	119	0	11	8 carb, 5 fat
Mocha Blast	med	440	17	3	12	0	60	95	80	2	7	5 1/2 carb, 3 fat
Mocha Blast	lg	690	22	3	15	0	75	130	137	3	10	9 carb, 3 fat
Peach Smoothie	med	310	1	0	0	0	10	115	69	4	4	4 1/2 carb

✔ = Healthiest Bets

(Continued)

BLASTS & SMOOTHIES *(Continued)*	Amount	Cal.	Fat (g)	% Cal. Fat	Sat. Fat (g)	Trans Fat (g)	Chol. (mg)	Sod. (mg)	Carb. (g)	Fiber (g)	Pro. (g)	Choices/Exchanges
Peach Smoothie	lg	470	1	0	0	0	15	170	104	7	7	7 carb
Strawberry Smoothie	med	310	1	0	0	0	10	110	66	3	4	4 1/2 carb
Strawberry Smoothie	lg	470	1	0	0	0	15	160	100	4	7	6 1/2 carb
Vanilla Blast	med	540	17	3	12	0	60	100	104	0	6	7 carb, 2 fat
Vanilla Blast	lg	760	21	2	15	0	75	130	152	0	8	10 carb, 3 fat
Wildberry Smoothie	med	380	7	2	5	0	35	110	71	3	4	4 1/2 carb, 1 fat
Wildberry Smoothie	lg	530	8	1	5	0	40	160	104	4	7	7 carb, 1 fat
BREADS												
Artisan Baguette	sandwich size	310	2	1	1	0	0	740	62	3	10	4 starch, 1/2 fat
✔Artisan Baguette	salad size	240	2	1	0	0	0	560	47	2	8	3 starch, 1/2 fat

Artisan Honey Multigrain Baguette	sandwich size	340	4	1	0	0	0	670	66	6	11	4 starch, 1/2 fat
✔Artisan Honey Multigrain Baguette	salad size	250	3	1	0	0	0	500	49	5	8	3 starch
✔Artisan Multigrain	1 srvg	280	3	1	0	0	0	670	53	5	10	4 starch
✔Artisan Sundried Tomato	1 srvg	270	1	0	0	0	0	760	55	3	9	4 starch
✔Asiago Breadstick	1 srvg	180	4	2	3	0	10	340	28	0	8	2 starch, 1 fat
Bacon & Cheese Mini Loaf	1	570	33	5	9	0	440	860	52	1	15	3 starch, 6 1/2 fat
✔Basil Pesto Cheese Toasts	3 pcs	140	2	1	0	0	0	330	26	1	5	2 starch, 1/2 fat
Bread Bowl	1	620	3	0	1	0	0	1690	121	1	26	8 starch
✔Cheddar Jalapeno Breadstick	1	130	2	1	1	0	5	250	25	0	6	2 starch
Cheese Bread	1 srvg	300	8	2	4	0	50	750	57	3	15	4 starch, 1 fat
✔Ciabatta	sm	180	1	1	0	0	0	470	37	2	6	2 starch

✔ = Healthiest Bets

(*Continued*)

BREADS *(Continued)*	Amount	Cal.	Fat (g)	% Cal. Fat	Sat. Fat (g)	Trans Fat (g)	Chol. (mg)	Sod. (mg)	Carb. (g)	Fiber (g)	Pro. (g)	Choices/Exchanges
Ciabatta	lg	300	1	0	0	0	0	780	61	3	10	4 starch
✔Cinnamon Raisin Breadstick	1	180	0	0	0	0	0	220	40	1	6	3 starch
Country White Bread	1 srvg	270	1	0	0	0	0	660	56	2	9	4 starch
✔Everything Breadstick	1	170	3	2	0	0	0	490	31	0	7	2 starch, 1/2 fat
Farm House Rolls	1 srvg	320	6	2	1	0	0	670	57	3	10	4 starch, 1/2 fat
Focaccia	1 srvg	350	7	2	1	0	0	680	61	1	12	4 starch, 1 fat
Lahvash	1 srvg	280	4	1	1	0	0	660	56	4	9	4 starch, 1/2 fat
Rosemary Garlic Breadstick	1	280	4	1	1	0	0	660	56	4	9	4 starch, 1/2 fat
✔Sesame Bread Stick	1	180	4	2	1	0	0	220	30	1	7	2 starch, 1 fat
Soft Roll	1 srvg	410	11	2	4	0	45	740	65	2	12	4 starch, 2 fat
BREAKFAST SANDWICHES												
Bacon & Bagel	1	340	6	2	2	0	15	640	57	0	16	4 starch, 1 medium-fat meat

Bacon & Egg Melt on Ciabatta	1	500	26	5	14	0	185	1250	40	2	26	2 1/2 starch, 3 medium-fat meat, 2 fat
Breakfast Quesadilla Sandwich	1	550	24	4	8	0	95	1330	56	5	27	3 1/2 starch, 2 medium-fat meat, 2 fat
Egg on a Bagel	1	360	4	1	1	0	115	780	59	0	21	4 starch, 1 lean meat
Egg on a Bagel w/ Bacon	1	420	8	2	3	0	130	990	60	0	25	4 starch, 2 medium-fat meat
Egg on a Bagel w/ Bacon & Cheese	1	500	15	3	6	0	150	1120	59	0	30	4 starch, 3 medium-fat meat, 1/2 fat
Egg on a Bagel w/ Cheese	1	430	10	2	5	0	140	900	58	0	25	4 starch, 2 medium-fat meat
Mediterranean Spinach Breakfast Sandwich	1	520	15	3	5	0	20	1090	79	7	20	5 1/2 starch, 1 lean meat, 2 fat
Portobello, Egg & Cheddar	1	490	26	5	13	0	170	1140	41	3	22	2 1/2 starch, 2 lean meat, 4 fat

✔ = Healthiest Bets

(*Continued*)

BREAKFAST SANDWICHES *(Continued)*	Amount	Cal.	Fat (g)	% Cal. Fat	Sat. Fat (g)	Trans Fat (g)	Chol. (mg)	Sod. (mg)	Carb. (g)	Fiber (g)	Pro. (g)	Choices/Exchanges
Prosciutto & Egg on Asiago Bagel	1	530	17	3	7	0	160	1650	59	1	34	4 starch, 3 lean meat, 1 fat
Sausage, Egg & Cheddar on Asiago Bagel	1	810	47	5	23	0.5	220	1540	58	1	38	4 starch, 4 medium-fat meat, 5 fat
Smoked Salmon & Wasabi on Onion Dill Bagel	1	430	11	2	5	0	45	1090	64	1	23	4 1/2 starch, 1 lean meat, 1 fat
CAFÉ SANDWICHES												
Arizona Chicken Sandwich	1	750	29	3	11	0	120	1510	61	4	49	4 starch, 5 lean meat, 3 fat
Baja Turkey Sandwich	1	640	24	3	8	0	80	2040	63	4	42	4 starch, 4 lean meat, 3 fat
Caprese Sandwich	1	680	32	4	14	0	75	1180	66	4	30	4 1/2 starch, 2 lean meat, 5 fat
Chicken Pesto Sandwich	1	720	24	3	5	0	80	1420	66	2	45	4 1/2 starch, 5 lean meat, 3 fat

Chicken Tarragon Sandwich	1	740	31	4	5	0	85	1170	61	1	39	4 starch, 4 lean meat, 4 1/2 fat
Chilean Chicken Sandwich	1	790	29	3	11	0	115	1540	64	6	51	4 starch, 5 lean meat, 4 fat
Ham & Cheddar Sandwich on Ciabatta	1	650	20	3	9	0	95	2330	80	4	40	5 starch, 3 lean meat, 1 fat
The Montana	1	560	23	4	12	0	105	1370	62	4	40	4 starch, 4 lean meat, 1 fat
Mozzarella Chicken Sandwich	1	750	25	3	8	0	100	1300	67	2	50	4 1/2 starch, 5 lean meat, 2 1/2 fat
Portobello & Goat Cheese Sandwich	1	560	26	4	9	0	25	1300	61	6	18	4 starch, 1 lean meat, 4 fat
Prosciutto Mozzarella Sandwich	1	770	41	5	16	0	105	2270	64	4	39	4 1/2 starch, 4 lean meat, 5 fat
Roast Beef Caesar	1	680	27	4	9	0	90	1540	65	3	40	4 1/2 starch, 4 medium-fat meat, 1 fat

✔ = Healthiest Bets

(*Continued*)

CAFÉ SANDWICHES *(Continued)*	Amount	Cal.	Fat (g)	% Cal. Fat	Sat. Fat (g)	Trans Fat (g)	Chol. (mg)	Sod. (mg)	Carb. (g)	Fiber (g)	Pro. (g)	Choices/Exchanges
Smoke Turkey Club Sandwich Sandwich		1	780	43	5	13	0	1152330		56	2	43 3 1/2 starch, 5 lean meat, 5 fat
Spicy Tuna Sandwich	1	500	18	3	3	0	40	1130	59	6	30	4 starch, 3 lean meat, 1 fat
Turkey & Cranberry Chutney Sandwich	1	530	10	2	2	0	40	1960	77	4	30	5 starch, 2 lean meat
Turkey & Swiss on Baguette	1	650	24	3	8	0	75	2120	66	3	41	4 1/2 starch, 4 lean meat, 2 fat
COFFEE & ESPRESSO												
✔Caffe Americano	sm	5	0	0	0	0	0	15	1	0	0	Free
✔Caffe Latte	sm	200	11	5	7	0	45	170	17	0	11	1/2 carb, 1 milk, 2 fat
✔Cappuccino	sm	120	7	5	4	0	20	85	10	0	6	1 milk, 1 fat
Caramel Macchiato	sm	350	10	3	6	0	30	160	53	0	10	2 1/2 carb, 1 milk, 2 fat

Chai Latte	sm	290	11	3	7	0	30	130	38	0	11	1 1/2 carb, 1 milk, 2 fat
✔Iced Caffe Latte	sm	110	6	5	4	0	20	80	19	0	6	1/2 carb, 1 milk, 1/2 fat
Iced Caramel Macchiato	sm	290	7	2	5	0	25	125	49	0	7	2 1/2 carb, 1 milk, 1 fat
✔Iced Chai Latte	sm	190	5	2	4	0	15	65	31	0	5	1 1/2 carb, 1 milk, 1/2 fat
✔Iced Decaf French Roast Coffee	med	10	0	0	0	0	0	20	2	0	0	Free
✔Iced French Roast Coffee	med	10	0	0	0	0	0	20	2	0	0	Free
✔Iced French Vanilla Coffee	med	10	0	0	0	0	0	20	2	0	0	Free
Iced Mocha Latte	sm	210	11	5	7	0	35	70	27	1	6	1 carb, 1 milk, 2 fat
Iced Vanilla Latte	sm	240	5	2	3	0	15	65	44	0	5	2 carb, 1 milk, 1/2 fat
Iced White Chocolate Latte	sm	250	11	4	7	0	35	135	35	0	5	1 carb, 1 milk, 2 fat
Mocha Latte	sm	300	16	5	10	0	60	160	35	1	11	1 carb, 1 milk, 3 fat
Vanilla Latte	sm	320	9	3	6	0	30	120	50	0	5	2 carb, 1 milk, 2 fat
White Chocolate Latte	sm	310	14	4	9	0	45	180	41	0	9	2 carb, 1 milk, 3 fat

✔ = Healthiest Bets

(*Continued*)

	Amount	Cal.	Fat (g)	% Cal. Fat	Sat. Fat (g)	Trans Fat (g)	Chol. (mg)	Sod. (mg)	Carb. (g)	Fiber (g)	Pro. (g)	Choices/Exchanges
COOKIES & DESSERTS												
Banana Nut Pound Cake	1 pc	520	28	5	5	0	85	470	60	1	7	4 carb, 5 fat
Blondie	1	330	19	5	6	0	35	350	61	3	7	4 carb, 3 fat
Blueberry Tulip	1	370	20	5	4	0	65	300	44	1	4	3 carb, 3 fat
Cappuccino Poundcake	1 pc	530	26	4	5	0	85	490	68	1	3	4 1/2 carb, 4 fat
Chocolate Bundt Cake	1 pc	440	21	4	8	0	45	340	61	1	3	4 carb, 3 fat
Chocolate Cheesecake Brownie	1	370	14	3	4	0	75	260	58	1	5	4 carb, 2 fat
Chocolate Chip Brownie	1	380	17	4	5	0	75	390	62	1	5	4 carb, 2 fat
Chocolate Chip Cookie	1	260	12	4	6	0	25	220	37	1	2	2 1/2 carb, 2 fat
Chocolate Dipped Cranberry Almond Macaroon	1	320	16	5	8	0	0	190	42	3	4	3 carb, 3 fat
Chocolate Dipped Shortbread	1	350	20	5	9	0	25	280	38	1	3	2 1/2 carb, 4 fat

Chocolate Pound Cake	1 pc	500	29	5	6	0	100	580	58	3	7	4 carb, 5 fat
Chocolate Raspberry Tulip	1	430	21	4	5	0	70	410	55	1	5	3 1/2 carb, 4 fat
Confetti Cookie w/ M&M's	1	310	14	4	5	0	25	290	42	1	3	3 carb, 3 fat
Crème de Fleur	1	490	25	5	14	1	95	410	57	2	11	4 carb, 5 fat
Crumb Cake	1 pc	470	25	5	13	0	60	780	56	1	5	3 1/2 carb, 4 fat
English Toffee Cookie	1	210	11	5	4	0	20	240	26	1	2	1 1/2 carb, 2 fat
Hazelnut Crème Pastry	1	540	34	6	16	0	85	380	50	3	10	3 1/2 carb, 7 fat
Hazelnut Dream Cookie	1	390	24	6	10	0.5	50	250	41	2	4	2 1/2 carb, 5 fat
Hazelnut Fudge Cookie	1	290	16	5	6	0	40	150	34	3	4	2 1/2 carb, 3 fat
Hazelnut Mocha Brownie	1	430	21	4	5	0	65	360	58	3	6	4 carb, 3 fat
Hazelnut Monkey Bread	1 pc	510	28	5	12	0	6	330	57	2	8	4 carb, 5 fat
Iced Cinnamon Roll	1	400	15	3	8	0	50	270	60	2	8	4 carb, 2 fat
Key Lime Sugar Cookie	1	250	8	3	4	0	35	200	39	1	3	2 1/2 carb, 1 fat

✔ = Healthiest Bets

(Continued)

COOKIES & DESSERTS *(Continued)*	Amount	Cal.	Fat (g)	% Cal. Fat	Sat. Fat (g)	Trans Fat (g)	Chol. (mg)	Sod. (mg)	Carb. (g)	Fiber (g)	Pro. (g)	Choices/Exchanges
Key Lime Tulip	1	440	22	5	5	0	70	360	55	1	5	3 1/2 carb, 4 fat
Lemon Pound Cake	1 pc	520	27	5	6	0	85	480	64	0	5	4 1/2 carb, 5 fat
Marble Pound Cake	1 pc	490	27	5	5	0	90	520	59	1	6	4 carb, 5 fat
✔Mini Chocolate Chip Cookie	1	70	3	4	2	0	5	55	9	0	1	1/2 carb, 1/2 fat
✔Mini Oatmeal Raisin Cookie	1	60	2	3	1	0	10	50	9	1	1	1/2 carb, 1/2 fat
Mint Chocolate Pound Cake	1 pc	530	28	5	6	0	95	590	65	3	7	4 1/2 carb, 5 fat
Oatmeal Raisin Cookie	1	230	8	3	4	0	35	190	36	2	3	2 1/2 carb, 1 fat
Palmier	1	440	23	5	15	0	60	330	53	1	1	3 1/2 carb, 4 fat
Pecan Roll	1	630	32	5	11	0	30	330	80	3	10	5 1/2 carb, 6 fat
Rocky Road Brownie	1	410	17	4	5	0	70	430	62	2	6	4 carb, 3 fat
Shortbread Cookie	1	310	18	5	8	0	25	270	34	1	3	2 1/2 carb, 3 fat
White Chocolate Chunk Macadamia Nut Cookie	1	280	15	5	7	0	30	240	34	1	3	2 1/2 carb, 2 fat

CROISSANTS												
Almond	1	600	38	6	14	0.5	115	300	55	4	13	4 starch, 7 fat
Apple	1	270	11	4	6	0	40	180	44	3	5	3 starch, 2 fat
Chocolate	1	430	22	5	13	0	45	210	58	3	7	4 starch, 4 1/2 fat
Ham & Cheese	1	400	20	5	11	0	80	690	38	2	16	2 1/2 starch, 1 lean meat, 3 1/2 fat
Plain	1	300	17	5	9	0	55	220	31	1	6	2 starch, 3 1/2 fat
Raspberry Cheese	1	320	15	4	8	0	50	250	41	2	7	3 starch, 3 fat
Spinach & Cheese	1	290	16	5	9	0	55	320	28	2	10	2 starch, 3 fat
Sweet Cheese	1	380	19	5	10	0.5	75	310	48	2	9	3 starch, 3 fat
DANISH												
Cherry	1	420	20	4	10	0	70	310	54	2	7	3 1/2 carb, 3 fat
Lemon	1	440	20	4	10	0	75	330	57	2	7	4 carb, 3 fat

✔ = Healthiest Bets

(*Continued*)

	Amount	Cal.	Fat (g)	% Cal. Fat	Sat. Fat (g)	Trans Fat (g)	Chol. (mg)	Sod. (mg)	Carb. (g)	Fiber (g)	Pro. (g)	Choices/Exchanges
HARVEST RICE BOWLS												
Cajun Shrimp	1	520	17	3	8	0	145	1660	69	2	16	4 1/2 starch, 3 1/2 fat
Cajun Shrimp w/ Brown Rice	1	560	2	0	7	0	145	1660	73	5	14	5 starch, 1 lean meat, 2 fat
Mayan Chicken	1	490	14	3	3	0	70	1430	67	4	25	4 1/2 starch, 2 lean meat, 2 fat
Mayan Chicken w/ Brown Rice	1	540	16	3	3	0	70	1430	71	7	23	4 1/2 starch, 1 lean meat, 2 fat
Steak Teriyaki	1	540	15	3	3	0	55	1670	76	2	29	5 starch, 2 medium-fat meat, 1/2 fat
Steak Teriyaki w/ Brown Rice	1	590	18	3	3	0	55	1670	80	5	27	5 1/2 starch, 2 medium-fat meat, 1 fat
HOT ENTREES												
Cheese Tortellini Primavera	1 srvg	580	30	5	16	0	70	1530	54	4	23	3 1/2 starch, 2 medium-fat meat, 4 fat

Chicken Penne Alfredo	1 srvg	700	31	4	15	0	130	1550	47	5	47	3 starch, 5 lean meat, 3 fat
Macaroni & Cheese	med	440	26	5	17	0	95	1280	31	2	19	2 starch, 2 medium-fat meat, 3 1/2 fat
Macaroni & Cheese	lg	590	34	5	22	0	130	1710	43	2	25	3 starch, 2 medium-fat meat, 4 1/2 fat
Meat Lasagna	1 srvg	480	28	5	13	0	75	1640	29	2	28	2 starch, 3 lean meat, 3 1/2 fat
✔Penne Marinara w/ Vegetables	1 srvg	350	11	3	5	0	20	780	52	7	15	3 starch, 2 veg, 1 lean meat, 1 fat
Penne w/ Chicken & Fire Roasted Pepper Sauce	1 srvg	620	19	3	8	0	100	1630	58	7	42	4 starch, 4 lean meat, 1 1/2 fat
✔Quinoa	1 oz/ 2 Tbsp	25	0	0	0	0	0	75	4	1	1	1/2 starch
✔Roasted Carrots	1 oz/ 2 Tbsp	15	0	0	0	0	0	60	3	1	0	1 veg

✔ = Healthiest Bets

(*Continued*)

HOT ENTREES *(Continued)*	Amount	Cal.	Fat (g)	% Cal. Fat	Sat. Fat (g)	Trans Fat (g)	Chol. (mg)	Sod. (mg)	Carb. (g)	Fiber (g)	Pro. (g)	Choices/Exchanges
✔Roasted Green Beans w/ Almonds	1 oz/ 2 Tbsp	20	1	5	0	0	0	60	2	1	1	1 veg
✔Roasted Vegetable	1 oz/ 2 Tbsp	15	1	6	0	0	0	110	2	1	1	1 veg
Spinach & Artichoke Lasagna	1 srvg	410	16	4	8	0	75	1540	43	5	24	2 1/2 starch, 1 veg, 2 medium-fat meat, 1 fat
Spinach & Artichoke Pizzetta	1 srvg	520	27	5	8	0	25	850	56	6	13	3 starch, 1 veg, 1 medium-fat meat, 5 fat
Three Cheese Pizzetta	1 srvg	700	41	5	18	0	75	1110	55	5	26	3 1/2 starch, 2 medium-fat meat, 6 fat
Tomato, Mozzarella & Basil Pizzetta	1 srvg	620	38	6	10	0	40	680	54	5	16	3 1/2 starch, 1 lean meat, 7 fat

HOT SANDWICHES & MELTS

BBQ Chicken on Farmhouse Roll	1	860	31	3	12	0	110	1650	78	4	50	5 starch, 5 lean meat, 4 fat
Cajun Shrimp Hot Wrap	1	660	20	3	7	0	85	1680	95	5	20	6 1/2 starch, 3 1/2 fat
Eggplant & Mozzarella Sandwich	1	670	31	4	12	0	60	1480	70	6	26	4 1/2 starch, 2 lean meat, 5 fat
Mayan Chicken Hot Wrap	1	590	15	2	3	0	35	1390	92	6	24	6 starch, 1 lean meat, 2 fat
Steak Teriyaki Hot Wrap	1	620	15	2	3	0	60	1410	96	5	26	6 1/2 starch, 1 medium-fat meat, 1 fat
Steakhouse on Ciabatta	1	720	31	4	10	0	85	1840	71	4	43	4 1/2 starch, 4 medium-fat meat, 1 fat
Tuna Melt	1	670	30	4	9	0	80	1200	62	5	40	4 starch, 4 lean meat, 3 fat
Turkey Melt	1	780	34	4	13	0	100	2370	73	3	45	5 starch, 4 lean meat, 3 1/2 fat

✔ = Healthiest Bets

(*Continued*)

	Amount	Cal.	Fat (g)	% Cal. Fat	Sat. Fat (g)	Trans Fat (g)	Chol. (mg)	Sod. (mg)	Carb. (g)	Fiber (g)	Pro. (g)	Choices/Exchanges
KIDS												
✔All Natural Grilled Chicken Sandwich	1	490	14	3	3	0	35	950	59	2	24	4 starch, 2 lean meat, 2 fat
✔Chicken Nuggets	1 srvg	180	7	4	1	0	30	470	14	0	14	1 starch, 2 lean meat, 1/2 fat
Grilled Cheese	1	670	41	6	25	0.5	105	1060	55	2	20	3 1/2 starch, 1 medium-fat meat, 7 fat
✔Kids Buttered Penne Pasta	1 srvg	260	12	4	7	0	30	95	31	1	6	2 starch, 2 fat
✔Macaroni & Cheese	1 srvg	220	14	6	9	0	50	650	15	0	9	1 starch, 1 medium-fat meat, 2 fat
Smoked Turkey Sandwich	1	450	13	3	3	0	20	1350	59	2	21	4 starch, 1 lean meat, 2 fat
MUFFINS												
Blueberry	1	450	17	3	2	0	20	500	66	3	8	4 1/2 carb, 3 fat

Carrot Walnut	1	520	25	4	6	0	55	800	66	4	8	4 1/2 carb, 4 fat
Corn	1	460	16	3	3	0	60	550	69	2	9	4 1/2 carb, 2 fat
Cranberry Walnut	1	500	23	4	2	0	20	450	61	4	9	4 carb, 4 fat
Double Chocolate Chunk	1	570	23	4	7	0	20	450	80	4	10	5 1/2 carb, 4 fat
Low-fat Triple Berry	1	290	2	1	0	0	15	490	67	2	3	4 1/2 carb
Mushroom, Gorgonzola, Red Pepper	1	490	28	5	6	0	80	540	50	1	8	3 1/2 starch, 5 1/2 fat
Pumpkin	1	530	19	3	4	0	65	570	81	3	9	5 1/2 carb, 3 fat
Raisin Bran	1	480	11	2	2	0	30	600	85	10	12	5 1/2 carb, 1 fat
Southwest Jalapeno	1	560	30	5	6	0	95	610	64	1	8	4 starch, 5 fat
OATMEAL												
✔Small	1 srvg	150	3	2	0	0	0	10	28	4	6	2 starch, 1/2 fat
✔Medium	1 srvg	210	4	2	1	0	0	10	38	5	8	3 starch, 1/2 fat
Large	1 srvg	270	5	2	1	0	0	15	50	7	10	3 starch, 1/2 fat

✔ = Healthiest Bets

(*Continued*)

	Amount	Cal.	Fat (g)	% Cal. Fat	Sat. Fat (g)	Trans Fat (g)	Chol. (mg)	Sod. (mg)	Carb. (g)	Fiber (g)	Pro. (g)	Choices/Exchanges
OTHER BEVERAGES												
Homestyle Lemonade	med	310	0	0	0	0	0	0	82	0	0	5 1/2 carb
Hot Chocolate	sm	350	11	3	7	0	30	125	58	3	12	2 1/2 carb, 1 milk, 2 fat
✔Peach Iced Tea	med	120	0	0	0	0	0	35	30	0	0	2 carb
SALAD DRESSING												
✔Balsamic Vinaigrette	2.25 oz	190	16	8	3	0	0	430	11	0	0	1/2 carb, 3 fat
Blue Cheese	1.75 oz	230	24	9	5	0	20	550	2	0	2	5 fat
Caesar	2.0 oz	280	28	9	5	0	20	400	4	0	2	1/2 carb, 5 1/2 fat
✔Fat Free Raspberry Vinaigrette	2.25 oz	70	0	0	0	0	0	150	17	0	0	1 carb
Hazelnut Vinaigrette	2.25 oz	330	31	8	5	0	0	210	10	1	2	1/2 carb, 6 fat
✔Light Olive Oil Vinaigrette	2.25 oz	130	10	7	2	0	0	630	9	0	0	1/2 carb, 2 fat

✔Light Ranch	2.25 oz	150	15	9	3	0	15	470	3	0	2	3 fat
✔Lite Honey Mustard	2.25 oz	180	11	6	2	0	10	590	21	1	1	1 1/2 carb, 2 fat
Sesame Ginger	2.25 oz	280	25	8	4	0	0	840	13	0	1	1 carb, 5 fat
Thai Peanut	2.25 oz	230	13	5	2	0	0	840	24	1	5	1 1/2 carb, 2 1/2 fat
SALADS - NO DRESSING												
✔Caesar Asiago Salad	1 side srvg	120	6	5	3	0	15	260	11	2	6	2 veg, 1 lean meat, 1/2 fat
✔Caesar Asiago Salad	1 srvg	210	12	5	6	0	25	470	18	3	11	1/2 starch, 2 veg, 1 lean meat, 1 1/2 fat
Chefs Salad	1 srvg	250	15	5	7	0	65	1130	8	3	23	1 veg, 3 lean meat, 1 fat
✔Chickpea & Cucumber Salad	1 srvg	230	12	5	5	0	20	810	23	7	11	1 starch, 1 veg, 1 lean meat, 1 1/2 fat
✔Garden Salad	1 side srvg	50	2	4	0	0	0	60	8	2	2	2 veg
✔Garden Salad	1 srvg	70	2	3	0	0	0	80	12	3	4	2 veg, 1/2 fat
✔Green Bean & Beet Salad	1 srvg	210	8	3	4	0	20	660	27	5	8	1 starch, 2 veg, 1 1/2 fat

✔ = Healthiest Bets

(Continued)

SALADS - NO DRESSING *(Continued)*	Amount	Cal.	Fat (g)	% Cal. Fat	Sat. Fat (g)	Trans Fat (g)	Chol. (mg)	Sod. (mg)	Carb. (g)	Fiber (g)	Pro. (g)	Choices/Exchanges
✔Grilled Chicken Caesar Asiago	1 srvg	340	13	3	6	0	65	680	19	3	29	1/2 starch, 2 veg, 4 lean meat, 1 fat
✔Mandarin Sesame Chicken Salad	1 srvg	350	18	5	1	0	35	370	30	3	21	1 starch, 2 veg, 3 lean meat, 2 fat
Mediterranean Chicken Salad	1 srvg	330	16	4	6	0	60	1170	12	3	24	2 veg, 3 lean meat, 2 fat
✔Riviera Salad	1 srvg	260	7	2	30	0	15	250	46	5	7	2 starch, 2 veg, 1 1/2 fat
✔Thai Peanut Chicken Salad	1 srvg	240	8	3	0	0	40	280	19	4	22	1/2 starch, 2 veg, 3 lean meat
✔Tuna Garden Salad	1 srvg	250	13	5	2	0	40	410	14	4	21	3 veg, 3 lean meat, 1/2 fat
✔Turkey Medallion Cobb Salad	1 srvg	340	19	5	8	0	260	980	15	4	27	3 veg, 4 lean meat, 1 1/2 fat
✔Turkey Spinach Sonoma Salad	1 srvg	230	11	4	6	0	45	920	16	5	19	3 veg, 3 lean meat, 1/2 fat

SCONES												
Cinnamon	1	530	27	5	16	0	140	400	60	2	9	4 starch, 5 fat
Orange	1	470	23	4	13	0	150	420	57	1	10	4 starch, 4 fat
SIDE DISHES												
✔Apples, Blue Cheese & Cranberries	1 srvg	200	10	5	4	0	20	290	27	3	4	2 fruit, 2 fat
✔Asparagus & Almonds	1 srvg	70	6	8	0	0	0	55	5	2	3	1 veg, 1 fat
✔BBQ Chicken	1 srvg	170	2	1	0	0	40	340	13	1	17	1 starch, 2 lean meat
✔Brie, Fruit & Crackers	1 srvg	190	10	5	5	0	25	250	17	1	6	1 starch, 2 fat
✔Cheddar, Fruit & Crackers	1 srvg	190	11	5	5	0	30	260	17	1	8	1/2 starch, 1/2 fruit, 1 medium-fat meat, 1 1/2 fat
✔Chickpea & Tomato Salad	1 srvg	100	1	1	0	0	0	200	19	6	5	1/2 starch, 1 veg, 1 lean meat
✔Herb Cheese, Fruit & Crackers	1 srvg	180	11	6	6	0	25	430	19	1	4	1 1/2 starch, 2 fat

✔ = Healthiest Bets

(*Continued*)

SIDE DISHES *(Continued)*	Amount	Cal.	Fat (g)	% Cal. Fat	Sat. Fat (g)	Trans Fat (g)	Chol. (mg)	Sod. (mg)	Carb. (g)	Fiber (g)	Pro. (g)	Choices/Exchanges
✔Honey Mustard Chicken	1 srvg	170	2	1	0	0	40	260	12	1	17	1 starch, 2 lean meat
✔Hummus & Cucumber	1 srvg	130	8	6	0	0	0	460	10	3	3	1/2 starch, 1 1/2 fat
✔Mediterranean Tuna Salad	1 srvg	120	8	6	2	0	20	250	4	1	10	1/2 starch, 1 lean meat, 1 fat
Mozzarella & Tomato	1 srvg	190	15	7	7	0	35	290	5	1	10	1/2 starch, 1 medium-fat meat, 1 1/2 fat
Mozzarella, Olive, Roasted Peppers & Tomato	1 srvg	180	14	7	7	0	35	390	4	1	10	1/2 starch, 1 medium-fat meat, 1 1/2 fat
✔Smoked turkey, Asparagus, Cranberry Chutney & Gorgonzola	1 srvg	140	5	3	3	0	35	760	10	1	15	1/2 starch, 2 lean meat
✔Thai Peanut Chicken & Snow Peas	1 srvg	200	7	3	2	0	40	400	7	1	19	1/2 starch, 3 medium-fat meat
SNACKS												
✔The 19th Hole Snack	1.1 oz	160	9	5	1	0	0	200	15	1	4	1 starch, 1 1/2 fat

Assorted Nuts	4 oz	730	64	8	7	0	0	130	24	10	21	1 1/2 starch, 2 medium-fat meat, 10 fat
Chocolate Covered Almonds	1.5 oz	220	14	6	5	0	0	35	24	2	3	1 1/2 starch, 3 fat
Chocolate Covered Pretzels	5 pcs	140	6	4	3	0	2	114	20	0	2	1 starch, 1 fat
✔Chocolate Covered Strawberry	1 berry	30	2	6	0	0	0	5	4	0	0	1/2 fat
Chocolate Nonpareils	1.4 oz	190	12	6	7	0	0	15	25	3	2	1 carb, 2 1/2 fat
Dark Chocolate Cranberries	1.4 oz	170	9	5	5	0	0	0	27	3	1	1 carb, 1 fruit, 1 1/2 fat
✔Fruit Cup	sm	70	0	0	0	0	0	10	16	1	1	1 fruit
✔Fruit Cup	lg	140	1	1	0	0	0	20	32	2	2	2 fruit
Fruit Sours	4 oz	400	0	0	0	0	0	15	105	0	0	7 carb
Jell-O	8 oz	140	0	0	0	0	0	150	34	0	2	2 carb
Kookaburra Red Licorice	1.4 oz	140	1	1	1	0	0	20	30	0	1	2 carb
✔MaJuKa Fruit Trail Mix	1.1 oz	140	7	5	2	0	0	0	17	2	2	1 carb, 1 1/2 fat

✔ = Healthiest Bets

(*Continued*)

SNACKS *(Continued)*	Amount	Cal.	Fat (g)	% Cal. Fat	Sat. Fat (g)	Trans Fat (g)	Chol. (mg)	Sod. (mg)	Carb. (g)	Fiber (g)	Pro. (g)	Choices/Exchanges
Maple Roasted Cashews	4 oz	650	49	7	10	0	0	120	45	4	16	3 starch, 1 medium-fat meat, 8 fat
Muesli	8 oz	390	8	2	2	0	5	50	76	7	11	5 starch, 1 fat
✔New Trail Mix	1.1 oz	120	5	4	1	0	0	5	20	2	2	1 1/2 starch, 1 fat
Peach Gummies	1.2 oz	150	0	0	0	0	0	0	36	0	2	2 carb
Summit Blend	4 oz	500	27	5	7	0	0	135	63	7	10	4 starch, 5 fat
Tamari Almonds	1.1 oz	180	14	7	1	0	0	160	5	3	9	1/2 starch, 1 medium-fat meat, 1 1/2 fat
Tamari Roast	4 oz	770	61	7	6	0	0	530	41	20	28	3 starch, 3 medium-fat meat, 8 fat
✔Turkish Apricots	1.4 oz	120	0	0	0	0	0	10	29	4	1	2 veg
Walnuts	4 oz	740	74	9	7	0	0	0	16	8	17	1 starch, 2 medium-fat meat, 12 fat

SOUPS & STEWS												
Baked Stuffed Potato	med	350	21	5	10	0	60	990	30	2	9	2 starch, 4 fat
Baked Stuffed Potato	lg	470	28	5	13	0	80	1320	39	3	12	3 starch, 5 1/2 fat
Beef Stew	med	300	16	5	3	0	55	1070	25	3	18	1 1/2 starch, 2 medium-fat meat, 1 1/2 fat
Beef Stew	lg	410	21	5	3	0	70	1430	33	4	24	2 starch, 2 medium-fat meat, 1 1/2 fat
✔Broccoli Cheddar	med	310	21	6	10	0	50	1000	20	2	11	1 1/2 starch, 1 medium-fat meat, 3 fat
Broccoli Cheddar	lg	410	28	6	13	0	70	1330	27	3	15	2 starch, 1 medium-fat meat, 4 fat
✔Carrot Ginger	med	130	5	3	0	0	0	920	21	3	7	1 starch, 1 veg, 1 fat
Carrot Ginger	lg	170	6	3	1	0	0	1220	28	4	9	1 starch, 2 veg, 1 fat
Chicken & Dumpling	med	210	7	3	3	0	50	1280	28	2	11	2 starch, 1 lean meat, 1 fat

✔ = Healthiest Bets

(*Continued*)

SOUPS & STEWS *(Continued)*	Amount	Cal.	Fat (g)	% Cal. Fat	Sat. Fat (g)	Trans Fat (g)	Chol. (mg)	Sod. (mg)	Carb. (g)	Fiber (g)	Pro. (g)	Choices/Exchanges
Chicken & Dumpling	lg	290	9	3	4	0	70	1710	28	2	14	2 starch, 1 lean meat, 2 fat
Chicken Florentine	med	240	13	5	6	0	35	1030	25	1	8	1 1/2 starch, 2 1/2 fat
Chicken Florentine	lg	320	17	5	7	0	50	1380	34	2	11	2 1/2 starch, 1 lean meat, 3 fat
✔Chicken Gumbo	med	200	9	4	1	0	10	910	24	2	7	1 1/2 starch, 2 fat
Chicken Gumbo	lg	270	12	4	2	0	15	1210	32	2	9	2 starch, 2 1/2 fat
Chicken Noodle	med	130	3	2	1	0	15	1000	20	2	9	1 1/2 starch, 1 lean meat
Chicken Noodle	lg	180	4	2	1	0	20	1330	26	2	12	1 1/2 starch, 1 lean meat
✔Chicken Vegetable Stew	med	290	17	5	5	0	40	930	26	3	11	1 1/2 starch, 1 lean meat, 3 fat

Chicken Vegetable Stew	lg	380	23	5	6	0	55	1250	34	4	16	2 starch, 1 lean meat, 3 1/2 fat
Clam Chowder	med	320	18	5	7	0	55	1020	27	1	9	1 1/2 starch, 1 milk, 3 fat
Clam Chowder	lg	450	24	5	10	0	75	1360	37	2	13	1 1/2 starch, 2 milk, 4 fat
Corn & Green Chili Bisque	med	250	14	5	7	0	35	1450	29	3	5	2 starch, 3 fat
Corn & Green Chili Bisque	lg	340	19	5	9	0	45	2050	38	3	7	3 starch, 3 fat
Corn Chowder	med	350	18	5	8	0	50	1120	40	3	9	3 starch, 3 fat
Corn Chowder	lg	460	23	5	11	0	65	1500	53	4	11	4 starch, 4 fat
Cream of Chicken & Wild Rice	med	260	15	5	5	0	35	990	24	1	7	1 1/2 starch, 3 fat
Cream of Chicken & Wild Rice	lg	340	20	5	7	0	50	1320	32	2	9	2 starch, 4 fat
Curried Rice & Lentil	med	150	2	1	0	0	0	1260	30	8	9	2 starch, 1/2 fat
Curried Rice & Lentil	lg	190	3	1	0	0	0	1670	40	11	11	2 1/2 starch, 1/2 fat

✔ = Healthiest Bets

(Continued)

SOUPS & STEWS *(Continued)*	Amount	Cal.	Fat (g)	% Cal. Fat	Sat. Fat (g)	Trans Fat (g)	Chol. (mg)	Sod. (mg)	Carb. (g)	Fiber (g)	Pro. (g)	Choices/Exchanges
French Moroccan Tomato Lentil	med	180	2	1	0	0	0	1050	32	8	10	2 starch, 1 lean meat
French Moroccan Tomato Lentil	lg	240	3	1	0	0	0	1400	43	11	14	3 starch, 1 lean meat
French Onion	med	130	5	3	3	0	10	1310	19	2	4	1 starch, 1 fat
French Onion	lg	170	6	3	3	0	15	1740	25	3	5	2 starch, 1 fat
Garden Vegetable	med	80	2	2	0	0	0	1010	14	3	3	3 veg, 1/2 fat
Garden Vegetable	lg	100	2	2	0	0	0	1340	18	3	4	4 veg, 1/2 fat
Gazpacho	med	90	5	5	0	0	0	1560	12	3	2	2 veg, 1 fat
Gazpacho	lg	120	6	5	1	0	0	2080	16	4	2	3 veg, 1 fat
✔Hearty Cabbage	med	110	5	4	1	0	10	910	14	3	4	3 veg, 1 fat
Hearty Cabbage	lg	140	6	4	2	0	10	1220	18	3	6	4 veg, 1 fat

Italian Wedding	med	170	7	4	3	0	15	1300	19	2	8	1 1/2 starch, 1 lean meat, 1 fat
Italian Wedding	lg	230	9	4	4	0	20	1730	26	3	11	1 1/2 starch, 1 lean meat, 1 1/2 fat
✔Jamaican Black Bean	med	180	1	1	0	0	0	460	45	25	16	3 starch, 1 lean meat
✔Jamaican Black Bean	lg	240	2	1	0	0	0	610	61	33	22	4 starch, 1 lean meat
✔Mediterranean Pepper	med	100	3	3	0	0	0	580	18	5	5	3 veg, 1/2 fat
✔Mediterranean Pepper	lg	140	4	3	0	0	0	770	24	7	7	5 veg, 1 fat
✔Old Fashioned Tomato Rice	med	120	1	1	0	0	0	340	24	3	4	2 starch
✔Old Fashioned Tomato Rice	lg	170	2	1	0	0	0	460	32	4	6	2 starch, 1/2 fat
✔Pasta E Fagioli	med	240	8	3	2	0	5	930	36	9	11	2 starch, 1 1/2 fat
Pasta E Fagioli	lg	320	11	3	3	0	5	1240	49	12	15	3 starch, 2 fat
Portuguese Kale	med	120	7	5	2	0	5	1510	20	4	7	1/2 starch, 2 veg, 1 fat
Portuguese Kale	lg	160	7	4	2	0	5	1540	20	4	7	1/2 starch, 3 veg, 1 1/2 fat

✔ = Healthiest Bets

(*Continued*)

SOUPS & STEWS *(Continued)*	Amount	Cal.	Fat (g)	% Cal. Fat	Sat. Fat (g)	Trans Fat (g)	Chol. (mg)	Sod. (mg)	Carb. (g)	Fiber (g)	Pro. (g)	Choices/Exchanges
Potato Cheese	med	250	14	5	8	0	50	1340	25	2	7	1 1/2 starch, 3 fat
Potato Cheese	lg	330	18	5	11	0	65	1790	33	2	9	2 starch, 3 1/2 fat
Potato Leek	med	300	20	6	11	0	60	1000	28	2	5	2 starch, 4 fat
Potato Leek	lg	400	26	6	14	0	80	1330	37	3	7	2 starch, 5 fat
Red Beans, Italian Sausage & Rice	med	200	5	2	2	0	10	1140	38	16	15	2 1/2 starch, 1 lean meat
Red Beans, Italian Sausage & Rice	lg	270	7	2	2	0	15	1520	51	22	19	3 1/2 starch, 1 lean meat
✔Southern Black-Eyed Pea	med	180	2	1	0	0	5	950	31	12	12	2 starch, 1 lean meat
Southern Black-Eyed Pea	lg	250	2	1	1	0	10	1260	42	16	16	3 starch, 1 lean meat
Southwest Tortilla	med	200	11	5	3	0	10	1290	24	4	4	2 starch, 2 fat
Southwest Tortilla	lg	260	14	5	4	0	15	1720	31	6	5	2 starch, 3 fat

✔Southwest Vegetable	med	100	3	3	0	0	0	370	17	3	4	3 veg, 1/2 fat
✔Southwest Vegetable	lg	140	4	3	0	0	0	490	23	4	5	5 veg, 1 fat
Split Pea w/ Ham	med	210	2	1	0	0	5	1190	42	15	18	3 starch, 1 lean meat
Split Pea w/ Ham	lg	280	2	1	0	0	10	1590	56	19	24	3 1/2 starch, 2 lean meat
Thai Coconut Curry	med	150	7	4	2	0	0	1150	20	2	3	1 starch, 1 1/2 fat
Thai Coconut Curry	lg	200	9	4	3	0	0	1530	27	3	5	2 starch, 2 fat
✔Tomato Basil Bisque	med	210	8	3	5	0	25	490	29	5	6	1 starch, 3 veg, 1 fat
✔Tomato Basil Bisque	lg	280	11	4	7	0	35	660	39	7	8	1 starch, 3 veg, 2 fat
Tomato Cheddar	med	240	15	6	6	0	25	1040	17	2	12	1 starch, 1 medium-fat meat, 2 fat
Tomato Cheddar	lg	320	21	6	7	0	35	1390	23	2	16	1 1/2 starch, 2 medium-fat meat, 2 fat
Tomato Florentine	med	120	3	2	1	0	5	1390	19	2	5	1/2 starch, 2 veg, 1/2 fat
Tomato Florentine	lg	160	4	2	1	0	10	1850	25	3	7	1 starch, 2 veg, 1 fat

✔ = Healthiest Bets

(*Continued*)

SOUPS & STEWS *(Continued)*	Amount	Cal.	Fat (g)	% Cal. Fat	Sat. Fat (g)	Trans Fat (g)	Chol. (mg)	Sod. (mg)	Carb. (g)	Fiber (g)	Pro. (g)	Choices/Exchanges
Tuscan Vegetable	med	170	5	3	2	0	10	1170	24	3	7	1 starch, 2 veg, 1 fat
Tuscan Vegetable	lg	230	7	3	3	0	10	1570	32	4	9	1 starch, 3 veg, 1 1/2 fat
✔Vegetable Beef Barley	med	140	3	2	2	0	20	1000	21	4	9	1 1/2 starch, 1 medium-fat meat
Vegetable Beef Barley	lg	190	4	2	2	0	30	1340	28	5	12	2 starch, 1 medium-fat meat
Vegetarian Chili	med	230	3	1	0	0	0	1000	40	11	12	2 1/2 starch, 1 lean meat, 1/2 fat
Vegetarian Chili	lg	300	3	1	0	0	0	1330	53	14	16	3 1/2 starch, 1 lean meat
Vegetarian Lentil	med	140	2	1	0	0	0	1260	32	11	10	1 starch, 3 veg
Vegetarian Lentil	lg	190	2	1	0	0	0	1680	42	15	14	2 starch, 3 veg
Vegetarian Minestrone	med	120	2	2	0	0	0	1120	21	4	5	1/2 starch, 3 veg, 1/2 fat

Vegetarian Minestrone	lg	160	2	1	0	0	0	1490	28	6	6	1 starch, 3 veg, 1/2 fat
✔Wild Mushroom Bisque	med	190	9	4	2	0	10	1010	23	2	5	2 starch, 2 fat
Wild Mushroom Bisque	lg	250	13	5	3	0	15	1350	31	3	6	2 starch, 2 1/2 fat
SPREADS												
✔Artichoke Aioli	1 oz	70	7	9	1	0	0	180	1	0	1	1 1/2 fat
Basil Pesto	1 oz	120	12	9	2	0	5	220	1	0	2	2 1/2 fat
Chili Dijon	1 oz	120	12	9	2	0	10	130	3	1	1	2 1/2 fat
Herb Bagel Spread	2 oz	130	11	8	7	0	35	470	5	0	4	1/2 carb, 2 fat
Herb Mayonnaise	1 oz	210	23	10	4	0	20	210	1	0	0	4 1/2 fat
Honey Mustard	2.5 oz	210	13	6	2	0	15	650	23	1	1	1 1/2 carb, 2 1/2 fat
Honey Pecan Cream Cheese	2 oz	120	10	8	7	0	35	340	5	0	4	1/2 carb, 2 fat
✔Jalapeno Mayonnaise	1 oz	60	6	9	1	0	0	250	1	0	2	1 fat
✔Lite Cream Cheese	2 oz	120	9	7	6	0	30	280	5	0	4	1/2 carb, 2 fat

✔ = Healthiest Bets

(*Continued*)

SPREADS *(Continued)*	Amount	Cal.	Fat (g)	% Cal. Fat	Sat. Fat (g)	Trans Fat (g)	Chol. (mg)	Sod. (mg)	Carb. (g)	Fiber (g)	Pro. (g)	Choices/Exchanges
✔Mayonnaise	1 oz	90	8	8	1	0	0	140	1	0	0	1 1/2 fat
✔Mediterranean Spread	1 oz	120	11	8	3	0	5	430	2	1	2	2 fat
✔Mustard	1 tsp	0	0	0	0	0	0	70	0	0	0	Free
✔Plain Cream Cheese	2 oz	170	16	8	11	0.5	50	290	4	0	3	1/2 carb, 3 fat
✔Strawberry Cream Cheese	2 oz	180	15	8	10	0.5	45	250	9	0	3	1/2 carb, 3 fat
✔Sun-Dried Tomato Cream Cheese	2 oz	120	10	8	7	0	35	340	5	0	4	1/2 carb, 2 fat
✔Sun-Dried Tomato Spread	.5 oz	45	4	8	0	0	0	70	1	0	0	1 fat
✔Vegetable Cream Cheese	2 oz	170	16	8	10	0.5	45	270	3	0	3	3 fat
STRUDEL												
Apple	1 pc	430	24	5	13	0	0	270	48	1	5	3 carb, 4 fat
Cherry	1 pc	460	26	5	16	0	0	270	49	2	5	3 1/2 carb, 5 fat

WRAPS												
Cajun Hot Shrimp	1	660	20	3	7	0	85	1680	95	5	20	6 1/2 starch, 4 fat
Chicken Caesar Asiago Wrap	1	660	28	4	9	0	75	1400	62	5	36	4 starch, 3 lean meat, 3 1/2 fat
Chopped Turkey Cobb Wrap	1	620	31	5	9	0	165	1660	63	6	29	4 starch, 2 lean meat, 4 fat
Fields & Feta Wrap	1	480	8	2	6	0	20	1190	67	6	17	4 starch, 1 veg, 1 lean meat, 2 fat
Mayan Chicken Hot Wrap	1	590	15	2	3	0	35	1390	92	6	24	6 starch, 1 lean meat, 2 fat
Mediterranean Wrap	1	610	29	4	7	0	20	1770	73	8	18	5 starch, 5 fat
Southwest Tuna Wrap	1	760	42	5	13	0	95	1410	65	7	40	4 1/2 starch, 4 lean meat, 5 fat
Steak Teriyaki Hot Wrap	1	620	15	2	3	0	30	1510	96	5	26	6 1/2 starch, 1 medium-fat meat, 1 fat

✔ = Healthiest Bets

(*Continued*)

WRAPS *(Continued)*	Amount	Cal.	Fat (g)	% Cal. Fat	Sat. Fat (g)	Trans Fat (g)	Chol. (mg)	Sod. (mg)	Carb. (g)	Fiber (g)	Pro. (g)	Choices/Exchanges
Thai Peanut Chicken Wrap	1	620	22	3	3	0	40	1240	76	6	32	5 starch, 2 lean meat, 2 fat
Turkey Spinach Sonoma Wrap	1	530	13	2	5	0	40	1480	83	7	26	5 1/2 starch, 1 lean meat, 1 fat
YOGURT												
Blueberry w/ Fruit	sm	220	2	1	2	0	10	120	44	0	6	1 carb, 1 fruit, 1 milk, 1/2 fat
✔Blueberry w/ Fruit	lg	440	4	1	3	0	20	240	88	1	12	3 carb, 1 fruit, 2 milk, 1/2 fat
Blueberry w/ Granola & Fruit	sm	310	6	2	2	0	10	130	56	2	10	2 carb, 1 fruit, 1 milk, 1/2 fat
Blueberry w/ Granola & Fruit	lg	620	13	2	4	0	20	260	112	5	20	5 carb, 1 fruit, 2 milk, 1 fat

Strawberry w/ Granola & Blueberries	sm	310	6	2	2	0	10	130	56	2	10	2 carb, 1 fruit, 1 milk, 1 fat
Strawberry w/ Granola & Blueberries	lg	620	13	2	4	0	20	260	112	5	20	5 carb, 1 fruit, 2 milk, 1/2 fat
✔Strawberry Yogurt w/ Blueberries	sm	220	2	1	2	0	10	120	44	0	6	1 carb, 1 fruit, 1 milk, 1/2 fat
✔Strawberry Yogurt w/ Blueberries	lg	440	4	1	3	0	20	240	88	1	12	3 carb, 1 fruit, 2 milk, 1 fat
Vanilla w/ Granola & Blueberries	sm	310	6	2	2	0	10	130	56	2	10	1 1/2 carb, 1 fruit, 1 milk, 1 fat
Vanilla w/ Granola & Blueberries	lg	622	13	2	4	0	20	260	112	5	20	5 carb, 1 fruit, 2 milk, 1 fat
✔Vanilla Yogurt w/ Blueberries	sm	190	2	1	1	0	10	160	32	0	10	1 fruit, 1 milk, 1 fat
Vanilla Yogurt w/ Blueberries	lg	390	4	1	3	0	25	320	64	1	20	1 1/2 carb, 1 fruit, 2 milk, 1 fat

✔ = Healthiest Bets

Blimpie Subs and Salads
(www.blimpie.com)

Light 'n Lean Choice

Grande Chili with Beans and Beef
Chef Salad with
Dijon Honey Mustard dressing *(2 T)*

Calories	561	Cholesterol (mg)	97
Fat (g)	21	Sodium (mg)	2,195
% calories from fat	34	Carbohydrate (g)	46
Saturated fat (g)	11	Fiber (g)	20
Trans fat (g)	0	Protein (g)	37

Exchanges: 2 starch, 2 veg, 4 lean meat, 2 1/2 fat

Healthy 'n Hearty Choice

Harvest Vegetable Soup
Club Sandwich *(6 inch)*
Potato Salad *(side)*

Calories	716	Cholesterol (mg)	57
Fat (g)	23	Sodium (mg)	2,473
% calories from fat	29	Carbohydrate (g)	96
Saturated fat (g)	7	Fiber (g)	9
Trans fat (g)	0	Protein (g)	32

Exchanges: 5 starch, 3 veg, 2 medium-fat meat, 3 fat

(*Continued*)

Blimpie

	Amount	Cal.	Fat (g)	% Cal. Fat	Sat. Fat (g)	Trans Fat (g)	Chol. (mg)	Sod. (mg)	Carb. (g)	Fiber (g)	Pro. (g)	Choices/Exchanges
BREAKFAST: BISCUIT												
Bacon, Egg, & Cheese	1	432	24	5	17	0	158	1579	37	1	17	2 1/2 starch, 1 medium-fat meat, 3 1/2 fat
Egg & Cheese	1	385	21	5	15	0	150	1377	37	1	14	2 1/2 starch, 1 medium-fat meat, 3 1/2 fat
Ham, Egg, & Cheese	1	420	21	5	16	0	165	1655	39	1	19	2 1/2 starch, 2 lean meat, 3 fat
Plain	1	263	11	4	10	0	1	830	34	1	6	2 1/2 starch, 2 1/2 fat
Sausage, Egg, & Cheese	1	535	35	6	20	0	180	1687	37	1	20	2 1/2 starch, 2 medium-fat meat, 4 fat

✔ = Healthiest Bets

(*Continued*)

	Amount	Cal.	Fat (g)	% Cal. Fat	Sat. Fat (g)	Trans Fat (g)	Chol. (mg)	Sod. (mg)	Carb. (g)	Fiber (g)	Pro. (g)	Choices/Exchanges
BREAKFAST: BLUFFIN												
✔Bacon, Egg, & Cheese	1	293	14	4	7	0	157	973	27	2	16	2 starch, 2 medium-fat meat, 1 fat
✔Egg & Cheese	1	245	10	4	5	0	149	771	27	2	13	2 starch, 1 medium-fat meat, 1 fat
Ham, Egg, & Cheese	1	280	11	4	6	0	164	1049	29	2	18	2 starch, 2 lean meat, 1 fat
✔Plain	1	129	1	1	0	0	0	242	25	2	5	1 1/2 starch
Sausage, Egg, & Cheese	1	395	24	5	10	0	179	1081	27	2	19	2 starch, 2 medium-fat meat, 3 fat
BREAKFAST: BURRITO												
Bacon, Egg, & Cheese	1	553	24	4	12	0	8	2095	56	5	31	3 1/2 starch, 3 medium-fat meat, 1 fat

Egg & Cheese	1	506	20	4	11	0	0	1892	56	5	28	3 1/2 starch, 2 medium-fat meat, 1 fat
Ham, Egg, & Cheese	1	559	21	3	11	0	23	2310	58	5	36	4 starch, 3 lean meat, 2 fat
Sausage, Egg, & Cheese	1	656	34	5	16	0	30	2202	56	5	34	3 1/2 starch, 3 medium-fat meat, 3 fat
BREAKFAST: CROISSANT												
Bacon, Egg, & Cheese	1	396	15	3	12	0	165	1026	30	1	16	2 starch, 1 medium-fat meat, 2 fat
✔Egg & Cheese	1	349	15	4	11	0	157	823	30	1	12	2 starch, 1 medium-fat meat, 3 fat
Ham, Egg, & Cheese	1	384	20	5	11	0	172	1102	31	1	17	2 starch, 2 lean meat, 3 fat
Plain	1	233	12	5	6	0	8	295	28	1	5	2 starch, 2 1/2 fat
Sausage, Egg, & Cheese	1	499	35	6	16	0	187	1133	30	1	18	2 starch, 2 medium-fat meat, 5 1/2 fat

✔ = Healthiest Bets

(Continued)

	Amount	Cal.	Fat (g)	% Cal. Fat	Sat. Fat (g)	Trans Fat (g)	Chol. (mg)	Sod. (mg)	Carb. (g)	Fiber (g)	Pro. (g)	Choices/Exchanges
BREAKFAST: PANINI												
4"	1 srvg	494	14	3	5	0	181	1408	67	2	26	4 1/2 starch, 2 medium-fat meat, 1 fat
6"	1 srvg	773	24	3	9	0	360	2368	96	3	43	6 1/2 starch, 3 medium-fat meat, 1 fat
BREAKFAST: ROLL												
Cinnamon Roll	1	449	20	4	9	0	30	729	60	2	9	4 carb, 3 fat
CHIPS												
Cheddar Sour Cream	1 srvg	240	15	6	5	0	0	285	21	2	3	1 1/2 starch, 3 fat
✔Cheetos Crunchy	1 srvg	160	10	6	3	0	0	290	15	1	2	1 starch, 2 fat
Doritos Cooler Ranch	1 srvg	245	12	4	3	0	0	297	32	2	4	2 starch, 2 fat
Doritos Nacho Cheese	1 srvg	245	12	4	3	0	0	332	30	2	4	2 starch, 2 fat
Fritos	1 srvg	320	20	6	2	0	0	210	30	2	4	2 starch, 4 fat

KC Master BBQ	1 srvg	240	15	6	5	0	0	300	23	2	3	1 1/2 starch, 3 fat
✔KC Master BBQ Baked	1 srvg	135	3	2	0	0	0	236	25	2	2	1 1/2 starch
✔Multigrain Harvest Cheddar	1 srvg	210	9	4	2	0	0	285	29	3	3	2 starch, 2 fat
✔Multigrain Original	1 srvg	209	9	4	1	0	0	139	29	4	3	2 starch, 2 fat
✔Potato Baked	1 srvg	124	2	1	0	0	0	169	26	2	2	1 1/2 starch, 1/2 fat
Potato Regular	1 srvg	225	15	6	5	0	0	270	23	2	3	1 1/2 starch, 3 fat
DESSERTS: BROWNIE												
✔Brownie	1	182	7	3	3	0	15	115	28	1	2	2 carb, 1 fat
DESSERTS: COOKIES												
✔Chocolate Chunk	1	196	10	5	4	0	13	153	25	0	2	1 1/2 carb, 2 fat
✔Oatmeal Raisin Walnut	1	170	7	4	3	0	9	142	26	1	2	1 1/2 carb, 1 fat
Peanut Butter	1	198	12	5	5	0	9	161	20	1	3	1 1/2 carb, 2 1/2 fat
Sugar	1	327	17	5	6	0	29	286	41	1	3	2 1/2 carb, 3 fat

✔ = Healthiest Bets

(*Continued*)

DESSERTS: COOKIES *(Continued)*	Amount	Cal.	Fat (g)	% Cal. Fat	Sat. Fat (g)	Trans Fat (g)	Chol. (mg)	Sod. (mg)	Carb. (g)	Fiber (g)	Pro. (g)	Choices/Exchanges
White Chocolate Macadamia Nut	1	198	12	5	5	0	9	161	20	1	3	1 1/2 carb, 2 1/2 fat
DESSERTS: TURNOVER												
Apple	1 srvg	340	21	6	10	0	0	190	35	1	4	2 1/2 carb, 4 fat
Cherry	1 srvg	350	21	5	10	0	0	190	35	1	4	2 1/2 carb, 4 fat
DRESSINGS												
Blue Cheese	1.5 oz.	230	24	9	5	0	25	440	2	na	2	5 fat
Buttermilk Ranch	1.5 oz.	230	24	9	4	0	10	380	2	na	1	5 fat
Creamy Caesar	1.5 oz.	210	21	9	4	0	10	520	2	na	1	4 1/2 fat
✔Creamy Italian	1.5 oz.	180	18	9	3	0	0	420	4	0	0	4 fat
Dijon Honey Mustard	1.5 oz.	180	17	9	3	0	15	240	8	na	1	1/2 carb, 3 1/2 fat
✔Fat-Free Italian	1.5 oz.	25	0	0	*	0	0	390	5	0	0	1/2 carb
✔Light Buttermilk Ranch	1.5 oz.	70	4	5	1	0	0	310	8	na	1	1/2 carb, 1 fat

✔Light Italian	1.5 oz.	20	1	5	0	0	0	770	2	na	0	Free
✔Special	0.7 oz.	70	7	9	1	0	0	0	0	na	0	1 1/2 fat
Thousand Island	1.5 oz.	210	20	9	3	0	15	350	6	0	0	1/2 carb, 4 fat
KID'S MEALS												
✔3" Ham & American Cheese	1 srvg	262	9	3	5	0	15	901	32	2	15	2 starch, 1 lean meat, 1 fat
✔3" Tuna	1 srvg	277	11	4	2	0	27	457	30	2	14	2 starch, 1 lean meat, 1 fat
✔3" Turkey	1 srvg	187	2	1	0	0	12	598	31	2	10	2 starch, 1 lean meat
SALADS												
Antipasto Salad w/ Dressing	1 srvg	423	32	7	8	0	59	2042	16	4	20	1/2 starch, 1 veg, 3 lean meat, 5 fat
✔Chef Salad, Regular	1 srvg	176	7	4	4	0	47	805	10	2	18	2 veg, 3 lean meat
Chicken Caesar Salad w/ Dressing	1 srvg	400	29	7	7	0	72	978	8	3	26	2 veg, 4 lean meat, 3 1/2 fat

✔ = Healthiest Bets

(*Continued*)

SALADS *(Continued)*	Amount	Cal.	Fat (g)	% Cal. Fat	Sat. Fat (g)	Trans Fat (g)	Chol. (mg)	Sod. (mg)	Carb. (g)	Fiber (g)	Pro. (g)	Choices/Exchanges
✔Cole Slaw Side Salad	1 srvg	160	9	5	2	0	5	240	20	2	1	1/2 starch, 2 veg, 2 fat
✔Garden Salad	1 srvg	29	0	0	0	0	0	16	6	3	2	1 veg
Macaroni Side Salad	1 srvg	330	22	6	5	0	15	790	28	2	5	2 starch, 4 1/2 fat
Northwest Potato Side Salad	1 srvg	260	17	6	4	0	25	390	22	3	3	1 1/2 starch, 3 1/2 fat
Potato Side Salad	1 srvg	230	12	5	3	0	10	490	28	3	3	2 starch, 2 fat
✔Seafood Salad, Regular	1 srvg	122	4	3	1	0	19	582	17	3	6	1 starch, 1 fat
Tuna Salad, Regular	1 srvg	272	18	6	3	0	55	517	7	2	18	2 veg, 3 lean meat, 2 fat
Ultimate Club Salad w/ Dressing	1 srvg	514	40	7	12	0	82	1571	12	3	25	2 veg, 4 lean meat, 6 fat
SANDWICHES: 4"												
✔Blimpie Best	1	268	8	3	4	0	34	910	33	2	16	2 starch, 1 lean meat, 1 fat

✔Club	1	254	6	2	3	0	32	743	33	2	16	2 starch, 1 lean meat, 1/2 fat
✔Ham & Swiss	1	257	6	2	3	0	33	724	33	2	16	2 starch, 1 lean meat, 1/2 fat
✔Roast Beef & Provolone	1	262	7	2	3	0	39	676	31	2	20	2 starch, 2 lean meat
✔Tuna	1	282	11	4	2	0	27	458	31	2	14	2 starch, 1 lean meat, 1 1/2 fat
✔Turkey & Provolone	1	247	6	2	2	0	26	858	33	2	16	2 starch, 1 lean meat
SANDWICHES: 6"												
Blimpie Best, Regular	1	420	14	3	6	0	55	1371	49	3	25	3 1/2 starch, 2 lean meat, 1 1/2 fat
Blimpie Best, Super Stacked	1	523	19	3	8	0	95	2128	52	3	37	3 1/2 starch, 4 lean meat, 1 fat
Blimpie Trio, Super Stacked	1	488	12	2	5	0	93	1773	52	3	41	3 1/2 starch, 4 lean meat

✔ = Healthiest Bets

(*Continued*)

SANDWICHES: 6" *(Continued)*	Amount	Cal.	Fat (g)	% Cal. Fat	Sat. Fat (g)	Trans Fat (g)	Chol. (mg)	Sod. (mg)	Carb. (g)	Fiber (g)	Pro. (g)	Choices/Exchanges
✔BLT, Regular	1	346	11	3	3	0	17	872	46	3	15	3 starch, 1 medium-fat meat, 1 fat
Chicken Cheddar Bacon Ranch, Regular	1	642	34	5	10	0	89	1648	48	3	36	3 starch, 4 medium-fat meat, 2 1/2 fat
Chicken Teriyaki, Regular	1	428	9	2	4	0	58	1315	50	1	35	3 1/2 starch, 4 lean meat
Club, Regular	1	386	10	2	4	0	47	1063	49	3	25	3 starch, 2 medium-fat meat
Cuban, Regular	1	413	11	2	5	0	65	1628	43	1	29	3 starch, 3 medium-fat meat
Ham & Swiss, Regular	1	391	10	2	5	0	50	1026	50	3	25	3 1/2 starch, 2 lean meat, 1/2 fat
Ham, Salami & Cheese, Regular	1	443	16	3	7	0	56	1306	49	3	25	3 1/2 starch, 2 medium-fat meat, 1/2 fat

Meatball, Regular	1	607	32	5	14	0	82	2072	51	4	28	3 1/2 starch, 3 medium-fat meat, 3 fat
Pastrami, Regular	1	454	17	3	7	0	61	1375	48	3	30	3 starch, 3 medium-fat meat
Philly Steak & Onion, Regular	1	499	24	4	10	0	72	1233	45	1	26	3 starch, 2 medium-fat meat, 2 fat
Reuben, Regular	1	571	24	4	7	0	75	1221	54	3	34	3 1/2 starch, 3 medium-fat meat, 1 fat
Roast Beef & Provolone, Regular	1	408	11	2	5	0	62	1051	47	3	31	3 starch, 3 lean meat
Roast Beef, Turkey & Cheddar, Regular	1	571	30	5	9	0	74	1769	48	3	27	3 starch, 2 lean meat, 4 fat
✔Seafood, Regular	1	333	7	2	1	0	19	840	56	4	13	3 1/2 starch, 1 fat
Tuna, Regular	1	483	21	4	3	0	55	776	46	3	25	3 starch, 2 lean meat, 3 fat

✔ = Healthiest Bets

(*Continued*)

SANDWICHES: 6" *(Continued)*	Amount	Cal.	Fat (g)	% Cal. Fat	Sat. Fat (g)	Trans Fat (g)	Chol. (mg)	Sod. (mg)	Carb. (g)	Fiber (g)	Pro. (g)	Choices/Exchanges
Turkey & Provolone, Regular	1	393	10	2	4	0	46	1405	49	3	26	3 1/2 starch, 2 lean meat
Turkey Bacon, SS	1	582	24	4	11	0	65	2622	48	2	40	3 starch, 4 lean meat, 2 fat
Veggie Supreme	1	553	28	5	16	0	36	1415	48	3	29	3 starch, 1 veg, 3 lean meat, 3 fat
VegiMax	1	522	20	3	6	0	15	1272	56	5	28	3 starch, 2 veg, 3 lean meat, 2 fat
SANDWICHES: 12"												
Blimpie Best, Regular	1	840	28	3	12	0	110	2743	99	6	50	6 1/2 starch, 4 lean meat, 2 fat
Blimpie Best, Super Stacked	1	1045	37	3	16	0	189	4256	104	6	73	7 starch, 7 lean meat, 2 fat

Blimpie Trio, Super Stacked	1	970	24	2	10	0	187	3542	102	6	82	6 1/2 starch, 8 lean meat, 1 fat
BLT, Regular	1	692	22	3	7	0	34	1744	93	6	31	6 starch, 2 medium-fat meat, 2 fat
Chicken Cheddar Bacon Ranch, Regular	1	967	44	4	15	0	108	2485	94	6	50	6 1/2 starch, 4 medium-fat meat, 3 fat
Chicken Teriyaki, Regular	1	838	18	2	9	0	115	2446	96	3	69	6 1/2 starch, 6 lean meat
Club, Regular	1	773	20	2	9	0	95	2127	99	6	49	6 1/2 starch, 4 lean meat, 1 fat
Cuban, Regular	1	827	21	2	9	0	131	3256	86	3	59	5 1/2 starch, 6 lean meat, 1/2 fat
Ham & Swiss, Regular	1	783	21	2	9	0	101	2052	99	6	49	6 1/2 starch, 4 lean meat, 1 fat
Ham, Salami & Cheese, Regular	1	887	32	3	15	0	112	2612	99	6	50	6 1/2 starch, 4 medium-fat meat, 1 fat

✔ = Healthiest Bets

(*Continued*)

SANDWICHES: 12" *(Continued)*	Amount	Cal.	Fat (g)	% Cal. Fat	Sat. Fat (g)	Trans Fat (g)	Chol. (mg)	Sod. (mg)	Carb. (g)	Fiber (g)	Pro. (g)	Choices/Exchanges
Meatball, Regular	1	1185	62	5	26	0	157	4007	101	8	55	6 1/2 starch, 5 medium-fat meat, 6 fat
Pastrami, Regular	1	908	33	3	15	0	122	2749	96	6	61	6 1/2 starch, 6 medium-fat meat
Philly Steak & Onion, Regular	1	981	46	4	19	0	139	2415	90	3	50	6 starch, 5 medium-fat meat, 4 fat
Reuben, Regular	1	1143	48	4	14	0	151	2442	107	6	67	7 starch, 7 medium-fat meat, 2 fat
Roast Beef & Provolone, Regular	1	817	22	2	9	0	124	2102	93	6	61	6 starch, 5 medium-fat meat
Roast Beef, Turkey & Cheddar, Regular	1	1142	60	5	19	0	149	3537	95	5	54	6 1/2 starch, 5 medium-fat meat, 6 fat
Seafood, Regular	1	666	14	2	3	0	38	1680	111	7	25	7 1/2 starch, 2 fat

Tuna, Regular	1	965	42	4	6	0	109	1551	92	6	50	6 starch, 5 lean meat, 5 fat
Turkey & Provolone, Regular	1	787	20	2	9	0	91	2810	99	6	52	6 1/2 starch, 5 lean meat
Turkey Bacon, Super Stacked	1	1165	48	4	21	0	129	5244	96	5	80	6 1/2 starch, 9 lean meat, 4 fat
Veggie Supreme	1	1106	56	5	33	0	73	2831	96	6	58	5 starch, 3 veg, 6 lean meat, 6 fat
SANDWICHES: CIABATTA												
Buffalo Chicken	1	583	27	4	7	0	69	2050	50	3	32	3 1/2 starch, 3 lean meat, 3 fat
Grilled Chicken Caesar	1	617	24	4	6	0	65	1584	63	3	34	4 starch, 3 lean meat, 3 fat
Roast Beef, Turkey & Cheddar	1	588	30	5	9	0	74	1941	51	3	28	3 1/2 starch, 3 medium-fat meat, 3 fat
Sicilian	1	637	25	4	7	0	71	2520	68	3	33	4 1/2 starch, 3 medium-fat meat, 1 fat

✔ = Healthiest Bets

(Continued)

SANDWICHES: CIABATTA *(Continued)*	Amount	Cal.	Fat (g)	% Cal. Fat	Sat. Fat (g)	Trans Fat (g)	Chol. (mg)	Sod. (mg)	Carb. (g)	Fiber (g)	Pro. (g)	Choices/Exchanges
Turkey Italiano	1	502	11	2	4	0	50	2164	64	3	30	4 1/2 starch, 2 medium-fat meat
Tuscan	1	600	23	3	7	0	55	2150	65	3	29	4 1/2 starch, 2 medium-fat meat, 2 fat
Ultimate Club	1	480	21	4	6	0	60	1538	47	2	27	3 starch, 3 lean meat, 2 1/2 fat
SNACKS												
Pretzels Classic Thin Style	1 srvg	223	2	1	0	0	0	na	47	2	4	3 starch
SOUPS												
Bean w/ Ham	1 srvg	140	1	1	0	0	0	1070	23	11	8	1 1/2 starch, 1/2 fat
✔Beef Steak & Noodle	1 srvg	120	3	2	2	0	30	780	14	0	8	1 starch, 1 medium-fat meat
✔Beef Stew	1 srvg	170	4	2	2	0	45	890	18	2	17	1 starch, 2 lean meat

✔Captain's Corn Chowder	1 srvg	210	7	3	3	0	5	890	29	4	6	2 starch, 1 1/2 fat
✔Chicken & Dumpling	1 srvg	170	5	3	3	0	50	970	19	3	11	1 1/2 starch, 1 lean meat, 1/2 fat
Chicken Gumbo	1 srvg	90	2	2	0	0	10	1280	13	2	6	1 starch, 1/2 fat
Chicken Noodle	1 srvg	130	4	3	1	0	30	1040	18	2	7	1 starch, 1 fat
Chicken w/ White & Wild Rice	1 srvg	250	10	4	3	0	30	1030	15	4	14	1 starch, 2 lean meat, 2 fat
✔Cream of Broccoli w/ Cheese	1 srvg	190	8	4	5	0	15	940	15	3	6	1 starch, 1 veg, 2 fat
✔Cream of Potato	1 srvg	190	9	4	3	0	5	860	24	3	5	1 1/2 starch, 2 fat
French Onion	1 srvg	80	4	5	1	0	0	1020	11	1	2	1/2 starch, 1 fat
Grande Chili w/ Bean & Beef	1 srvg	250	9	3	5	0	40	1230	30	18	18	2 starch, 2 lean meat
✔Harvest Vegetable	1 srvg	100	1	1	0	0	0	920	19	3	4	3 veg, 1 fat
✔Italian Style Wedding	1 srvg	130	4	3	2	0	10	900	17	0	7	1 starch, 1 medium-fat meat, 1/2 fat

✔ = Healthiest Bets

(*Continued*)

SOUPS *(Continued)*	Amount	Cal.	Fat (g)	% Cal. Fat	Sat. Fat (g)	Trans Fat (g)	Chol. (mg)	Sod. (mg)	Carb. (g)	Fiber (g)	Pro. (g)	Choices/Exchanges
Minestrone	1 srvg	90	3	3	0	0	0	1150	14	4	4	1 starch, 1/2 fat
New England Clam Chowder	1 srvg	170	3	2	2	0	25	1060	28	2	7	2 starch, 1/2 fat
✔Pasta Fagioli w/Sausage	1 srvg	150	5	3	2	0	20	910	22	4	7	1 1/2 starch, 1 fat
✔Pilgrim Turkey Vegetables w/ Rice	1 srvg	110	2	2	1	0	20	800	19	2	4	1 1/2 starch, 1/2 fat
✔Seafood Gumbo	1 srvg	100	2	2	1	0	20	850	16	2	4	1 starch, 1/2 fat
Split Pea w/ Ham	1 srvg	130	2	1	0	0	5	1090	21	6	8	1 1/2 starch, 1 lean meat
✔Tomato Basil w/ Raviolini	1 srvg	110	1	1	0	0	10	720	22	0	4	1/2 starch, 3 veg
✔Yankee Pot Roast	1 srvg	80	2	2	1	0	10	750	12	2	5	1 starch

WRAPS

Chicken Caesar, Regular	1	607	29	4	9	0	61	1586	56	4	30	3 1/2 starch, 3 lean meat, 4 fat
Roast Beef & Cheddar, Regular	1	684	36	5	12	0	85	1928	59	6	32	4 starch, 3 medium-fat meat, 4 fat
Southwestern, Regular	1	530	22	4	6	0	54	1771	61	4	23	4 starch, 2 lean meat, 3 fat
Steak & Onion, Regular	1	774	47	5	15	0	84	1795	62	6	28	4 starch, 2 medium-fat meat, 6 fat
Zesty, Regular	1	569	26	4	10	0	69	1979	59	6	28	4 starch, 2 lean meat, 3 fat

✓ = Healthiest Bets

Panera Bread

(www.panerabread.com)

Light 'n Lean Choice

Low-Fat Garden Vegetable Soup ***(8 oz)***
Asian Sesame Chicken Salad,
dressing included ***(1/2 serving)***
Whole-Grain Loaf Bread (***1 slice*****)**

Calories	440	Cholesterol (mg)	35
Fat (g)	13	Sodium (mg)	1,780
% calories from fat	27	Carbohydrate (g)	60
Saturated fat (g)	1.5	Fiber (g)	7
Trans fat (g)	0	Protein (g)	25

Exchanges: 3 starch, 2 veg, 2 lean meat, 1 fat

Healthy 'n Hearty Choice

Low-Fat Vegetarian Black Bean Soup ***(8 oz)***
Mediterranean Veggie Sandwich on
Tomato Basil Bread ***(1/2)***
Nutty Oatmeal Raisin Cookie ***(2)***

Calories	620	Cholesterol (mg)	25
Fat (g)	15	Sodium (mg)	1,780
% calories from fat	22	Carbohydrate (g)	103
Saturated fat (g)	4.5	Fiber (g)	13
Trans fat (g)	0.5	Protein (g)	21

Exchanges: 5 starch, 1 1/2 carb, 1 veg, 3 fat

Panera Bread

	Amount	Cal.	Fat (g)	% Cal. Fat	Sat. Fat (g)	Trans Fat (g)	Chol. (mg)	Sod. (mg)	Carb. (g)	Fiber (g)	Pro. (g)	Choices/Exchanges
ARTISAN BREADS												
Ciabatta	1 loaf	460	5	1	1	0	0	760	84	3	16	6 starch, 1 fat
✔Country Loaf	1 slice	140	1	1	0	0	0	310	27	1	5	2 starch
✔Country Miche	1 slice	130	1	1	0	0	0	300	26	1	5	2 starch
✔Focaccia	1 slice	160	3	2	0	0	0	330	29	1	5	2 starch, 1/2 fat
✔Focaccia w/ Asiago Cheese	1 slice	160	5	3	1.5	0	5	230	23	1	5	2 starch, 1 fat
✔French Baguette	1 slice	150	1	1	0	0	0	370	29	1	5	2 starch
✔French Miche	1 slice	130	1	1	0	0	0	330	26	1	5	2 starch
✔Sesame Semolina Loaf	1 slice	140	1	1	0	0	0	350	29	1	4	2 starch
✔Sesame Semolina Miche	1 slice	130	1	1	0	0	0	330	27	1	4	2 starch

✔ = Healthiest Bets

(*Continued*)

ARTISAN BREADS *(Continued)*	Amount	Cal.	Fat (g)	% Cal. Fat	Sat. Fat (g)	Trans Fat (g)	Chol. (mg)	Sod. (mg)	Carb. (g)	Fiber (g)	Pro. (g)	Choices/Exchanges
✔Stone-Milled Rye Loaf	1 slice	120	1	1	0	0	0	340	25	2	4	2 starch
✔Stone-Milled Rye Miche	1 slice	120	1	1	0	0	0	340	25	2	4	2 starch
✔Three Cheese Demi	1 slice	140	2	1	1	0	5	300	26	1	6	2 starch, 1/2 fat
✔Three Cheese Loaf	1 slice	140	2	1	1	0	5	300	26	1	6	2 starch, 1/2 fat
✔Three Cheese Miche	1 slice	140	2	1	1	0	5	290	25	1	5	2 starch, 1/2 fat
✔Three Seed Demi	1 slice	150	3	2	0	0	0	290	26	2	5	2 starch, 1/2 fat
✔Whole Grain Baguette	1 slice	150	2	1	0	0	0	310	29	3	6	2 starch, 1/2 fat
✔Whole Grain Loaf	1 slice	140	2	1	0	0	0	300	27	2	5	2 starch, 1/2 fat
✔Whole Grain Miche	1 slice	150	2	1	0	0	0	300	29	3	6	2 starch, 1/2 fat
ARTISAN PASTRIES												
Caramel Apple	1	400	19	4	12	1	60	300	51	2	7	1 1/2 starch, 1 1/2 carb, 4 fat
Cheese	1	380	22	5	13	1	65	330	39	1	7	1 1/2 starch, 1 1/2 carb, 4 1/2 fat

Cherry	1	420	21	5	13	1	10	330	51	1	8	1 1/2 starch, 1 1/2 carb, 3 fat
Chocolate	1	340	20	5	12	0	10	230	37	2	6	1 starch, 1 carb, 3 1/2 fat
Chocolate Crumb	1	470	21	4	12	0	45	260	64	3	9	2 starch, 2 carb, 3 fat
Fresh Strawberry Citrus	1	310	16	5	10	0	10	270	37	1	6	1 starch, 1 carb, 3 fat
Pecan Braid	1	410	22	5	8	0	5	230	48	2	6	1 1/2 starch, 1 1/2 carb, 3 fat
BAKED EGG SOUFFLÉS												
Four Cheese	1	470	30	6	16	0	150	700	35	2	16	2 1/2 starch, 1 medium-fat meat, 4 1/2 fat
Spinach & Artichoke	1	490	32	6	18	0	130	830	36	2	18	2 1/2 starch, 2 medium-fat meat, 5 fat
Spinach & Bacon	1	560	36	6	20	0	140	990	37	2	21	2 1/2 starch, 2 medium-fat meat, 5 1/2 fat
Turkey Sausage & Potato	1	450	28	6	15	0	115	600	36	2	14	2 1/2 starch, 1 medium-fat meat, 4 1/2 fat

✔ = Healthiest Bets

(Continued)

	Amount	Cal.	Fat (g)	% Cal. Fat	Sat. Fat (g)	Trans Fat (g)	Chol. (mg)	Sod. (mg)	Carb. (g)	Fiber (g)	Pro. (g)	Choices/Exchanges
BROWNIES												
Caramel Pecan	1	470	24	5	6	0	80	170	59	2	5	4 carb, 4 fat
Very Chocolate	1	460	22	4	5	0	80	180	61	2	5	4 carb, 3 fat
CAFÉ SANDWICHES												
Chicken Salad on Sesame Semolina	1	680	25	3	4.5	0	20	1870	94	13	29	6 1/2 starch, 1 lean meat, 3 fat
Chicken Salad on Whole Grain	1	590	25	4	4.5	0	20	1570	71	16	29	4 1/2 starch, 2 lean meat, 3 fat
✔Half Chicken Salad on Sesame Semolina	1	340	12	3	2	0	10	930	44	7	15	3 starch, 1 lean meat, 2 fat
✔Half Chicken Salad on Whole Grain	1	290	13	4	2.5	0	10	790	35	8	15	2 1/2 starch, 1 lean meat, 1 fat
✔Half Smoked Ham & Swiss on Rye	1	350	18	5	7	0	55	940	28	2	20	2 starch, 2 lean meat, 2 1/2 fat

Half Smoked Ham & Swiss on Stone-Milled Rye	1	390	16	4	6	0	55	1200	38	3	22	2 1/2 starch, 2 lean meat, 2 fat
Half Smoked Turkey Breast on Country	1	310	9	3	1.5	0	30	1040	40	2	17	2 1/2 starch, 1 lean meat, 1 fat
✔Half Smoked Turkey Breast on Sourdough	1	240	9	3	1.5	0	30	840	25	1	15	1 1/2 starch, 1 lean meat, 1 fat
✔Half Tuna Salad on Honey Wheat	1	360	23	6	4	0	20	570	29	2	10	2 starch, 1 lean meat, 4 fat
Smoked Ham & Swiss on Rye	1	700	35	5	13	0	110	1890	55	4	40	3 1/2 starch, 4 lean meat, 4 fat
Smoked Ham & Swiss on Stone-Milled Rye	1	770	32	4	12	0	110	2400	76	6	44	5 starch, 4 lean meat, 3 fat
Smoked Turkey Breast on Country	1	620	18	3	2.5	0	60	2080	81	4	35	5 1/2 starch, 3 lean meat, 1 fat
Smoked Turkey Breast on Sourdough	1	470	17	3	2.5	0	60	1680	49	3	30	3 1/2 starch, 3 lean meat, 1 fat

✔ = Healthiest Bets

(Continued)

CAFÉ SANDWICHES *(Continued)*	Amount	Cal.	Fat (g)	% Cal. Fat	Sat. Fat (g)	Trans Fat (g)	Chol. (mg)	Sod. (mg)	Carb. (g)	Fiber (g)	Pro. (g)	Choices/Exchanges
Tuna Salad on Honey Wheat	1	720	45	6	8	0	45	1140	59	5	19	4 starch, 1 lean meat, 8 fat
COOKIES												
Chocolate Chipper	1	380	19	5	10	0	50	270	51	2	5	3 1/2 carb, 3 fat
Chocolate Duet w/ Walnuts	1	400	22	5	10	0	50	290	52	3	6	3 1/2 carb, 3 1/2 fat
Nutty Chocolate Chipper	1	430	24	5	10	0	50	270	51	3	5	3 1/2 carb, 4 fat
Nutty Oatmeal Raisin	1	340	14	4	6	0	45	270	50	3	5	3 1/2 carb, 2 fat
✔Petite - Chocolate Chipper	1	100	5	5	2.5	0	15	65	13	0	1	1 carb, 1 fat
✔Petite - Chocolate Duet w/ Walnuts	1	100	6	5	2.5	0	15	75	13	1	2	1 carb, 1 fat
✔Petite - Nutty Oatmeal Raisin	1	80	4	5	1.5	0	10	65	12	1	1	1 carb, 1/2 fat
Petite - Shortbread	1	180	12	6	7	0	30	90	16	0	2	1 carb, 2 1/2 fat
Shortbread	1	350	21	5	12	1	55	160	36	1	3	2 1/2 carb, 3 1/2 fat

CRISPANI												
✔BBQ Chicken	2 slices	380	15	4	6	0	50	970	42	2	20	3 starch, 2 lean meat, 2 fat
✔Italian Meat Classic	2 slices	390	18	4	7	0	40	990	38	2	17	2 1/2 starch, 1 medium-fat meat, 2 fat
✔Pepperoni	2 slices	390	18	4	8	0	30	870	38	2	17	2 1/2 starch, 1 medium-fat meat, 2 fat
✔Roasted Wild Mushroom	2 slices	350	16	4	6	0	30	600	38	2	13	2 1/2 starch, 1 medium-fat meat, 2 fat
✔Sausage & Roasted Peppers	2 slices	380	18	4	7	0	40	730	38	2	15	2 1/2 starch, 1 medium-fat meat, 2 fat
✔Three Cheese	2 slices	350	16	4	7	0	35	590	37	2	15	2 1/2 starch, 1 medium-fat meat, 2 fat
✔Tomato & Fresh Basil	2 slices	330	13	4	6	0	20	590	38	2	13	2 1/2 starch, 1 medium-fat meat, 2 fat

✔ = Healthiest Bets

(*Continued*)

	Amount	Cal.	Fat (g)	% Cal. Fat	Sat. Fat (g)	Trans Fat (g)	Chol. (mg)	Sod. (mg)	Carb. (g)	Fiber (g)	Pro. (g)	Choices/Exchanges
ESPRESSO DRINKS												
✔Caffe Latte	8.5 oz.	110	5	4	3	0	20	95	11	0	7	1 milk, 1 fat
Caffe Mocha	11.5 oz.	410	17	4	12	0	45	140	61	2	10	3 carb, 1 milk, 2 1/2 fat
✔Cappuccino	8.5 oz.	110	5	4	3	0	20	95	11	0	7	1 milk, 1 fat
Caramel Latte	11.5 oz.	430	18	4	12	0	55	180	53	0	9	2 1/2 carb, 1 milk, 3 1/2 fat
FLAVORFUL CREAM CHEESE SPREADS												
✔Plain	2 oz.	180	18	9	11	1	55	210	2	0	3	3 1/2 fat
✔Reduced Fat Hazelnut	2 oz.	140	11	7	6	0.5	35	210	6	1	5	1/2 carb, 2 fat
✔Reduced Fat Honey Walnut	2 oz.	150	11	7	6	0	30	200	8	1	5	1/2 carb, 2 fat
✔Reduced Fat Plain	2 oz.	130	12	8	7	0.5	35	230	2	1	5	2 1/2 fat
✔Reduced Fat Raspberry	2 oz.	130	10	7	6	0	30	200	7	1	4	1/2 carb, 2 fat
✔Reduced Fat Sun-Dried Tomato	2 oz.	130	11	8	7	0.5	35	220	4	1	5	1/2 carb, 2 fat

✔Reduced Fat Veggie	2 oz.	120	10	8	6	0.5	30	210	3	1	5	2 fat
FRESHLY BAKED BAGELS												
Asiago Cheese	1	370	6	1	3.5	0	10	630	61	2	15	4 starch, 1 fat
Blueberry	1	350	2	1	0	0	0	520	71	3	11	5 starch
Chocolate Chip Bagel	1	390	6	1	4.5	0	0	500	73	3	11	5 starch, 1/2 fat
Cinnamon Crunch	1	420	8	2	6	0	0	490	76	2	10	5 starch, 1 fat
Dutch Apple & Raisin	1	340	3	1	1	0	0	590	73	2	7	5 starch
Everything	1	310	2	1	0	0	0	610	61	2	11	4 starch, 1/2 fat
French Toast	1	390	5	1	2.5	0	0	680	74	2	11	5 starch, 1/2 fat
Plain	1	310	2	1	0	0	0	480	62	2	10	4 starch
Sesame	1	330	5	1	0.5	0	0	450	60	3	11	4 starch, 1/2 fat
Whole Grain	1	350	3	1	0.5	0	0	410	67	5	12	4 starch
FROZEN DRINKS: GRANDE												
Caramel	16.5 oz.	590	26	4	17	0	75	150	81	0	5	5 1/2 carb, 4 fat

✔ = Healthiest Bets

(*Continued*)

FROZEN DRINKS: GRANDE *(Continued)*	Amount	Cal.	Fat (g)	% Cal. Fat	Sat. Fat (g)	Trans Fat (g)	Chol. (mg)	Sod. (mg)	Carb. (g)	Fiber (g)	Pro. (g)	Choices/Exchanges
✔Frozen Lemonade	16 oz.	90	0	0	0	0	0	10	21	0	0	1 1/2 carb
Mango	15 oz.	290	0.5	0	0	0	0	20	73	1	1	5 carb
Mocha	16 oz.	550	25	4	16	1	60	140	78	2	7	5 carb, 3 1/2 fat
Strawberry Smoothie	18 oz.	240	1.5	1	0.5	0	5	190	51	3	1	3 1/2 carb
FROZEN DRINKS: LARGO												
Caramel	20 oz.	720	30	4	20	0.5	90	200	102	0	6	7 carb, 4 fat
✔Frozen Lemonade	20.25 oz.	120	0	0	0	0	0	15	29	0	1	2 carb
Mango	18.5 oz.	360	0.5	0	0	0	0	25	92	2	1	6 carb
Mocha	20 oz.	670	28	4	19	1	75	180	98	3	9	6 1/2 carb, 4 fat
Strawberry Smoothie	21.5 oz.	290	1.5	0	0.5	0	5	230	62	5	1	4 carb
GRILLED BREAKFAST SANDWICHES												
Bacon, Egg & Cheese	1	510	24	4	10	0.5	215	1060	44	2	28	3 starch, 3 medium-fat meat, 2 fat

✔Egg & Cheese	1	380	14	3	6	0	190	620	43	2	18	3 starch, 1 medium-fat meat, 1 1/2 fat
Sausage, Egg & Cheese	1	540	27	5	11	0	220	980	44	2	26	3 starch, 2 medium-fat meat, 3 fat
HAND-TOSSED SALADS												
✔Asian Sesame Chicken	1	410	19	4	3.5	0	65	900	31	5	32	1 starch, 3 veg, 4 lean meat, 1 fat
Caesar	1	400	27	6	8	0.5	50	620	26	4	13	1/2 starch, 3 veg, 2 lean meat, 4 1/2 fat
✔Classic Café	1	170	11	6	1.5	0	0	270	19	4	3	3 veg, 2 fat
Fandango	1	370	28	7	7	0	25	540	23	5	13	1/2 starch, 3 veg, 2 lean meat, 4 fat
Fandango w/ Chicken	1	490	29	5	7	0	95	830	25	5	37	1/2 starch, 3 veg, 5 lean meat, 3 fat
✔Fresh Fruit Cup - Large	1	150	0	0	0	0	0	30	37	2	2	2 1/2 veg

✔ = Healthiest Bets

(Continued)

HAND-TOSSED SALADS *(Continued)*	Amount	Cal.	Fat (g)	% Cal. Fat	Sat. Fat (g)	Trans Fat (g)	Chol. (mg)	Sod. (mg)	Carb. (g)	Fiber (g)	Pro. (g)	Choices/Exchanges
✔Fresh Fruit Cup - Small	1	70	0	0	0	0	0	15	19	1	1	1 veg
Greek	1	440	39	8	8	0.5	20	1370	15	6	10	3 veg, 1 lean meat, 7 fat
✔Greek - Half Portion	1	220	20	8	4	0	10	690	7	3	5	2 veg, 1 medium-fat meat, 4 fat
Grilled Chicken Caesar	1	510	28	5	8	0.5	120	1040	27	4	37	1/2 starch, 3 veg, 5 lean meat, 2 1/2 fat
✔Half Asian Sesame Chicken	1	210	10	4	1.5	0	35	450	16	2	16	1/2 starch, 1 veg, 2 lean meat, 1 fat
✔Half Caesar	1	200	14	6	4	0	25	310	13	2	6	1/2 starch, 1 veg, 3 fat
✔Half Classic Café	1	90	5	5	1	0	0	135	9	2	1	2 veg, 1 fat
✔Half Fandango	1	190	14	7	3.5	0	15	270	12	2	6	1/2 starch, 1 veg, 3 fat
✔Half Fandango w/ Chicken	1	240	14	5	3.5	0	45	410	12	2	19	1/2 starch, 1 veg, 3 lean meat, 1 1/2 fat

✔Half Grilled Chicken Caesar	1	250	14	5	4	0	60	520	13	2	18	1/2 starch, 1 veg, 2 lean meat, 1 1/2 fat
✔Half Strawberry Poppyseed	1	90	2	2	0	0	0	100	16	3	2	1 fruit, 1/2 fat
✔Half Strawberry Poppyseed w/ Chicken	1	150	2	1	0	0	35	240	16	3	14	1 fruit, 2 lean meat
Half Tomato & Fresh Mozzarella	1	440	24	5	10	0.5	35	830	42	3	18	2 starch, 2 veg, 2 lean meat, 3 fat
✔Strawberry Poppyseed Salad	1	190	3	1	0	0	0	200	31	6	4	2 fruit, 1/2 fat
✔Strawberry Poppyseed Salad w/ Chicken	1	300	4	1	0.5	0	65	480	33	6	29	2 fruit, 4 lean meat, 1 fat
Tomato & Fresh Mozzarella	1	890	47	5	19	1.5	75	1660	83	6	36	4 starch, 4 veg, 4 medium-fat meat, 5 fat
HOT DRINKS												
Chai Tea Latte	10 oz.	190	4	2	2.5	0	15	85	31	0	7	1 carb, 1 milk, 1 fat
Hot Chocolate	11.5 oz.	410	17	4	12	0	50	150	61	2	11	3 carb, 1 milk, 3 fat

✔ = Healthiest Bets

(*Continued*)

	Amount	Cal.	Fat (g)	% Cal. Fat	Sat. Fat (g)	Trans Fat (g)	Chol. (mg)	Sod. (mg)	Carb. (g)	Fiber (g)	Pro. (g)	Choices/Exchanges
HOT PANINI												
Chicken Bacon Dijon on Country	1	910	35	3	13	1	150	1900	91	4	58	6 starch, 6 lean meat, 3 fat
Chicken Bacon Dijon on French	1	780	36	4	14	1	155	1540	63	2	53	4 starch, 6 lean meat, 3 fat
Frontega Chicken on Focaccia	1	810	34	4	9	0.5	100	2140	79	5	45	5 1/2 starch, 4 lean meat, 4 fat
✔Half Chicken Bacon Dijon on Country	1	460	17	3	7	0	75	950	45	2	29	3 starch, 3 lean meat, 1 1/2 fat
✔Half Chicken Bacon Dijon on French	1	390	18	4	7	0	75	770	32	1	27	2 starch, 3 lean meat, 2 fat
Half Frontega Chicken on Focaccia	1	400	17	4	5	0	50	1070	39	2	23	2 1/2 starch, 2 lean meat, 2 fat
✔Half Portobello & Mozzarella on Focaccia	1	330	12	3	5	0	20	640	41	2	13	2 1/2 starch, 1 lean meat, 2 fat

Half Smokehouse Turkey on Focaccia	1	400	15	3	5	0	50	1310	40	2	26	2 1/2 starch, 3 lean meat, 1 1/2 fat
Half Smokehouse Turkey on Three Cheese	1	390	14	3	5	0	55	1320	40	2	27	2 1/2 starch, 3 lean meat, 1 fat
Half Turkey Artichoke on Focaccia	1	350	11	3	3	0	45	1170	44	3	20	3 starch, 2 lean meat, 1 fat
Portobello & Mozzarella on Focaccia	1	650	24	3	10	0.5	35	1270	82	5	27	5 1/2 starch, 2 lean meat, 3 fat
Smokehouse Turkey on Focaccia	1	800	30	3	9	0.5	105	2630	80	5	51	5 1/2 starch, 5 lean meat, 2 1/2 fat
Smokehouse Turkey on Three Cheese	1	790	29	3	11	1	115	2640	80	5	54	5 1/2 starch, 5 lean meat, 2 fat
Turkey Artichoke on Focaccia	1	700	22	3	6	0	85	2330	87	7	40	6 starch, 3 lean meat, 2 fat
ICED DRINKS: GRANDE												
✔Iced Green Tea	16 oz.	100	0	0	0	0	0	10	25	0	0	1 1/2 carb
✔Lemonade	16 oz.	90	0	0	0	0	0	10	22	0	0	1 1/2 carb

✔ = Healthiest Bets

(Continued)

ICED DRINKS: GRANDE *(Continued)*	Amount	Cal.	Fat (g)	% Cal. Fat	Sat. Fat (g)	Trans Fat (g)	Chol. (mg)	Sod. (mg)	Carb. (g)	Fiber (g)	Pro. (g)	Choices/Exchanges
ICED DRINKS: LARGO												
✔Iced Green Tea	20 oz.	130	0	0	0	0	0	10	30	0	0	2 carb
✔Lemonade	20 oz.	130	0	0	0	0	0	10	31	0	1	2 carb
ICED DRINKS: OTHER												
✔Iced Chai Tea Latte	16 oz.	150	3.5	2	2	0	15	75	25	0	6	1 1/2 carb, 1/2 fat
MINI BUNDT CAKES												
Lemon Poppyseed	1 pc	460	20	4	4	0	95	440	63	0	6	4 carb, 3 fat
Pineapple Upside-Down	1 pc	520	25	4	10	0	80	570	74	2	6	5 carb, 3 fat
MUFFIES												
Chocolate Chip	1	270	12	4	3	0	35	140	40	1	4	2 1/2 carb, 1 1/2 fat
✔Pumpkin	1	250	10	4	2	0	15	200	39	1	3	2 1/2 carb, 1 fat
MUFFINS												
Carrot Walnut	1	430	19	4	4	0	55	380	61	2	8	4 carb, 3 fat

Pumpkin	1	530	20	3	4	0	30	430	82	2	6	5 1/2 carb, 2 1/2 fat
✔Reduced Fat Wild Blueberry	1	360	10	3	2	0	55	220	61	1	6	4 carb, 1 fat
Wild Blueberry	1	400	16	4	3	0	60	240	59	1	6	4 carb, 2 fat
PANERA KIDS												
✔Deli Sandwich - Roast Beef	1	310	9	3	4.5	0	50	780	35	3	22	2 1/2 starch, 2 lean meat, 1/2 fat
Deli Sandwich - Smoked Ham	1	300	10	3	4.5	0	45	1230	34	3	20	2 1/2 starch, 2 lean meat, 1 fat
Deli Sandwich - Smoked Turkey	1	300	8	2	3.5	0	40	1150	36	3	20	2 1/2 starch, 2 lean meat, 1/2 fat
✔Grilled Cheese Sandwich	1	300	11	3	6	0	30	890	35	3	14	2 1/2 starch, 1 medium-fat meat, 1 fat
✔Peanut Butter & Jelly Sandwich	1	400	16	4	2	0	0	400	56	6	13	3 1/2 starch, 2 fat

✔ = Healthiest Bets

(*Continued*)

	Amount	Cal.	Fat (g)	% Cal. Fat	Sat. Fat (g)	Trans Fat (g)	Chol. (mg)	Sod. (mg)	Carb. (g)	Fiber (g)	Pro. (g)	Choices/Exchanges
SALAD DRESSINGS												
Balsamic Vinaigrette	1.5 oz.	130	10	7	1.5	0	0	240	9	0	0	1/2 carb, 2 fat
Caesar	1.5 oz.	150	16	10	2.5	0	35	190	2	0	1	3 fat
✔Fat-Free Half Poppyseed	0.75 oz.	10	0	0	0	0	0	75	3	1	0	Free
✔Fat-Free Poppyseed	1.5 oz.	25	0	0	0	0	0	150	5	1	0	1/2 carb
✔Fat-Free Raspberry	1.5 oz.	30	0	0	0	0	0	90	8	0	0	1/2 carb
Greek	1.5 oz.	220	24	10	3.5	0	0	380	1	0	0	5 fat
✔Half Balsamic Vinaigrette	0.75 oz.	60	5	8	1	0	0	120	4	0	0	1/2 carb, 1 fat
Half Caesar	0.75 oz.	80	8	9	1.5	0	15	95	1	0	0	1 1/2 fat
✔Half Fat-Free Raspberry	0.75 oz.	15	0	0	0	0	0	45	4	0	0	Free
Half Greek	0.75 oz.	110	12	10	2	0	0	190	1	0	0	2 1/2 fat
✔Half Light Buttermilk Ranch	0.75 oz.	40	2	5	0	0	0	170	4	0	0	1/2 carb, 1/2 fat

✔Half Meyer Lemon Vinaigrette	0.75 oz.	30	1	3	0	0	0	135	5	0	0	1/2 carb
✔Half Reduced-Sugar Asian Sesame Vinaigrette	0.75 oz.	45	4	8	0.5	0	0	190	3	0	0	1 fat
✔Half White Balsamic Apple Vinaigrette	0.75 oz.	80	6	7	1	0	0	160	6	0	0	1/2 carb, 1 fat
Light Buttermilk Ranch	1.5 oz.	80	4	5	0.5	0	0	350	9	1	1	1/2 carb, 1 fat
✔Meyer Lemon Vinaigrette	1.5 oz.	60	2	3	0	0	0	270	9	0	0	1/2 carb, 1/2 fat
Reduced-Sugar Asian Sesame Vinaigrette	1.5 oz.	90	8	8	1	0	0	390	6	0	0	1/2 carb, 1 1/2 fat
White Balsamic Apple Vinaigrette	1.5 oz.	150	12	7	2	0	0	310	11	0	0	1/2 carb, 2 1/2 fat
SCONES												
Cinnamon Chip	1	530	27	5	16	0	110	310	67	2	8	4 starch, 4 fat
Orange	1	460	20	4	11	0	110	290	65	1	8	4 starch, 3 fat

✔ = Healthiest Bets

(*Continued*)

SCONES *(Continued)*	Amount	Cal.	Fat (g)	% Cal. Fat	Sat. Fat (g)	Trans Fat (g)	Chol. (mg)	Sod. (mg)	Carb. (g)	Fiber (g)	Pro. (g)	Choices/Exchanges
Tart Cherry	1	380	16	4	10	0	65	370	58	2	9	4 starch, 2 fat
Wild Blueberry	1	410	15	3	10	0	60	360	63	2	6	4 starch, 2 fat
SIGNATURE SANDWICHES												
Asiago Roast Beef on Asiago Cheese	1	710	32	4	13	1	120	1280	57	3	47	4 starch, 5 medium-fat meat, 1 fat
Bacon Turkey Bravo on Tomato Basil	1	830	31	3	9	0.5	105	2920	86	4	51	5 1/2 starch, 5 lean meat, 3 fat
Chicken Caesar on Asiago Focaccia	1	810	34	4	8	0.5	125	1630	81	4	43	5 1/2 starch, 4 lean meat, 4 fat
Chicken Caesar on Three Cheese	1	770	32	4	9	0.5	135	1600	77	4	45	5 starch, 4 lean meat, 3 fat
Chipotle Chicken on Artisan French	1	1030	55	5	13	1	150	2540	79	4	54	5 1/2 starch, 5 lean meat, 7 fat
Chipotle Chicken on French	1	900	56	6	13	1	155	2090	53	3	49	3 1/2 starch, 5 lean meat, 7 fat

✔Half Asiago Roast Beef on Asiago Cheese	1	360	16	4	6	0	60	640	29	1	24	2 starch, 3 medium-fat meat, 1/2 fat
Half Bacon Turkey Bravo on Tomato Basil	1	410	15	3	4.5	0	55	1460	43	2	25	3 starch, 2 lean meat, 1 1/2 fat
✔Half Chicken Caesar on Asiago Focaccia	1	400	17	4	4	0	60	820	40	2	22	2 1/2 starch, 2 lean meat, 2 fat
✔Half Chicken Caesar on Three Cheese	1	380	16	4	4.5	0	70	800	39	2	22	2 1/2 starch, 2 lean meat, 2 fat
Half Chipotle Chicken on Artisan French	1	520	27	5	6	0	75	1270	40	2	27	2 1/2 starch, 3 lean meat, 4 fat
Half Chipotle Chicken on French	1	450	28	6	7	0	75	1050	26	2	25	1 1/2 starch, 3 lean meat, 4 fat
Half Italian Combo on Ciabatta	1	530	25	4	10	0	85	1500	47	2	30	3 starch, 3 medium-fat meat, 2 fat
✔Half Mediterranean Veggie on Tomato Basil	1	310	7	2	1.5	0	5	730	51	5	11	3 starch, 1 veg, 1 1/2 fat

✔ = Healthiest Bets

(*Continued*)

SIGNATURE SANDWICHES (Continued)	Amount	Cal.	Fat (g)	% Cal. Fat	Sat. Fat (g)	Trans Fat (g)	Chol. (mg)	Sod. (mg)	Carb. (g)	Fiber (g)	Pro. (g)	Choices/Exchanges
Half Sierra Turkey on Focaccia w/ Asiago Cheese	1	480	27	5	6	0	45	990	40	2	19	2 1/2 starch, 2 lean meat, 4 1/2 fat
Italian Combo on Ciabatta	1	1070	50	4	19	0.5	175	3010	93	5	59	6 starch, 6 medium-fat meat, 4 fat
Mediterranean Veggie on Tomato Basil	1	610	13	2	3	0	10	1450	102	9	22	6 starch, 2 veg, 1 lean meat, 2 1/2 fat
Sierra Turkey on Focaccia w/ Asiago Cheese	1	970	54	5	12	1	85	1970	80	4	39	5 1/2 starch, 3 lean meat, 8 fat
SOUPS												
Baked Potato	1 cup	230	14	5	9	0	45	720	21	2	5	1 starch, 3 fat
Broccoli Cheddar	1 cup	230	16	6	9	0	45	970	14	1	8	1 starch, 3 fat
Cream of Chicken & Wild Rice	1 cup	200	12	5	6	0	35	970	19	1	5	1 starch, 2 1/2 fat
French Onion w/ Cheese & Croutons	9.25 oz.	200	10	5	5	0	20	1780	23	2	8	2 starch, 2 fat

French Onion w/o Cheese & Croutons	1 cup	90	3	3	1.5	0	10	1560	13	1	2	1 starch, 1/2 fat
Low-Fat Chicken Noodle	1 cup	100	2	2	0	0	15	1110	16	1	6	1 starch, 1/2 fat
✔Low-Fat Vegetarian Black Bean	1 cup	150	1	1	0	0.5	0	920	28	6	8	2 starch
Low-Fat Vegetarian Garden Vegetable	1 cup	90	1	1	0	0	0	1030	17	3	4	1 starch, 1 veg
New England Clam Chowder	1 cup	320	28	8	18	0.5	100	740	11	1	6	1 starch, 5 1/2 fat
✔Turkey Chickpea Chili Soup	1 cup	180	5	3	1.5	0	25	800	22	7	10	1 1/2 starch, 1 lean meat, 1/2 fat
Vegetarian Summer Corn Chowder	1 cup	210	13	6	8	0	40	510	20	3	4	1 starch, 2 1/2 fat
SPECIALTY BREADS												
✔Asiago Cheese Demi	1 slice	160	4	2	2.5	0	10	320	22	1	7	1 starch, 1 fat

✔ = Healthiest Bets

(*Continued*)

SPECIALTY BREADS *(Continued)*	Amount	Cal.	Fat (g)	% Cal. Fat	Sat. Fat (g)	Trans Fat (g)	Chol. (mg)	Sod. (mg)	Carb. (g)	Fiber (g)	Pro. (g)	Choices/Exchanges
✔Asiago Cheese Loaf	1 slice	160	4	2	2.5	0	10	320	22	1	7	1 starch, 1 fat
✔Challah Bread	1 slice	180	3	2	1	0	10	290	34	1	6	2 starch, 1/2 fat
✔Cinnamon Raisin Loaf	1 slice	170	3	2	1.5	0	0	230	33	1	4	2 starch, 1/2 fat
✔French Baguette	1 slice	160	2	1	0	0	5	330	31	1	6	2 starch, 1/2 fat
✔French Loaf	1 slice	150	2	1	0	0	5	310	29	1	6	2 starch, 1/2 fat
✔French Roll	1	180	2	1	0	0	5	380	35	1	7	2 starch, 1/2 fat
✔Honey Wheat Loaf	1 slice	170	3	2	1	0	0	270	31	2	5	2 starch, 1/2 fat
✔Sourdough Baguette	1 slice	160	1	1	0	0	0	320	31	1	6	2 starch
✔Sourdough Loaf	1 slice	140	1	1	0	0	0	290	28	1	5	2 starch
✔Sourdough Roll	1	200	1	0	0	0	0	400	39	1	7	3 starch
Sourdough Soup Bowl	1 srvg	590	2.5	0	0	0	0	1210	117	4	22	8 starch
✔Sunflower Loaf	1 slice	180	6	3	1.5	0	0	280	27	2	6	2 starch, 1 fat
✔Tomato Basil Loaf	1 slice	140	1	1	0	0	0	330	27	1	5	2 starch

✔White Whole Wheat Loaf	1 slice	140	2	1	0	0	0	320	28	3	5	2 starch, 1/2 fat
✔XL French Loaf	1 slice	150	2	1	0	0	5	310	28	1	6	2 starch, 1/2 fat
✔XL Sourdough Loaf	1 slice	140	1	1	0	0	0	290	28	1	5	2 starch
SPECIALTY PASTRIES												
Bear Claw	1	460	27	5	14	1	85	310	49	2	10	1 1/2 starch, 1 1/2 carb, 4 1/2 fat
French Croissant	1	240	14	5	7	0	35	170	25	1	5	1 starch, 1 carb, 3 fat
Pastry Ring - Cherry Cheese	1	210	11	5	6	0	40	120	26	1	3	1 starch, 1 carb, 2 fat
SWEET ROLLS												
Cinnamon	1	610	27	4	15	1	80	340	90	5	9	3 starch, 3 carb, 3 fat
Cobblestone	1	590	12	2	3.5	0	0	510	107	3	6	3 1/2 starch, 3 1/2 carb, 1 1/2 fat
Pecan	1	620	35	5	8	1	45	270	72	2	9	2 1/2 starch, 2 1/2 carb, 5 fat

✔ = Healthiest Bets

Schlotzsky's (www.schlotzskys.com)

Light 'n Lean Choice

BLT Sandwich *(small)*
Pasta Salad

Calories	432	Cholesterol (mg)	28
Fat (g)	15	Sodium (mg)	844
% calories from fat	31	Carbohydrate (g)	62
Saturated fat (g)	3	Fiber (g)	3
Trans fat (g)	0	Protein (g)	14

Exchanges: 4 starch, 1 medium-fat meat, 2 fat

Healthy 'n Hearty Choice

Vegetarian Vegetable Soup *(bowl)*
Mozzarella & Portobello Panini
Oatmeal Raisin Cookie

Calories	752	Cholesterol (mg)	55
Fat (g)	18	Sodium (mg)	2,502
% calories from fat	22	Carbohydrate (g)	114
Saturated fat (g)	10	Fiber (g)	9
Trans fat (g)	0	Protein (g)	29

Exchanges: 7 1/2 starch, 1 veg, 2 lean meat, 2 1/2 fat

Schlotzsky's

	Amount	Cal.	Fat (g)	% Cal. Fat	Sat. Fat (g)	Trans Fat (g)	Chol. (mg)	Sod. (mg)	Carb. (g)	Fiber (g)	Pro. (g)	Choices/Exchanges
BEVERAGES												
✔Iced Tea	kid's	2	0	0	0	0	0	9	0	0	0	Free
✔Iced Tea	med	3	0	0	0	0	0	15	1	0	0	Free
✔Iced Tea	lg	4	0	0	0	0	0	24	1	0	0	Free
Lemonade	kid's	146	0	0	0	0	0	62	39	0	0	2 carb
Lemonade	med	243	0	0	0	0	0	103	45	0	0	3 carb
Lemonade	lg	388	0	0	0	0	0	164	104	0	0	7 carb
Raspberry Lemonade	kid's	146	0	0	0	0	0	62	39	0	0	2 carb
Raspberry Lemonade	med	243	0	0	0	0	0	103	45	0	0	3 carb
Raspberry Lemonade	lg	388	0	0	0	0	0	164	104	0	0	7 carb

✔ = Healthiest Bets

(Continued)

	Amount	Cal.	Fat (g)	% Cal. Fat	Sat. Fat (g)	Trans Fat (g)	Chol. (mg)	Sod. (mg)	Carb. (g)	Fiber (g)	Pro. (g)	Choices/Exchanges
CHIPS												
Barbeque	1 srvg	220	12	5	2	0	0	270	25	1	3	1 1/2 starch, 2 fat
Chili & Lime Tortilla Chips	1 srvg	250	12	4	1.5	0	0	280	32	3	3	2 starch, 2 fat
Cracker Pepper	1 srvg	220	12	5	2	0	0	310	25	1	3	1 1/2 starch, 2 fat
Jalapeno	1 srvg	220	12	5	2	0	0	220	25	1	3	1 1/2 starch, 2 fat
✔Mesquite BBQ Crisps	1 srvg	140	4	3	0.5	0	0	220	24	2	2	1 1/2 starch, 1/2 fat
✔Original Baked Crisps	1 srvg	140	4	3	0	0	0	210	26	2	2	1 1/2 starch, 1/2 fat
Original Kettle Crisps	1 srvg	190	11	5	1	0	0	200	18	2	2	1 starch, 2 fat
Regular (plain)	1 srvg	220	12	5	2	0	0	190	25	1	3	1 1/2 starch, 2 fat
Salt & Vinegar	1 srvg	220	12	5	2	0	0	310	25	1	3	1 1/2 starch, 2 fat
Sour Cream & Onion	1 srvg	220	12	5	2	0	0	220	25	1	3	1 1/2 starch, 2 fat

DESSERTS												
Brownie	1	414	24	5	9	0	55	151	47	3	6	3 starch, 4 fat
Carrot Cake	1 pc	717	42	5	6	0	74	767	80	3	7	5 1/2 starch, 8 fat
Cheesecake	1 pc	350	23	6	13	1	75	200	30	1	6	2 starch, 4 1/2 fat
✔Chocolate Fudge Cookie	1	160	7	4	3	0	11	48	24	1	2	1 1/2 starch, 1 fat
✔Fudge Chocolate Chip Cookie	1	162	7	4	4	0	12	57	23	1	2	1 1/2 starch, 1 fat
✔Oatmeal Raisin Cookie	1	145	5	3	2	0	10	48	24	1	2	1 1/2 starch, 1 fat
✔Sugar Cookie	1	150	6	4	3	0	14	121	23	1	2	1 1/2 starch, 1 fat
✔White Chocolate Macadamia Cookie	1	167	8	4	4	0	11	50	23	1	2	1 1/2 starch, 1 fat
KIDS												
Cheese Pizza	1 srvg	479	13	2	5	0	24	1060	73	3	18	5 starch, 2 1/2 fat
✔Cheese Sandwich	1	397	15	3	8	1	40	780	48	2	17	3 starch, 1 medium-fat meat, 2 fat

✔ = Healthiest Bets

(*Continued*)

KIDS *(Continued)*	Amount	Cal.	Fat (g)	% Cal. Fat	Sat. Fat (g)	Trans Fat (g)	Chol. (mg)	Sod. (mg)	Carb. (g)	Fiber (g)	Pro. (g)	Choices/Exchanges
Ham & Cheese Sandwich	1	427	16	3	8	1	50	1154	49	2	21	3 1/2 starch, 2 lean meat, 2 fat
Pepperoni Pizza	1 srvg	523	17	3	6	0	33	1246	73	3	20	5 starch, 1 medium-fat meat, 2 fat
✔Turkey Sandwich	1	303	5	1	1	0	20	754	49	2	13	3 1/2 starch, 1/2 fat
PANINI												
Classic Swiss & Tomato	1	624	26	4	15	1	78	1081	63	1	33	4 starch, 3 medium-fat meat, 2 fat
Grilled Chicken Romano	1	570	16	3	8	1	104	1567	62	1	70	4 starch, 8 lean meat
Mozzarella & Portobello	1	485	12	2	8	0	45	1158	63	2	24	4 starch, 2 lean meat, 1 1/2 fat
Panini Italiano	1	736	32	4	15	1	114	2406	67	2	43	4 1/2 starch, 4 medium-fat meat, 1 1/2 fat

Smoke Turkey & Guacamole	1	606	21	3	6	0	58	1812	68	4	32	4 1/2 starch, 3 lean meat, 2 fat
Smoked Ham Crostini	1	644	23	3	12	1	94	1978	67	2	39	4 1/2 starch, 4 lean meat, 2 fat
PIZZA												
Baby Spinach Salad	1 srvg	471	8	2	3	0	12	1255	83	4	18	5 starch, 1 veg, 1 1/2 fat
Bacon, Tomato & Portobello	1 srvg	614	22	3	9	1	53	1404	76	4	29	5 starch, 2 medium-fat meat, 2 fat
BBQ Chicken & Jalapeno	1 srvg	715	16	2	8	0	96	2447	99	3	69	6 1/2 starch, 7 lean meat
Combination Special	1 srvg	639	25	4	10	1	54	1690	76	4	27	5 starch, 2 medium-fat meat, 3 fat
Double Cheese	1 srvg	597	21	3	10	1	52	1373	74	3	27	5 starch, 2 medium-fat meat, 2 fat

✓ = Healthiest Bets

(Continued)

PIZZA ***(Continued)***	**Amount**	**Cal.**	**Fat (g)**	**% Cal. Fat**	**Sat. Fat (g)**	**Trans Fat (g)**	**Chol. (mg)**	**Sod. (mg)**	**Carb. (g)**	**Fiber (g)**	**Pro. (g)**	**Choices/Exchanges**
Fresh Tomato & Pesto	1 srvg	556	19	3	8	0	42	1334	73	3	25	5 starch, 1 lean meat, 3 fat
Grilled Chicken & Pesto	1 srvg	683	22	3	9	1	100	1891	75	4	72	5 starch, 8 lean meat
Mediterranean	1 srvg	560	20	3	9	0	51	1580	74	1	21	5 starch, 1 lean meat, 3 fat
Pepperoni & Double Cheese	1 srvg	685	30	4	13	1	71	1740	74	3	31	5 starch, 2 medium-fat meat, 3 fat
Smoked Turkey & Jalapeno	1 srvg	642	19	3	8	0	76	2204	78	4	39	5 starch, 3 lean meat, 2 fat
Thai Chicken	1 srvg	724	23	3	9	0	94	2008	85	4	71	5 1/2 starch, 8 lean meat
Vegetarian Special	1 srvg	540	17	3	7	0	36	1369	74	4	22	4 1/2 starch, 1 veg, 1 lean meat, 2 1/2 fat

SALADS - NO DRESSING												
✔Baby Spinach & Feta	1	197	15	7	5	0	27	447	10	4	10	1 veg, 1 lean meat, 2 fat
✔Caesar	1	103	5	4	2	0	6	289	10	3	6	2 veg, 1 fat
✔Chicken Salad	1	292	15	5	4	0	93	898	12	3	61	1 starch, 8 lean meat
✔Garden	1	51	1	2	0	0	0	291	12	4	3	1 veg
✔Greek	1	137	8	5	5	0	29	655	13	4	7	1/2 starch, 2 veg, 1 lean meat, 1 fat
✔Grilled Chicken Caesar	1	221	8	3	2	0	65	759	12	3	53	1/2 starch, 2 veg, 7 lean meat
Ham & Turkey Chef	1	254	13	5	6	0	60	1340	14	4	22	1/2 starch, 2 veg, 3 lean meat, 1 fat
✔Pasta Salad	1	68	3	4	0	0	0	293	12	1	0	1 starch, 1/2 fat
Potato Salad	1	242	13	5	3	0	11	515	29	3	3	2 starch, 2 fat
✔Side Salad	1	26	1	3	0	0	0	236	7	2	1	1 1/2 veg

✔ = Healthiest Bets

(*Continued*)

SALADS - NO DRESSING *(Continued)*	Amount	Cal.	Fat (g)	% Cal. Fat	Sat. Fat (g)	Trans Fat (g)	Chol. (mg)	Sod. (mg)	Carb. (g)	Fiber (g)	Pro. (g)	Choices/Exchanges
Turkey Chef	1	303	16	5	7	0	72	1132	15	4	26	3 veg, 4 lean meat, 2 fat
SANDWICHES												
Albuquerque Turkey	sm	693	37	5	12	1	97	1713	56	4	34	3 1/2 starch, 3 lean meat, 5 1/2 fat
Albuquerque Turkey	med	972	51	5	16	1	136	2432	80	6	48	5 1/2 starch, 5 lean meat, 7 fat
Angus Beef & Provolone	sm	503	19	3	6	0	50	1354	56	3	27	3 1/2 starch, 2 medium-fat meat, 1 fat
Angus Beef & Provolone	med	757	29	3	10	0	79	2009	80	4	41	5 1/2 starch, 4 medium-fat meat, 1 1/2 fat
Angus Corned Beef	sm	395	9	2	2	0	36	1568	53	4	27	3 1/2 starch, 2 lean meat
Angus Corned Beef	med	582	13	2	3	0	52	2351	77	6	40	5 starch, 4 lean meat

Angus Corned Beef Reuben	sm	629	28	4	13	1	95	1612	54	3	40	3 1/2 starch, 4 medium-fat meat, 1 fat
Angus Corned Beef Reuben	med	918	41	4	19	1	140	2291	78	5	59	5 starch, 6 medium-fat meat, 1 1/2 fat
Angus Pastrami & Swiss	sm	611	24	4	12	1	93	1657	56	4	43	3 1/2 starch, 5 medium-fat meat
Angus Pastrami & Swiss	med	905	36	4	18	1	138	2484	82	6	64	5 1/2 starch, 7 medium-fat meat
Angus Pastrami Rueben	sm	629	27	4	13	1	100	1592	54	3	41	3 1/2 starch, 4 medium-fat meat, 1/2 fat
Angus Pastrami Rueben	med	918	40	4	19	1	147	2261	78	5	61	5 starch, 6 medium-fat meat, 1 fat
Angus Roast Beef & Cheese	sm	536	22	4	11	1	85	1429	50	2	33	3 1/2 starch, 3 medium-fat meat, 1 fat
Angus Roast Beef & Cheese	med	781	33	4	15	1	119	2186	73	4	47	5 starch, 5 medium-fat meat, 2 fat

✓ = Healthiest Bets

(*Continued*)

SANDWICHES *(Continued)*	Amount	Cal.	Fat (g)	% Cal. Fat	Sat. Fat (g)	Trans Fat (g)	Chol. (mg)	Sod. (mg)	Carb. (g)	Fiber (g)	Pro. (g)	Choices/Exchanges
✔BLT	sm	364	12	3	3	0	28	551	50	2	14	3 1/2 starch, 1 medium-fat meat, 1 1/2 fat
✔BLT	med	543	18	3	5	0	44	801	74	4	22	5 starch, 1 medium-fat meat, 2 fat
Cheese	sm	565	28	4	15	1	79	1190	51	3	28	3 1/2 starch, 3 medium-fat meat, 2 1/2 fat
Cheese	med	788	38	4	20	1	105	1697	84	4	39	5 1/2 starch, 3 medium-fat meat, 3 fat
Chicken & Pesto	sm	387	9	2	1	0	48	1126	50	3	27	3 1/2 starch, 2 lean meat
Chicken & Pesto	med	564	14	2	2	0	70	1647	72	4	40	5 starch, 4 lean meat
Chicken Breast	sm	334	4	1	0	0	46	1343	52	3	26	3 1/2 starch, 1 lean meat
Chicken Breast	med	507	6	1	1	0	67	2035	77	5	38	5 starch, 2 lean meat

Chipotle Chicken	sm	379	10	2	2	0	56	1094	47	3	27	3 starch, 3 lean meat
Chipotle Chicken	med	551	14	2	3	0	81	1596	68	4	39	4 1/2 starch, 4 lean meat
Deluxe	sm	742	38	5	169	1	143	3132	55	3	43	3 1/2 starch, 5 medium-fat meat, 3 fat
Deluxe	med	953	46	4	18	1	160	4082	78	4	55	5 starch, 6 medium-fat meat, 3 fat
Dijon Chicken	sm	391	7	2	1	0	46	1539	54	5	30	3 1/2 starch, 2 lean meat
Dijon Chicken	med	576	11	2	1	0	67	2329	79	8	44	5 1/2 starch, 3 lean meat
✔Fresh Veggie	sm	354	10	3	5	0	23	774	52	4	14	3 starch, 1 veg, 1 1/2 fat
Fresh Veggie	med	482	12	2	5	0	23	1155	77	6	18	5 starch, 1 veg, 2 fat
Ham & Cheese	sm	511	19	3	9	1	80	2040	54	3	31	3 1/2 starch, 3 lean meat, 2 fat

✔ = Healthiest Bets

(*Continued*)

SANDWICHES *(Continued)*	Amount	Cal.	Fat (g)	% Cal. Fat	Sat. Fat (g)	Trans Fat (g)	Chol. (mg)	Sod. (mg)	Carb. (g)	Fiber (g)	Pro. (g)	Choices/Exchanges
Ham & Cheese	med	730	27	3	12	1	113	2979	78	4	44	5 starch, 4 lean meat, 2 fat
Homestyle Tuna	sm	388	11	3	2	0	46	1023	51	3	22	3 1/2 starch, 2 lean meat, 1 fat
Homestyle Tuna	med	563	16	3	3	0	67	1468	73	5	33	5 starch, 3 lean meat, 1 fat
Mediterranean Tuna	sm	343	5	1	1	0	29	1056	52	4	22	3 1/2 starch, 2 lean meat
Mediterranean Tuna	med	504	7	1	1	0	44	1618	76	6	33	5 starch, 3 lean meat
Santa Fe Chicken	sm	425	10	2	4	0	66	1452	53	4	31	3 1/2 starch, 3 lean meat
Santa Fe Chicken	med	619	15	2	7	0	98	2098	76	5	45	5 starch, 4 lean meat
Smoked Turkey Breast	sm	355	6	2	1	0	35	1074	53	2	20	3 1/2 starch, 1 lean meat, 1/2 fat

Smoked Turkey Breast	med	515	9	2	1	0	51	1561	76	4	19	5 starch, 1 lean meat, 2 fat
Smoked Turkey Reuben	sm	619	26	4	11	1	89	1587	58	3	35	4 starch, 3 lean meat, 3 fat
Smoked Turkey Reuben	med	904	39	4	17	1	132	2254	83	5	52	5 1/2 starch, 5 lean meat, 5 fat
Texas Schlotzsky's	sm	540	23	4	12	1	96	1976	51	2	32	3 1/2 starch, 3 medium-fat meat, 1 1/2 fat
Texas Schlotzsky's	med	756	31	4	15	1	119	2853	73	4	45	5 starch, 4 medium-fat meat, 2 fat
The Original	sm	562	26	4	12	1	85	1841	52	3	28	3 1/2 starch, 3 medium-fat meat, 2 fat
The Original	med	768	34	4	15	1	111	2632	76	4	40	5 starch, 4 medium-fat meat, 3 fat
Turkey	sm	605	27	4	11	1	96	1840	54	3	34	3 1/2 starch, 3 lean meat, 3 fat

✔ = Healthiest Bets

(Continued)

SANDWICHES *(Continued)*	Amount	Cal.	Fat (g)	% Cal. Fat	Sat. Fat (g)	Trans Fat (g)	Chol. (mg)	Sod. (mg)	Carb. (g)	Fiber (g)	Pro. (g)	Choices/Exchanges
Turkey	med	808	35	4	14	1	125	2528	78	4	47	5 starch, 4 lean meat, 4 fat
Turkey & Guacamole	sm	373	8	2	1	0	31	1123	54	4	20	3 1/2 starch, 1 lean meat, 1 fat
Turkey & Guacamole	med	564	13	2	1	0	45	1689	80	6	30	5 1/2 starch, 2 lean meat, 1 1/2 fat
Turkey Bacon Club	sm	573	24	4	9	1	86	1580	53	4	33	3 1/2 starch, 3 medium-fat meat, 1 fat
Turkey Bacon Club	med	784	31	4	12	1	114	2206	76	5	47	5 starch, 5 medium-fat meat, 1 fat
SOUPS												
Boston Clam Chowder	cup	217	11	5	3	3	11	1181	23	1	6	1/2 starch, 1 milk, 2 fat
Boston Clam Chowder	bowl	323	17	5	4	5	16	1750	34	2	9	1 starch, 1 1/2 milk, 3 1/2 fat

Broccoli Cheese Soup	cup	187	12	6	6	2	34	1063	13	1	4	1 starch, 2 1/2 fat
Broccoli Cheese Soup	bowl	303	20	6	9	3	40	1771	20	1	7	1 1/2 starch, 4 fat
Chicken Tortilla Soup	cup	150	6	4	3	0	30	1470	13	1	10	1 starch, 1 lean meat, 1/2 fat
Chicken Tortilla Soup	bowl	225	9	4	5	0	45	2205	20	1	15	1 1/2 starch, 2 lean meat, 1 fat
Hearty Vegetable Beef Soup	cup	109	5	4	2	0	15	1029	12	2	6	1 starch, 1 medium-fat meat, 1/2 fat
Hearty Vegetable Beef Soup	bowl	165	8	4	3	0	23	1563	18	3	9	1 starch, 1 medium-fat meat, 1 fat
Old Fashioned Chicken Noodle Soup	cup	90	2	2	1	0	55	1243	11	1	7	1/2 starch, 1 lean meat
Old Fashioned Chicken Noodle Soup	bowl	135	2	1	1	0	83	1865	17	1	11	1 starch, 1 lean meat

✔ = Healthiest Bets

(*Continued*)

SOUPS *(Continued)*	**Amount**	**Cal.**	**Fat (g)**	**% Cal. Fat**	**Sat. Fat (g)**	**Trans Fat (g)**	**Chol. (mg)**	**Sod. (mg)**	**Carb. (g)**	**Fiber (g)**	**Pro. (g)**	**Choices/Exchanges**
Potato with Bacon Soup	cup	182	9	4	2	3	4	1063	26	2	2	1 1/2 starch, 2 fat
Potato with Bacon Soup	bowl	271	13	4	3	4	6	1584	38	3	4	2 1/2 starch, 2 fat
✔Timberline Chile	cup	227	8	3	3	1	35	890	26	8	15	1 1/2 starch, 1 medium-fat meat
Timberline Chile	bowl	345	12	3	5	1	53	1335	39	12	23	2 1/2 starch, 2 medium-fat meat
Tomato Basil Soup	cup	302	27	8	16	0	87	942	14	4	4	1 starch, 5 fat
Tomato Basil Soup	bowl	453	40	8	23	0	130	1413	21	6	6	1 starch, 8 fat
✔Vegetarian Vegetable Soup	cup	85	1	1	0	0	0	900	19	4	2	1 starch, 1 veg
Vegetarian Vegetable Soup	bowl	122	1	1	0	0	0	1296	27	6	3	1 1/2 starch, 1 veg
Wisconsin Cheese Soup	cup	306	22	6	9	4	21	1214	24	1	6	1 1/2 starch, 4 fat
Wisconsin Cheese Soup	bowl	460	33	6	14	5	32	1821	36	2	18	2 1/2 starch, 6 fat

WRAPS												
Asian Chicken	1	537	11	2	3	0	59	2143	80	5	56	5 1/2 starch, 6 lean meat
Feta & Portobello	1	618	39	6	10	0	30	1631	55	4	14	3 1/2 starch, 7 1/2 fat
Grilled Chicken & Guacamole	1	695	36	5	1	0	91	1495	59	6	63	4 starch, 7 lean meat, 1 1/2 fat
Homestyle Tuna	1	457	17	3	4	0	44	1320	55	4	23	3 1/2 starch, 2 lean meat, 2 fat
Mediterranean Tuna	1	420	12	3	2	0	28	1300	57	5	22	4 starch, 2 lean meat, 1 fat
Parmesan Chicken Caesar	1	649	33	5	8	0	78	1698	56	5	62	3 1/2 starch, 7 lean meat, 1 fat

✔ = Healthiest Bets

Steak 'n' Shake (www.steaknshake.com)

Light 'n Lean Choice

The Original Steakburger Sandwich *(single)*
French Fries *(small)*
Apples & Grapes

Calories	570	Cholesterol (mg)	35
Fat (g)	22	Sodium (mg)	515
% calories from fat	35	Carbohydrate (g)	76
Saturated fat (g)	6	Fiber (g)	8
Trans fat (g)	1.5	Protein (g)	17

Exchanges: 4 starch, 1 1/2 fruit, 1 1/2 medium-fat meat, 2 1/2 fat

Healthy 'n Hearty Choice

Marinated Grilled Chicken Sandwich *(double)*
Garden Salad *(small)* with
Low-Fat Italian Dressing *(1 oz, 2 Tbsp)*
Premium Vanilla Ice Cream *(4 oz)*

Calories	663	Cholesterol (mg)	138
Fat (g)	25	Sodium (mg)	1,611
% calories from fat	34	Carbohydrate (g)	77
Saturated fat (g)	10	Fiber (g)	2
Trans fat (g)	0.5	Protein (g)	35

Exchanges: 3 starch, 2 carb, 1 veg, 3 lean meat, 3 fat

Steak 'n' Shake

	Amount	Cal.	Fat (g)	% Cal. Fat	Sat. Fat (g)	Trans Fat (g)	Chol. (mg)	Sod. (mg)	Carb. (g)	Fiber (g)	Pro. (g)	Choices/Exchanges
BEVERAGES: FOUNTAIN SYRUP ADDED TO DRINK												
✔Cherry, Jr.	0.5 oz.	43	0	0	0	0	0	4	11	0	0	1/2 carb
Cherry, regular	1.25 oz.	107	0	0	0	0	0	9	27	0	0	2 carb
Cherry, large	1.5 oz.	129	0	0	0	0	0	11	32	0	0	2 carb
✔Chocolate, Jr.	0.5 oz.	49	0	0	0	0	0	21	12	0	0	1 carb
Chocolate, regular	1.25 oz.	122	0	0	0	0	0	52	31	1	1	2 carb
Chocolate, large	1.5 oz.	146	0	0	0	0	0	62	37	1	1	2 1/2 carb
Hot Chocolate w/ Whipped Topping	7 oz.	160	5.5	3	2	0	5	218	28	1	2	2 carb, 1 fat
✔Sweetened Iced Tea	1 portion	87	0	0	0	0	0	12	23	0	0	1 1/2 carb

✔ = Healthiest Bets

(*Continued*)

BEVERAGES: FOUNTAIN SYRUP ADDED TO DRINK *(Continued)*	Amount	Cal.	Fat (g)	% Cal. Fat	Sat. Fat (g)	Trans Fat (g)	Chol. (mg)	Sod. (mg)	Carb. (g)	Fiber (g)	Pro. (g)	Choices/Exchanges
✔Vanilla, Jr.	0.5 oz.	42	0	0	0	0	0	1	11	0	0	1/2 carb
Vanilla, regular	1.25 oz.	105	0	0	0	0	0	2	27	0	0	2 carb
Vanilla, large	1.5 oz.	126	0	0	0	0	0	3	32	0	0	2 carb
BITS N PIECES MILK SHAKES												
Bits 'n Pieces Milkshake made w/ M&M's	reg	1050	37	3	23.5	1	78	318	164	3	18	11 carb, 7 fat
Bits 'n Pieces Milkshake made w/ M&M's	lg	1385	49.5	3	31.5	1	104	451	212	5	26	14 carb, 9 fat
Chocolate Chip Cookie Dough	reg	919	30	3	18	0.5	67	414	148	2	17	10 carb, 5 fat
Chocolate Chip Cookie Dough	lg	1203	40	3	24	1	89	587	190	3	25	12 1/2 carb, 3 fat
Cookies 'n Cream	reg	796	25	3	15	0.5	67	407	129	2	17	8 1/2 carb, 4 fat
Cookies 'n Cream	lg	1030	33	3	19.5	1	89	576	164	3	24	11 carb, 5 1/2 fat

Peanut Butter Cup	reg	995	40	4	24	1	73	352	144	3	19	9 1/2 carb, 7 fat
Peanut Butter Cup	lg	1310	54	4	32.5	1	98	500	186	4	28	12 1/2 carb, 10 fat
BREAKFAST												
Biscuit & Sausage Gravy	1 portion	656	38	5	14.5	10	35	1950	59	1	16	4 starch, 1 medium-fat meat, 7 fat
Breakfast Bacon Bagel	1	458	17	3	7	0	193	1102	51	2	25	3 1/2 starch, 2 medium-fat meat, 1 fat
Breakfast Sausage Bagel	1	576	30	5	11.5	0	212	1120	51	2	26	3 1/2 starch, 2 medium-fat meat, 3 fat
✔Breakfast Steakburger Bagel	1	460	16	3	7	0.5	205	795	50	2	27	3 1/2 starch, 2 medium-fat meat, 1/2 fat
Cheddar Scrambler	1 portion	1149	80	6	20.5	5.5	562	2315	72	9	38	5 starch, 3 medium-fat meat, 12 fat
Classic Stack 'O Cakes	4 pancakes	320	4	1	1	0	16	1220	62	2	10	4 starch, 1 fat

✔ = Healthiest Bets

(*Continued*)

BREAKFAST *(Continued)*	Amount	Cal.	Fat (g)	% Cal. Fat	Sat. Fat (g)	Trans Fat (g)	Chol. (mg)	Sod. (mg)	Carb. (g)	Fiber (g)	Pro. (g)	Choices/Exchanges
Sourdough Breakfast Bacon Melt	1	757	55	7	17	4	215	1493	35	0	29	2 1/2 starch, 3 medium-fat meat, 8 fat
Sourdough Breakfast Sausage Melt	1	1042	85	7	27	4	264	1694	35	0	35	2 1/2 starch, 4 medium-fat meat, 13 fat
Sourdough Breakfast Steakburger Melt	1	810	57	6	18	5	250	1050	33	0	37	2 starch, 4 medium-fat meat, 7 fat
BREAKFAST: A LA CARTE												
✔American Cheese	1 slice	60	5	8	3	0	10	200	0	0	3	1 fat
✔Apples & Grapes	sm	45	0	0	0	0	0	0	12	2	0	1 fruit
✔Apples & Grapes	reg	74	0	0	0	0	0	1	19	3	0	1 1/2 fruit
✔Bagel	1	240	1	0	0	0	0	400	49	2	9	3 starch
Biscuit & Sausage Gravy	1 portion	656	38	5	5	10	35	1950	59	1	16	4 starch, 1 medium-fat meat, 7 fat

Buttermilk Biscuit w/o Margarine	1	400	19	4	5	10	0	1230	47	1	9	3 starch, 4 fat
Caramel Dip	2 oz.	240	3	1	2	0	11	200	51	0	2	3 1/2 carb, 1/2 fat
✔Cholesterol Free Egg Product	1 egg equivalent	34	0	0	0	0	0	90	1	0	5	1 lean meat
✔Cholesterol Free Egg Product	2 egg equivalent	68	0	0	0	0	0	181	2	0	11	2 lean meat
✔Cottage Cheese	3.5 oz.	98	2	2	1	0	13	392	9	0	11	1 milk
✔Deluxe Bakery Bun, dry toasted	1	190	3	1	0.5	0	0	350	35	1	7	2 starch, 1/2 fat
Extra Shredded Cheese	2 oz.	180	16	8	9	0.5	50	260	2	0	10	1 medium-fat meat, 2 fat
Four Bacon Strips	4 strips	196	14	6	5	0	45	685	2	0	14	2 medium-fat meat, 1 fat
Hash Browns	6 pcs	256	16	6	2.5	0.5	30	525	25	8	3	2 starch, 3 fat

✔ = Healthiest Bets

(Continued)

BREAKFAST: A LA CARTE *(Continued)*	Amount	Cal.	Fat (g)	% Cal. Fat	Sat. Fat (g)	Trans Fat (g)	Chol. (mg)	Sod. (mg)	Carb. (g)	Fiber (g)	Pro. (g)	Choices/Exchanges
✔One Fresh Egg	1 egg	74	5	6	1.5	0	212	70	0	0	6	1 medium-fat meat
One Sausage Patty	1 patty	216	20	8	7	0	42	360	1	0	8	1 medium-fat meat, 3 fat
✔One Scrambled Egg	1 egg	60	4	6	1.5	0	160	160	1	0	6	1 medium-fat meat
One Thick Cut Bacon Strip	1 strip	72	5	6	2	0	16	237	0	0	5	1 medium-fat meat, 1/2 fat
Pepperjack Cheese	1 slice	70	6	8	3.5	0	10	220	1	0	4	1 medium-fat meat, 1/2 fat
Rye Toast w/ Margarine	2 slices	275	17	6	2.5	2	0	400	26	2	4	2 starch, 3 1/2 fat
✔Rye Toast w/o Margarine	2 slices	140	2	1	0	0	0	400	26	2	4	2 starch, 1/2 fat
Sausage Gravy	5 oz.	256	19	7	9.5	0	35	720	12	0	7	1 starch, 1 medium-fat meat, 3 fat
Sourdough Toast w/ Margarine	2 slices	295	16	5	2.5	2	0	420	32	0	6	2 starch, 3 fat

✔Sourdough Toast w/o Margarine	2 slices	160	1	1	0	0	0	420	32	0	6	2 starch
✔Steakburger Bun, dry toasted	1	150	4	2	1	0	0	350	26	1	6	1 1/2 starch, 1/2 fat
✔Steakburger Patty	1 patty	100	6	5	2.5	0.5	35	35	0	0	9	1 medium-fat meat
✔Steakburger Patties	2 patties	200	12	5	5	1	70	70	0	0	18	3 medium-fat meat
Swiss Cheese	1 slice	80	6	7	3.5	0	20	44	0	0	6	1 medium-fat meat, 1/2 fat
Two Bacon Strips	2 strips	98	7	6	2.5	0	23	342	1	0	7	1 medium-fat meat, 1/2 fat
✔Two Buttermilk Pancakes	2 pancakes	160	2	1	2	0	8	610	31	1	5	2 starch, 1/2 fat
Two Fresh Eggs	2 eggs	148	10	6	3	0	423	140	1	0	12	2 medium-fat meat, 1/2 fat
Two Sausage Patties	2 patties	432	40	8	14	0	84	714	2	0	16	2 medium-fat meat, 5 1/2 fat

✔ = Healthiest Bets

(Continued)

BREAKFAST: A LA CARTE *(Continued)*	Amount	Cal.	Fat (g)	% Cal. Fat	Sat. Fat (g)	Trans Fat (g)	Chol. (mg)	Sod. (mg)	Carb. (g)	Fiber (g)	Pro. (g)	Choices/Exchanges
Two Scrambled Eggs	2 eggs	120	7	5	2.5	0	320	320	3	0	12	2 medium-fat meat
Two Thick Cut Bacon Strips	2 strips	143	10	6	3.5	0	32	473	1	0	10	1 medium-fat meat, 1/2 fat
Wheat Toast w/ Margarine	2 slices	275	17	6	2.5	2	0	270	26	2	6	2 starch, 3 1/2 fat
✔Wheat Toast w/o Margarine	2 slices	140	2	1	0	0	0	270	26	2	6	2 starch, 1/2 fat
White Toast w/ Margarine	2 slices	335	17	5	2.5	2	0	400	40	0	6	3 starch, 3 1/2 fat
✔White Toast w/o Margarine	2 slices	200	2	1	0	0	0	400	40	0	6	3 starch, 1/2 fat
BREAKFAST: CONDIMENTS												
✔Coffee Creamer	0.4 oz.	15	1	6	0.5	0	5	10	0	0	0	Free
✔Cream Cheese	1 oz.	90	9	9	7	0	30	95	2	0	2	2 fat
✔Grape Jelly	0.75 oz.	53	0	0	0	0	0	0	14	0	0	1 carb
Honey	0.75 oz.	68	0	0	0	0	0	0	18	0	0	1 carb
✔Margarine Cup	0.2 oz.	20	2	9	0.5	0	0	0	0	44	0	1/2 fat

Pancake Syrup	1.5 oz.	120	0	0	0	0	0	0	31	30	0	2 carb
Strawberry Jelly	0.75 oz.	53	0	0	0	0	0	0	14	0	0	1 carb
Sugar	1 packet	12	0	0	0	0	0	0	3	0	0	Free
BREAKFAST: FRUIT SMOOTHIES												
Banana	1	491	11	2	6	0.5	41	246	83	4	11	5 1/2 carb, 1 1/2 fat
Raspberry	1	476	11	2	6	0.5	41	246	83	6	12	5 1/2 carb, 1 1/2 fat
Strawberry	1	548	11	2	6	0.5	41	246	102	5	11	7 carb, 1 fat
Strawberry Banana	1	519	11	2	6	0.5	41	246	93	4	11	6 carb, 1 fat
BREAKFAST: HOT CHOCOLATE												
✔Hot Chocolate	7 oz.	140	4	3	1	0	0	215	27	1	2	2 carb, 1/2 fat
✔Whipped Topping	0.25 oz.	20	2	9	1	0	5	3	1	0	0	1/2 fat
BREAKFAST: ITEMS AVAILABLE IN LIMITED MARKETS ONLY												
✔Cinnamon Swirl French Toast	3 slices	256	7	2	1.5	0.5	85	320	40	2	9	3 starch, 1 fat

✔ = Healthiest Bets

(*Continued*)

BREAKFAST: ITEMS AVAILABLE IN LIMITED MARKETS ONLY *(Continued)*	Amount	Cal.	Fat (g)	% Cal. Fat	Sat. Fat (g)	Trans Fat (g)	Chol. (mg)	Sod. (mg)	Carb. (g)	Fiber (g)	Pro. (g)	Choices/Exchanges
Country Scrambler	1 portion	790	52	6	19.5	0.5	567	2068	42	8	35	3 starch, 4 medium-fat meat, 6 1/2 fat
Strawberry French Toast	1 portion	467	12	2	4.5	0.5	98	329	81	4	10	5 starch, 2 fat
The Strawberry Stack	1 portion	451	8	2	4	0	25	924	88	3	9	6 starch, 1 fat
BREAKFAST: SPECIALS												
Biscuits, Gravy n Hash Browns	1 portion	1567	91	5	31	20.5	100	4425	143	10	35	9 1/2 starch, 1 medium-fat meat, 17 1/2 fat
English Muffin w/ Margarine	1 muffin	275	17	6	2.5	2	0	300	27	1	6	2 starch, 3 fat
✔English Muffin w/o Margarine	1 muffin	140	2	1	0	0	0	300	27	1	6	2 starch, 1/2 fat
✔The Number 1 (two scrambled eggs only)	1 portion	120	7	5	2.5	0	320	320	3	0	12	2 medium-fat meat

The Number 2 (Steak-burger, egg n cheese on a toasted bun, silver dollar hash browns)	1 portion	626	34	5	11	1	235	1270	53	9	27	3 1/2 starch, 2 medium-fat meat, 4 fat
The Number 3 (Two scrambled eggs and one buttermilk biscuit w/ sausage gravy)	1 portion	776	45	5	17	10	355	2270	62	1	28	4 starch, 2 medium-fat meat, 6 fat
The Number 4 (two scrambled eggs and silver dollar hash browns)	1 portion	376	23	6	5	0.5	350	845	29	8	15	2 starch, 1 medium-fat meat, 3 fat
The Number 5 (One butter-milk biscuit, sausage gravy and silver dollar hash browns)	1 portion	912	54	5	16.5	10.5	65	2475	84	9	19	5 1/2 starch, 10 fat

✔ = Healthiest Bets

(*Continued*)

BREAKFAST: SPECIALS *(Continued)*	Amount	Cal.	Fat (g)	% Cal. Fat	Sat. Fat (g)	Trans Fat (g)	Chol. (mg)	Sod. (mg)	Carb. (g)	Fiber (g)	Pro. (g)	Choices/Exchanges
✔The Number 6 (Two scrambled eggs only)	1 portion	120	7	5	2.5	0	320	320	3	0	12	2 medium-fat meat
The Number 7 (Egg sandwich w/ bacon & silver dollar hash browns)	1 portion	565	30	5	7	0.5	213	1377	54	9	22	3 1/2 starch, 2 medium-fat meat, 4 1/2 fat
The Number 7 (Egg sandwich w/ sausage & silver dollar hash browns)	1 portion	682	43	6	11.5	0.5	232	1392	54	9	23	3 1/2 starch, 2 medium-fat meat, 7 fat
The Number 8 (Sausage n biscuit sandwich and silver dollar hash browns)	1 portion	872	55	6	14.5	10.5	72	2112	73	9	20	5 starch, 1 medium-fat meat, 9 1/2 fat
The Number 9 (Egg sandwich w/ two bacon strips & melted American cheese on a toasted bagel)	1 portion	458	16.5	3	7	0	193	1102	51	2	26	3 1/2 starch, 2 medium-fat meat, 1 fat

CONDIMENTS N TOPPINGS												
Bacon Strips	2 strips	98	7	6	2.5	0	23	342	1	0	7	1 medium-fat meat, 1/2 fat
Cheddar Cheese	1 slice	85	7	7	4	0	21	143	0	0	5	1 medium-fat meat, 1/2 fat
Cheddar Cheese Sauces	2 oz.	84	7	8	2.5	1.5	9	530	3	0	3	1 1/2 fat
✔Cream Cheese	1 oz.	90	9	9	7	0	30	95	2	0	2	2 fat
Frisco Sauce	1.5 oz.	210	18	8	3	0	15	465	10	0	0	1/2 starch, 3 1/2 fat
✔Grilled Green Peppers	1.5 oz.	40	4	9	0.5	0.5	0	0	2	1	0	1/2 fat
Grilled Onions	1.5 oz.	80	7	8	1	1	0	0	4	0	0	1 veg, 1 1/2 fat
✔Jalapeno Slices	2 oz.	10	0	0	0	0	0	960	2	0	0	Free
✔Lettuce	1 large leaf	2	0	0	0	0	0	0	0	0	0	Free
✔Mushroom Topping	2 oz.	48	4	8	1	0.5	0	289	3	1	1	1 veg, 1 fat
✔Oyster Crackers	1 pkg	65	2	3	0	0	0	37	12	0	1	1 starch

✔ = Healthiest Bets

(Continued)

CONDIMENTS N TOPPINGS *(Continued)*	Amount	Cal.	Fat (g)	% Cal. Fat	Sat. Fat (g)	Trans Fat (g)	Chol. (mg)	Sod. (mg)	Carb. (g)	Fiber (g)	Pro. (g)	Choices/Exchanges
Pickles	2 slices	2	0	0	0	0	0	280	0	0	0	Free
✔Portobello Mushrooms	3 oz.	32	0	0	0	0	1	97	5	1	2	1 veg
✔Premium Grilled Onions	1 oz.	20	1	5	0	0	0	88	3	1	0	1 veg
Romano Cheese	0.2 oz.	32	2	6	1	0	3	95	1	0	2	1 fat
✔Salsa	2 oz.	28	0	0	0	0	0	506	6	0	0	1 veg
✔Saltine Crackers	2 crackers	25	1	4	0	0	0	80	5	0	0	Free
✔Sliced Onion	1 slice	7	0	0	0	0	0	0	2	0	0	Free
✔Sliced Tomato	2 slices	6	0	0	0	0	0	2	1	0	0	Free
✔Sour Cream	1 oz.	56	5	8	3	0	20	23	2	0	1	1 fat
Thick Cut Bacon Strips	2 strips	143	10	6	4	0	32	473	1	0	10	1 medium-fat meat, 1/2 fat

DESSERTS												
Berry Berry Cobbler a La Mode	1 portion	650	28.5	4	14	0	47	456	92	4	8	6 carb, 4 1/2 fat
Berry Berry Cobbler w/o Ice Cream	1 portion	468	18	3	7	0	0	396	72	4	5	5 carb, 3 1/2 fat
Brownie Fudge Sundae	1 portion	864	43.5	5	23	0.5	86	377	112	4	10	7 1/2 carb, 7 1/2 fat
Hot Fudge Sundae	1 sundae	566	29	5	19	0.5	69	247	71	1	7	4 1/2 carb, 5 fat
Outrageous Parfait	1 portion	827	43	5	28	1	124	313	103	2	11	7 carb, 7 1/2 fat
Premium Vanilla Ice Cream	4 oz.	243	14	5	9	0.5	63	80	26	0	4	1 1/2 carb, 3 fat
Root Beer Float	1 float	531	21	4	14	0.5	94	156	85	0	5	5 1/2 carb, 3 fat
Strawberry Shortcake	1 portion	577	27	4	14	5.5	65	687	76	2	8	5 carb, 4 1/2 fat
Strawberry Sundae	1 sundae	354	20	5	10	0.5	68	111	40	1	5	2 1/2 carb, 3 fat
FREEZES												
Orange	reg	686	20	3	14	0.5	67	275	113	1	14	7 1/2 carb, 3 fat

✔ = Healthiest Bets

(Continued)

FREEZES *(Continued)*	Amount	Cal.	Fat (g)	% Cal. Fat	Sat. Fat (g)	Trans Fat (g)	Chol. (mg)	Sod. (mg)	Carb. (g)	Fiber (g)	Pro. (g)	Choices/Exchanges
Orange	lg	851	26	3	17	0.5	86	375	138	2	20	9 carb, 4 fat
FROZEN YOGURT MILK SHAKES												
Chocolate Frozen Yogurt Milk Shake	reg	723	15.5	2	9	0.5	56	388	133	3	16	9 carb, 2 fat
Chocolate Frozen Yogurt Milk Shake	lg	931	21	2	12	1	78	518	167	4	22	11 carb, 3 fat
Vanilla Frozen Yogurt Milk Shake	reg	696	15.5	2	8	0.5	56	310	126	1	14	8 1/2 carb, 2 fat
Vanilla Frozen Yogurt Milk Shake	lg	904	21	2	12	1	78	440	160	1	20	10 1/2 carb, 3 fat
FRUIT N FROZEN YOGURT MILK SHAKES												
Banana Fruit 'n Frozen Yogurt	1	487	13	2	7	0.5	46	248	77.5	1	11	5 carb, 2 fat

Black Cherry Fruit 'n Frozen Yogurt	1	681	11.5	2	7	0.5	45	272	129	0	13	8 1/2 carb, 2 fat
Peach Fruit 'n Frozen Yogurt	1	587	11.5	2	7	0.5	45	272	104	1	13	7 carb, 2 fat
Raspberry Fruit 'n Frozen Yogurt	1	473	13	2	7	0.5	46	248	77	3	12	5 carb, 2 fat
Strawberry Banana Fruit 'n Frozen Yogurt	1	516	13	2	7	0.5	46	248	87	2	11	6 carb, 2 fat
Strawberry Fruit 'n Frozen Yogurt	1	545	13	2	7	0.5	46	248	97	2	11	6 1/2 carb, 2 fat
HALLOWEEN MILK SHAKES												
Popping Candy	reg	875	32	3	24	0.5	68	302	135	1	15	9 carb, 5 1/2 fat
Popping Candy	lg	1108	41	3	31	1	88	412	169	2	21	11 1/2 carb, 7 fat
HOLIDAY MILK SHAKES												
Chocolate w/ Chocolate Turtle Bark	reg	1042	39	3	27	1	76	477	159	4	21	10 1/2 carb, 7 fat

✓ = Healthiest Bets

(*Continued*)

HOLIDAY MILK SHAKES *(Continued)*	Amount	Cal.	Fat (g)	% Cal. Fat	Sat. Fat (g)	Trans Fat (g)	Chol. (mg)	Sod. (mg)	Carb. (g)	Fiber (g)	Pro. (g)	Choices/Exchanges
Chocolate w/ Chocolate Turtle Bark	lg	1346	52	3	36	1	98	629	201	5	28	13 1/2 carb, 9 1/2 fat
Vanilla w/ Chocolate Turtle Bark	reg	1015	39	3	27	1	76	399	152	2	20	10 carb, 7 fat
Vanilla w/ Chocolate Turtle Bark	lg	1319	52	4	35	1	98	550	194	3	27	13 carb, 7 1/2 fat
KIDS MENU: JR. BITS 'N PIECES MILK SHAKES												
Jr. Bits 'n Pieces Milkshake Made w/ M&M's	1	568	20	3	12	0	38	173	90	2	10	6 carb, 3 fat
Jr. Chocolate Chip Cookie Dough	1	491	15	3	9	0	32	232	81	1	9	5 1/2 carb, 2 fat
Jr. Cookies 'n Cream	1	416	12	3	7	0	32	226	70	1	9	4 1/2 carb, 2 fat
Jr. Peanut Butter Cup	1	537	22	4	12.5	0	36	194	79	1	11	5 1/2 carb, 4 fat

KIDS MENU: JR. BREAKFAST												
Bacon 'n Scrambled Egg	1 portion	203	16	7	4.5	0.5	183	502	3	0	13	2 medium-fat meat, 1 1/2 fat
✔French Toast 'n Syrup	1 portion	176	5	3	1	0	57	214	28	1	6	2 carb, 1 fat
Hot Chocolate w/ Whipped Topping	7 oz.	160	6	3	2	0	5	218	28	1	2	2 carb, 1 fat
✔Pancakes 'n Syrup	2 pancakes	250	12	4	2	1.5	8	610	31	1	5	2 carb, 2 fat
✔Scrambled Egg, Bacon, 'n Toast (Toast facts not included in nutrition facts)	1 portion	158	11	6	4	0	183	502	2	0	13	2 medium-fat meat, 1/2 fat
KIDS MENU: JR. FREEZES												
Orange	1	368	10	2	6.5	0	34	160	63	1	8	4 carb, 1 fat
KIDS MENU: JR. FROZEN YOGURT MILK SHAKES												
Chocolate	1	432	10.5	2	5.5	0	36	232	77	2	10	5 carb, 1 fat

✔ = Healthiest Bets

(*Continued*)

KIDS MENU: JR. FROZEN YOGURT MILK SHAKES *(Continued)*	Amount	Cal.	Fat (g)	% Cal. Fat	Sat. Fat (g)	Trans Fat (g)	Chol. (mg)	Sod. (mg)	Carb. (g)	Fiber (g)	Pro. (g)	Choices/Exchanges
Vanilla	1	420	10.5	2	5.5	0	36	193	73	0	9	5 carb, 1 fat
KIDS MENU: JR. FRUIT 'N FROZEN YOGURT MILK SHAKES												
Banana	1	363	10	2	5.5	0	36	191	57	0	9	4 carb, 2 fat
Raspberry	1	356	10	3	5.5	0	36	191	57	2	9	4 carb, 1 fat
Strawberry	1	392	10	2	5.5	0	36	191	67	1	9	4 1/2 carb, 1 fat
Strawberry Banana	1	389	10	2	5.5	0	36	191	65	1	9	4 1/2 carb, 1 fat
KIDS MENU: JR. HALLOWEEN MILK SHAKES												
Popping Candy	1	472	17	3	12.5	0	33	165	75	1	8	5 carb, 3 fat
KIDS MENU: JR. HOLIDAY MILK SHAKES												
Chocolate w/ Chocolate Turtle Bark	1	578	21	3	14	0.5	40	276	90	2	12	6 carb, 3 fat
Vanilla w/ Chocolate Turtle Bark	1	565	21	3	14	0.5	40	236	86	1	11	5 1/2 carb, 3 fat

KIDS MENU: JR. MILK SHAKES												
Banana	1	393	11	3	7	0	39	199	65	1	10	4 1/2 carb, 1 fat
Chocolate	1	405	11	2	7	0	39	223	68	2	11	4 1/2 carb, 1 fat
Chocolate Mint	1	408	11.5	3	7	0	39	224	68	2	11	4 1/2 carb, 2 fat
Dark Chocolate	1	397	12	3	7	0	39	208	65	2	11	4 1/2 carb, 2 fat
Malt flavor added to any shake	1 oz.	91	0	0	0	0	0	184	22	0	0	1 1/2 carb
Mocha	1	395	11	3	7	0	39	254	66	1	10	4 1/2 carb, 1 fat
Strawberry	1	387	11	3	7	0	39	186	63	1	10	4 carb, 1 fat
Vanilla	1	391	11	3	7	0	39	184	64	1	10	4 1/2 carb, 1 fat
KIDS MENU: JR. SIPPABLE SUNDAE MILK SHAKES												
Banana Split	1	541	18	3	10	0	32	239	88	1	10	6 carb, 3 fat
Double Chocolate Fudge	1	555	18	3	14	0	32	255	91	2	10	6 carb, 3 fat

✔ = Healthiest Bets

(*Continued*)

KIDS MENU: JR. SIPPABLE SUNDAE MILK SHAKES *(Continued)*	Amount	Cal.	Fat (g)	% Cal. Fat	Sat. Fat (g)	Trans Fat (g)	Chol. (mg)	Sod. (mg)	Carb. (g)	Fiber (g)	Pro. (g)	Choices/Exchanges
Turtle Caramel Nut	1	623	20	3	11	0	37	339	104	1	11	7 carb, 3 fat
KIDS MENU: LUNCH/DINNER												
✔Apples & Grapes	sm	45	0	0	0	0	0	0	12	2	0	1 fruit
✔Jr. Chicken Fingers 'n Fries	1 portion	330	20	5	3	1	15	272	29	2	8	2 starch, 4 fat
✔Jr. Chili Mac Plate	1 portion	433	19	4	7	0	44	928	49	4	17	3 1/2 starch, 1 medium-fat meat, 3 fat
✔Jr. Fries	1 portion	155	8	5	1.5	0.5	0	82	20	2	1	1 1/2 starch, 1 fat
Jr. Grilled Cheese 'n Fries	1 portion	805	55	6	16	5.5	30	1082	60	2	17	4 starch, 1 medium-fat meat, 10 fat
✔Jr. Steakburger Sandwich 'n Fries	1 portion	405	18	4	5	1	35	467	46	3	16	3 starch, 1 medium-fat meat, 2 fat

Jr. Steakburger w/ Cheese 'n Fries	1 portion	465	23	4	8	1	45	667	46	3	19	3 starch, 1 medium-fat meat, 3 fat
MELTS												
Chicken Melt	1	936	64	6	14.5	4	130	2025	46	0	41	3 starch, 5 medium-fat meat, 8 fat
Frisco Melt	1	980	72	7	20	5	115	1199	42	0	33	3 starch, 4 medium-fat meat, 11 fat
Patty Melt	1	810	61	7	18	6	90	870	30	2	28	2 starch, 3 medium-fat meat, 9 fat
Pepperjack Melt	1	958	73	7	20.5	6.5	100	1002	39	0	32	2 1/2 starch, 3 medium-fat meat, 11 fat
Turkey Melt	1	914	64	6	14.5	4	96	2048	47	0	34	3 starch, 4 lean meat, 10 fat
MILK SHAKES 'N MALTS												
Banana	reg	721	22	3	14.5	0.5	74	339	116	1	17	7 1/2 carb, 3 1/2 fat

✔ = Healthiest Bets

(Continued)

MILK SHAKES 'N MALTS *(Continued)*	Amount	Cal.	Fat (g)	% Cal. Fat	Sat. Fat (g)	Trans Fat (g)	Chol. (mg)	Sod. (mg)	Carb. (g)	Fiber (g)	Pro. (g)	Choices/Exchanges
Banana	lg	901	28	3	18	0.5	96	453	142	2	24	9 1/2 carb, 4 1/2 fat
Caramel added to any shake	2 oz.	240	3.5	1	2	0	11	200	51	0	2	3 1/2 carb, 1/2 fat
Chocolate	reg	744	22	3	15	0.5	74	388	122	3	19	8 carb, 3 1/2 fat
Chocolate	lg	924	28	3	18.5	0.5	96	502	148	4	25	10 carb, 4 1/2 fat
Chocolate Mint	reg	750	23	3	14.5	0.5	74	389	122	3	19	8 carb, 3 1/2 fat
Chocolate Mint	lg	930	29	3	18	0.5	96	503	148	4	25	10 carb, 5 fat
Dark Chocolate	reg	729	24	3	15	0.5	74	357	117	5	20	8 carb, 4 fat
Dark Chocolate	lg	909	30	3	19	0.5	96	471	143	5	26	9 1/2 carb, 5 fat
Hot Fudge added to any shake	2 oz.	250	9	3	8.5	0	1	135	41	1	3	2 1/2 carb, 1 fat
Malt flavor added to any shake	1 oz.	91	0	0	0	0	0	184	22	0	0	1 1/2 carb

Mocha	reg	724	22	3	14.5	0.5	74	448	117	2	18	8 carb, 3 1/2 fat
Mocha	lg	904	28	3	18.5	0.5	96	563	144	2	24	9 1/2 carb, 4 1/2 fat
Strawberry	reg	709	22	3	14.5	0.5	74	313	113	1	17	7 1/2 carb, 3 1/2 fat
Strawberry	lg	889	28	3	18.5	0.5	96	427	139	2	24	9 1/2 carb, 4 1/2 fat
Vanilla	reg	717	22	3	14.5	0.5	74	309	115	1	17	7 1/2 carb, 3 1/2 fat
Vanilla	lg	897	28	3	18	0.5	96	423	141	2	24	9 1/2 carb, 4 1/2 fat
NEW & IMPROVED SALADS												
Classic Grilled Chicken Salad Make It Lighter	1	277	10	3	1	0	72	1201	21	2	26	3 veg, 4 lean meat
Improved Beef Taco Salad	1	1000	69	6	20	4	90	1910	66	8	29	3 starch, 3 veg, 4 medium-fat meat, 9 fat
✔Improved Deluxe Garden Salad	1	198	11	5	4.5	0	25	359	17	3	8	3 veg, 1 lean meat, 1 1/2 fat
Improved Fried Chicken Salad	1	698	53	7	18	0	101	931	20	1	33	1/2 starch, 2 veg, 5 lean meat, 8 fat

✔ = Healthiest Bets

(*Continued*)

NEW & IMPROVED SALADS *(Continued)*	Amount	Cal.	Fat (g)	% Cal. Fat	Sat. Fat (g)	Trans Fat (g)	Chol. (mg)	Sod. (mg)	Carb. (g)	Fiber (g)	Pro. (g)	Choices/Exchanges
Improved Grilled Chicken Taco Salad	1	922	57	6	15	4	117	2232	64	6	37	3 starch, 3 veg, 4 lean meat, 9 fat
✔New Apple Walnut Grilled Chicken Salad	1	337	10	3	0	0	72	804	38	5	25	1 starch, 3 veg, 3 lean meat
New Classic Grilled Chicken Salad	1	466	25	5	8	0	120	1675	23	2	38	1/2 starch, 3 veg, 5 lean meat, 2 fat
OUR GENUINE CHILI												
Chili 3-Way	1 portion	823	45	5	17.5	0	108	2048	65	11	38	4 1/2 starch, 4 medium-fat meat, 5 fat
Chili 5-Way	1 portion	1120	69	6	31	1.5	184	2445	74	12	54	5 starch, 6 medium-fat meat, 7 fat
Chili Deluxe	1 cup	538	38	6	17	0.5	102	1319	21	7	29	1 1/2 starch, 4 medium-fat meat, 4 fat

Chili Deluxe	1 bowl	946	68	6	31	1.5	183	2264	37	12	51	2 1/2 starch, 6 medium-fat meat, 7 fat
Chili Mac	1 portion	827	38	4	14.5	0	88	1828	89	8	33	6 starch, 2 medium-fat meat, 5 fat
Chili Mac Supreme	1 portion	1124	62	5	28	1	164	2225	98	9	49	6 1/2 starch, 4 medium-fat meat, 7 fat
Genuine Chili	1 cup	389	26	6	10	0	64	1120	17	7	21	1 starch, 3 medium-fat meat, 2 1/2 fat
Genuine Chili	1 bowl	650	44	6	17	0	107	1867	28	12	35	2 starch, 4 medium-fat meat, 4 fat
PREMIUM TOPPING STEAKBURGER SANDWICH												
BBQ Bacon Ranch	1	633	31	4	10	1	107	1613	46	2	35	3 starch, 4 medium-fat meat, 2 1/2 fat
Black Peppercorn Bacon	1	620	31	5	12.5	1	112	1395	40	1	39	2 1/2 starch, 4 medium-fat meat, 1 1/2 fat

✓ = Healthiest Bets

(Continued)

PREMIUM TOPPING STEAKBURGER SANDWICH *(Continued)*	Amount	Cal.	Fat (g)	% Cal. Fat	Sat. Fat (g)	Trans Fat (g)	Chol. (mg)	Sod. (mg)	Carb. (g)	Fiber (g)	Pro. (g)	Choices/Exchanges
Grilled Mushroom 'n Onion	1	504	23	4	9	1	80	1135	40	2	28	2 1/2 starch, 3 medium-fat meat, 1 1/2 fat
Hickory Smoked Thick Bacon	1	610	30	4	12	1	112	1375	39	1	38	2 1/2 starch, 4 medium-fat meat, 1 1/2 fat
✔Portobello & Swiss	1	512	21	4	9	1	91	843	41	2	33	2 1/2 starch, 4 medium-fat meat, 1/2 fat
SALAD DRESSINGS												
Bleu Cheese	2 oz.	320	34	10	7	0	30	480	2	0	2	7 fat
Caesar	2 oz.	240	24	9	4	0	20	620	2	0	2	5 fat
✔Fat Free Raspberry Vinaigrette	2 oz.	50	0	0	0	0	0	80	12	2	0	1 carb
Honey Mustard	2 oz.	320	30	8	5	8	30	280	10	0	2	1/2 carb, 6 fat
✔Light Ranch	2 oz.	160	16	9	8	0	10	380	2	0	0	3 fat

Low Fat Italian	2 oz.	60	3	5	0	0	0	580	8	0	0	1/2 carb, 1/2 fat
✔Ranch	2 oz.	200	20	9	3	0	20	720	4	0	2	1/2 carb, 4 fat
Thousand Island	2 oz.	280	24	8	4	0	20	620	14	0	0	1 carb, 5 fat
SIPPABLE SUNDAE MILK SHAKES												
Banana Split	reg	904	29	3	17	0.5	67	364	147	2	17	10 carb, 5 fat
Banana Split	lg	1084	35	3	21	1	89	479	174	3	23	11 1/2 carb, 6 fat
Double Chocolate Fudge	reg	1020	33	3	26	0.5	68	488	166	5	20	11 carb, 5 1/2 fat
Double Chocolate Fudge	lg	1200	39	3	30	1	90	602	193	5	26	13 carb, 7 fat
Turtle Caramel Nut	reg	949	31	3	18	0.5	72	464	154	1	18	10 1/2 carb, 5 fat
Turtle Caramel Nut	lg	1129	37	3	22	1	94	579	181	2	24	12 carb, 6 1/2 fat
SOUPS 'N SIDES												
✔Apples & Grapes	sm	45	0	0	0	0	0	0	12	2	0	1 fruit
✔Apples & Grapes	reg	74	0	0	0	0	0	1	19	3	0	1 1/2 fruit
✔Broccoli Cheese Soup	1 cup	90	5	5	2.5	0.5	10	830	10	1	3	1/2 starch, 1 fat

✔ = Healthiest Bets

(*Continued*)

SOUPS 'N SIDES *(Continued)*	Amount	Cal.	Fat (g)	% Cal. Fat	Sat. Fat (g)	Trans Fat (g)	Chol. (mg)	Sod. (mg)	Carb. (g)	Fiber (g)	Pro. (g)	Choices/Exchanges
Broccoli Cheese Soup	1 bowl	180	9	5	5	1	20	1660	20	2	6	1 1/2 starch, 2 fat
Cheddar Cheese Fries	sm	330	19	5	5	2.5	9	659	34	4	5	2 starch, 4 fat
Cheddar Cheese Fries	reg	616	36	5	10	5.5	19	1296	64	7	9	4 starch, 6 fat
Cheddar Cheese Fries	lg	816	47	5	11.5	6.5	19	1402	89	11	10	6 starch, 9 fat
✔Chicken Gumbo Soup	1 cup	80	2	2	0.5	0	10	880	14	1	5	1 starch, 1/2 fat
Chicken Gumbo Soup	1 bowl	160	4	2	1	0	20	1760	28	2	10	2 starch, 1 lean meat
✔Chicken Noodle Soup	1 cup	80	2	2	0.5	0	5	690	10	1	4	1 starch, 1/2 fat
Chicken Noodle Soup	1 bowl	160	3	2	1	0	10	1380	20	2	8	1 1/2 starch, 1 lean meat, 1/2 fat
✔Cottage Cheese	1 srvg	98	2	2	1	0	13	392	9	0	11	1 milk
Creamy Coleslaw	1 srvg	300	24	7	4	0	45	410	20	2	1	1 starch, 1 veg, 5 fat
✔French Fries	sm	246	13	5	2.5	1	0	129	31	4	2	2 starch, 2 fat
French Fries	reg	447	23	5	4.5	2	0	235	57	7	3	4 starch, 4 fat

French Fries	lg	647	34	5	6	3	0	341	82	11	4	5 starch, 6 fat
Genuine Chili	1 cup	389	26	6	10	0	64	1120	17	7	21	1 starch, 3 medium-fat meat, 2 1/2 fat
Old-Fashioned Baked Beans	1 crock	352	0	0	0	0	0	1212	74	12	14	5 starch
Onion Rings	sm	350	18	5	3	1	0	750	41	3	6	3 starch, 3 fat
Onion Rings	reg	700	36	5	6.5	2	0	1500	82	6	12	5 starch, 6 fat
✔Small Garden Salad	1	53	2	3	0	0	0	114	8	1	2	2 veg
✔Vegetable Beef Soup	1 cup	60	2	3	0	0	0	680	12	1	2	1 starch, 1/2 fat
Vegetable Beef Soup	1 bowl	120	3	2	0	0	0	1360	24	2	4	1 1/2 starch, 1/2 fat
SPECIALTIES												
Bacon, Lettuce & Tomato	1	504	27	5	7	0	55	1157	43	0	20	3 starch, 2 medium-fat meat, 4 fat
Black Peppercorn Bacon Chicken Sandwich	1	550	23	4	8	0	117	1820	41	1	43	2 1/2 starch, 5 lean meat, 1 fat

✔ = Healthiest Bets

(Continued)

SPECIALTIES *(Continued)*	Amount	Cal.	Fat (g)	% Cal. Fat	Sat. Fat (g)	Trans Fat (g)	Chol. (mg)	Sod. (mg)	Carb. (g)	Fiber (g)	Pro. (g)	Choices/Exchanges
Breaded Chicken Sandwich (double)	1	581	23	4	4.5	1	53	1835	60	1	31	4 starch, 3 lean meat, 3 fat
Breaded Chicken Sandwich (single)	1	366	15.5	4	3.5	0	28	1105	39	1	18	2 1/2 starch, 1 lean meat, 2 fat
✔Chicken Fingers	3 strips	262	18	6	2	1	23	285	14	0	11	1 starch, 1 lean meat, 3 fat
Chicken Fingers 'n Fries	1 portion	508	31	5	4.5	2	23	414	45	4	13	3 starch, 1 lean meat, 6 fat
Fish Fillet	1	398	17	4	3.5	0.5	58	1105	43	2	21	3 starch, 2 lean meat, 2 fat
Fish Fillet w/ Cheese	1	457	22	4	6.5	1	68	1306	43	2	24	3 starch, 2 lean meat, 3 fat

Fish Fillets	2 fillets	456	23	5	4	1.5	110	1420	32	2	30	2 starch, 3 lean meat, 2 fat
Grilled Cheese	1	650	47	7	14.5	5	30	1000	40	0	16	2 1/2 starch, 1 medium-fat meat, 8 fat
Grilled Cheese 'n Bacon	1	748	54	6	17	5	53	1342	41	0	23	2 1/2 starch, 2 medium-fat meat, 8 fat
✔Marinated Grilled Chicken Sandwich (single)	1	241	7	3	1.5	0	39	751	29	1	17	2 starch, 2 lean meat, 1/2 fat
Marinated Grilled Chicken Sandwich (double)	1	337	7	2	1	0	75	1127	39	1	29	2 1/2 starch, 3 lean meat
Spicy Breaded Chicken Sandwich (single)	1	351	14	4	3.5	0	33	1345	37	2	20	2 1/2 starch, 2 lean meat, 1 fat
Spicy Breaded Chicken Sandwich (double)	1	551	20	3	4.5	0.5	63	2315	56	3	35	3 1/2 starch, 3 lean meat, 2 fat
Turkey Club	1	567	30	5	6	0	78	1636	46	0	28	3 starch, 3 lean meat, 4 fat

✔ = Healthiest Bets

(Continued)

	Amount	Cal.	Fat (g)	% Cal. Fat	Sat. Fat (g)	Trans Fat (g)	Chol. (mg)	Sod. (mg)	Carb. (g)	Fiber (g)	Pro. (g)	Choices/Exchanges
STEAKBURGER SANDWICH												
Bacon 'n Cheese Double	1	508	28	5	11.5	1	103	962	27	1	34	2 starch, 4 medium-fat meat, 1 1/2 fat
Cheddar 'n Bacon Steakburger	1	572	28	4	10.5	2.5	102	1292	39	1	35	2 1/2 starch, 4 medium-fat meat, 1 1/2 fat
The Mushroom 'n Swiss	1	586	29	4	13.5	1	110	725	38	2	38	2 1/2 starch, 4 medium-fat meat, 1 1/2 fat
✔The Original Single	1	250	10	4	3.5	0.5	35	385	26	1	15	1 1/2 starch, 1 medium-fat meat, 1/2 fat
✔The Original Single w/ Cheese	1	310	15	4	6.5	0.5	45	585	26	1	18	1 1/2 starch, 2 medium-fat meat, 1 fat
✔The Original Double	1	350	16	4	6	1	70	420	26	1	24	1 1/2 starch, 3 medium-fat meat, 1/2 fat

✔The Original Double w/ Cheese	1	410	21	5	9	1	80	620	26	1	27	1 1/2 starch, 3 medium-fat meat, 1 fat
Philadelphia Steakburger	1	594	32	5	9.5	4	79	950	44	2	28	3 starch, 3 medium-fat meat, 3 1/2 fat
Triple Steakburger Sandwich	1	450	22	4	8.5	1.5	105	455	26	1	33	1 1/2 starch, 4 medium-fat meat, 1/2 fat
Triple Steakburger Sandwich w/ Cheese	1	570	32	5	14.5	1.5	125	855	26	1	40	1 1/2 starch, 5 medium-fat meat, 1 1/2 fat

✔ = Healthiest Bets

Exclusive Web Content

Be sure to visit the following restaurants online at http://www.diabetes.org/healthyrestaurant

Carvel
Del Taco
El Pollo Loco
Frëshens
Godfather's
Jersey Mike's
Jimmy John's
Tim Hortons
Whataburger
Wienerschnitzel
Zaxby's

Subway

(www.subway.com)

Light 'n Lean Choice

Minestrone Soup *(8 oz)*
Ham Sandwich *(4")*
Oatmeal Raisin Cookie *(1)*

Calories	460	Cholesterol (mg)	25
Fat (g)	12	Sodium (mg)	2,005
% calories from fat	23	Carbohydrate (g)	75
Saturated fat (g)	5.5	Fiber (g)	9
Trans fat (g)	0	Protein (g)	18

Exchanges: 2 1/2 starch, 2 carb, 1 veg, 1 lean meat, 1 1/2 fat

Healthy 'n Hearty Choice

Chili Con Carne *(10 oz)*
Turkey Breast and Ham Sub *(6")*
Berry 'Lichus Fruizie Express *(small)*

Calories	690	Cholesterol (mg)	50
Fat (g)	13	Sodium (mg)	2,230
% calories from fat	17	Carbohydrate (g)	110
Saturated fat (g)	5	Fiber (g)	18
Trans fat (g)	0	Protein (g)	40

Exchanges: 5 1/2 starch, 2 carb, 1 veg, 2 1/2 medium-fat meat

Subway

	Amount	Cal.	Fat (g)	% Cal. Fat	Sat. Fat (g)	Trans Fat (g)	Chol. (mg)	Sod. (mg)	Carb. (g)	Fiber (g)	Pro. (g)	Choices/Exchanges
4" SANDWICHES												
✔Ham	1	180	3	2	1	0	10	710	30	4	11	2 starch, 1 lean meat
✔Roast Beef	1	190	3.5	2	1.5	0	15	600	30	4	13	2 starch, 1 lean meat
✔Tuna w/Cheese	1	320	18	5	4.5	0	30	690	30	4	13	2 starch, 1 lean meat, 3 fat
✔Turkey Breast	1	190	3	1	1	0	15	670	30	4	12	2 starch, 1 lean meat
6" DOUBLE SUBS (DOUBLE MEAT)												
Chicken & Bacon Ranch (includes cheese)	1	710	35	4	13	1	160	1890	48	6	55	3 starch, 6 medium-fat meat
Cold Cut Combo (includes cheese)	1	550	28	5	10	1	110	2360	49	5	31	3 1/2 starch, 3 medium-fat meat, 2 fat

✔ = Healthiest Bets

(*Continued*)

6" DOUBLE SUBS (DOUBLE MEAT) *(Continued)*	Amount	Cal.	Fat (g)	% Cal. Fat	Sat. Fat (g)	Trans Fat (g)	Chol. (mg)	Sod. (mg)	Carb. (g)	Fiber (g)	Pro. (g)	Choices/Exchanges
Ham	1	350	7	2	2.5	0	50	2020	49	5	28	3 1/2 starch, 2 lean meat
Italian BMT (includes cheese)	1	630	35	5	14	0	100	2850	49	5	34	3 1/2 starch, 3 medium-fat meat, 3 fat
Meatball Marinara (includes cheese)	1	860	42	4	18	2	85	2480	82	11	37	5 1/2 starch, 3 medium-fat meat, 5 fat
Oven Roasted Chicken Breast	1	400	8	2	2.5	0	45	1160	51	6	38	3 1/2 starch, 3 lean meat
Roast Beef	1	360	7	2	3.5	0	40	1300	46	5	29	3 starch, 3 lean meat
Steak & Cheese	1	540	18	3	8	1	105	1510	52	7	46	3 1/2 starch, 4 medium-fat meat
Subway Club	1	420	8	2	3.5	0	65	2080	50	5	39	3 1/2 starch, 3 lean meat
Subway Melt (includes cheese)	1	490	17	3	8	0	80	2500	51	5	40	3 1/2 starch, 3 medium-fat meat
Sweet Onion Chicken Teriyaki	1	480	7	1	2	0	100	1820	65	6	43	4 1/2 starch, 3 lean meat

Turkey Breast	1	330	5	1	1.5	0	40	1500	48	5	28	3 starch, 2 lean meat
Turkey Breast & Ham	1	360	7	2	2	0	50	1930	50	5	31	3 1/2 starch, 2 lean meat
6" JARED SANDWICHES W/ 6G OF FAT OR LESS												
Ham	1	290	5	2	1.5	0	25	1260	47	5	18	3 starch, 1 lean meat, 1/2 fat
✔Oven Roasted Chicken Breast	1	310	5	1	1.5	0	25	830	48	6	24	3 starch, 1 lean meat
✔Roast Beef	1	290	5	2	2	0	20	900	45	5	19	3 starch, 1 lean meat
Subway Club	1	320	6	2	2	0	35	1290	47	5	24	3 starch, 2 lean meat
Sweet Onion Chicken Teriyaki	1	370	5	1	1.5	0	50	1200	59	5	26	4 starch, 1 lean meat
✔Turkey Breast	1	280	5	2	1.5	0	20	1000	46	5	18	3 starch, 1 lean meat
Turkey Breast & Ham	1	290	5	2	1.5	0	25	1210	47	5	20	3 starch, 1 lean meat
✔Veggie Delite	1	230	3	1	1	0	0	500	44	5	9	3 starch, 1/2 fat
6" LIMITED TIME OFFER/REGIONAL SUBS												
Barbecue Chicken	1	310	6	2	2	0	35	1090	52	6	16	3 1/2 starch, 1 lean meat

✔ = Healthiest Bets

(*Continued*)

6" LIMITED TIME OFFER/ REGIONAL SUBS *(Continued)*	Amount	Cal.	Fat (g)	% Cal. Fat	Sat. Fat (g)	Trans Fat (g)	Chol. (mg)	Sod. (mg)	Carb. (g)	Fiber (g)	Pro. (g)	Choices/Exchanges
✔Barbecue Rib Patty	1	420	19	4	6	0	50	810	47	5	20	3 starch, 2 medium-fat meat, 2 fat
Big Philly Cheese steak (double meat)	1	520	19	3	10	0	100	1390	50	6	40	3 1/2 starch, 4 medium-fat meat
✔BLT (includes cheese)	1	350	13	3	6	0	30	940	43	5	18	3 starch, 1 medium-fat meat, 1 fat
Buffalo Chicken	1	380	18	4	4	0	55	1490	46	5	25	3 starch, 2 lean meat, 1 fat
The Feast (includes cheese)	1	590	25	4	10	0	105	3120	52	5	44	3 1/2 starch, 4 medium-fat meat
Pastrami (double meat)	1	580	30	5	10	0	14	1860	48	5	33	3 starch, 3 medium-fat meat, 2 fat
Subway Seafood Sensation (includes cheese)	1	450	22	4	6	1	25	1130	51	6	16	3 1/2 starch, 1 lean meat, 3 fat

Veggie Patty	1	390	8	2	1.5	0	10	1080	56	8	24	3 1/2 starch, 2 lean meat
6" SANDWICHES												
Chicken & Bacon Ranch	1	580	30	5	11	1	99	1390	47	6	36	3 starch, 4 lean meat, 3 fat
Cold Cut Combo	1	410	17	4	7	0.5	60	1530	47	5	21	3 starch, 2 medium-fat meat, 1 fat
Italian BMT	1	450	21	4	8	0	55	1770	47	5	23	3 starch, 2 medium-fat meat, 2 fat
Meatball Marinara	1	560	24	4	11	1	45	1590	63	8	24	4 starch, 2 medium-fat meat, 3 fat
Spicy Italian	1	480	25	5	9	0	55	1660	45	5	21	3 starch, 2 medium-fat meat, 3 fat
Steak & Cheese	1	400	12	3	6	0.5	60	1110	48	6	29	3 starch, 2 medium-fat meat
Subway Melt	1	380	12	3	5	0	45	1600	48	5	25	3 starch, 2 medium-fat meat

✓ = Healthiest Bets

(*Continued*)

6" SANDWICHES *(Continued)*	Amount	Cal.	Fat (g)	% Cal. Fat	Sat. Fat (g)	Trans Fat (g)	Chol. (mg)	Sod. (mg)	Carb. (g)	Fiber (g)	Pro. (g)	Choices/Exchanges
Tuna	1	530	31	5	7	0.5	45	1010	44	5	22	3 starch, 2 lean meat, 5 fat
8" PIZZA												
Cheese	1	680	22	3	9	0	40	1070	96	4	32	6 1/2 starch, 1 medium-fat meat, 2 fat
Cheese & Veggies	1	740	25	3	11	0	50	1210	100	5	36	6 starch, 1 veg, 3 medium-fat meat, 2 fat
Pepperoni	1	790	32	4	13	0	60	1350	96	4	38	6 1/2 starch, 3 medium-fat meat, 3 fat
Sausage	1	820	34	4	14	0	68	1420	97	4	39	6 1/2 starch, 3 medium-fat meat, 3 fat
BREAKFAST SANDWICHES ON 6" BREAD												
Cheese	1	420	18	4	8	0	190	1010	44	5	23	3 starch, 2 medium-fat meat, 1 fat

Chipotle Steak & Cheese	1	600	32	5	11	0.5	220	1470	49	6	34	3 1/2 starch, 3 medium-fat meat, 2 fat
Double Bacon & Cheese	1	510	25	4	11	0.5	210	1380	45	5	30	3 starch, 3 medium-fat meat, 1 fat
Honey Mustard Ham & Cheese	1	470	19	4	8	0	200	1500	52	5	28	3 1/2 starch, 3 lean meat, 2 fat
Western w/ Cheese	1	450	19	4	8	0	200	1390	46	5	28	3 starch, 3 medium-fat meat, 1/2 fat
BREAKFAST WRAPS												
Cheese	1	520	23	4	9	1	190	1260	55	2	25	3 1/2 starch, 2 medium-fat meat, 2 fat
Chipotle Steak & Cheese	1	700	37	5	12	1	220	1720	60	3	35	4 starch, 3 medium-fat meat, 3 fat
Double Bacon & Cheese	1	610	30	4	13	1	210	1630	56	2	30	3 1/2 starch, 3 medium-fat meat, 3 fat

✓ = Healthiest Bets

(Continued)

BREAKFAST WRAPS *(Continued)*	Amount	Cal.	Fat (g)	% Cal. Fat	Sat. Fat (g)	Trans Fat (g)	Chol. (mg)	Sod. (mg)	Carb. (g)	Fiber (g)	Pro. (g)	Choices/Exchanges
Honey Mustard Ham & Cheese	1	580	25	4	10	1	200	1750	64	2	30	4 1/2 starch, 2 lean meat, 3 fat
Western w/ Cheese	1	550	24	4	10	1	200	1640	58	2	30	4 starch, 3 lean meat, 2 fat
CHEESE (AMOUNT ON 6" SUB, WRAP, OR SALAD)												
✔American, Processed	1 srvg	40	4	9	2	0	10	200	1	0	2	1 fat
✔Monterey Cheddar, Shredded	1 srvg	50	5	9	3	0	15	90	1	0	3	1 fat
✔Natural Cheddar	1 srvg	60	5	8	3	0	15	95	0	0	4	1 medium-fat meat, 1/2 fat
✔Pepperjack	1 srvg	50	4	7	2.5	0	15	140	0	0	3	1 fat
✔Provolone	1 srvg	50	4	7	2	0	10	125	0	0	4	1 medium-fat meat
✔Swiss	1 srvg	50	5	9	2.5	0	15	30	0	0	4	1 medium-fat meat, 1/2 fat

DESSERTS

Apple Pie	1 srvg	250	10	4	2	0	0	290	37	1	0	2 1/2 carb, 2 fat
✔Apple Slices	1 pkg	35	0	0	0	0	0	0	9	2	0	1/2 veg
✔Chocolate Chip Cookie	1	210	10	4	6	0	15	150	30	1	2	2 carb, 2 fat
✔Chocolate Chunk Cookie	1	220	10	4	5	0	10	100	30	<1	2	2 carb, 2 fat
✔Double Chocolate Chip Cookie	1	210	10	4	5	0	15	170	30	1	2	2 carb, 2 fat
M & M Cookie	1	210	10	4	5	0	10	100	32	<1	2	2 carb, 2 fat
✔Oatmeal Raisin Cookie	1	200	8	4	4	0	15	170	30	1	3	2 carb, 1 1/2 fat
Peanut Butter Cookie	1	220	12	5	5	0	15	200	26	1	4	1 1/2 carb, 2 1/2 fat
✔Raisins	1 pkg	140	0	0	0	0	0	0	33	2	2	2 veg
Sugar Cookie	1	220	12	5	6	0	15	140	28	<1	2	2 carb, 2 1/2 fat
White Chip Macadamia Nut Cookie	1	220	11	5	5	0	15	160	29	<1	2	2 carb, 2 fat

✔ = Healthiest Bets

(*Continued*)

DESSERTS *(Continued)*	Amount	Cal.	Fat (g)	% Cal. Fat	Sat. Fat (g)	Trans Fat (g)	Chol. (mg)	Sod. (mg)	Carb. (g)	Fiber (g)	Pro. (g)	Choices/Exchanges
✔Yogurt - Dannon All Natural Strawberry	4 oz.	110	1	1	0.5	0	5	65	20	0	5	1/2 carb, 1 milk
FRUIZLE EXPRESS												
✔Berry Lishus	sm	110	0	0	0	0	0	30	28	1	1	2 carb
Berry Lishus w/Banana	sm	140	0	0	0	0	0	30	35	2	1	2 1/2 carb
✔Peach Pizzazz	sm	100	0	0	0	0	0	25	26	0	0	1 1/2 carb
Pineapple Delight	sm	130	0	0	0	0	0	25	33	1	1	2 carb
Pineapple Delight w/Banana	sm	160	0	0	0	0	0	25	40	2	1	2 1/2 carb
✔Sunrise Refresher	sm	120	0	0	0	0	0	20	29	1	1	2 carb
JARED LOW FAT FOOTLONG SANDWICHES												
Ham	1	570	10	2	3.5	0	50	2520	93	11	37	6 starch, 2 lean meat
Oven Roasted Chicken Breast	1	630	11	2	3.5	0	45	1660	95	11	47	6 1/2 starch, 3 lean meat

Roast Beef	1	580	10	2	4.5	0	40	1800	90	11	38	6 starch, 2 lean meat, 1 fat
Subway Club	1	640	12	2	4.5	0	65	2580	94	11	48	6 1/2 starch, 3 lean meat
Sweet Onion Chicken Teriyaki	1	750	10	1	3	0	100	2400	118	11	52	8 starch, 3 lean meat
Turkey Breast	1	560	9	1	2.5	0	40	2000	92	11	37	6 starch, 2 lean meat
Turkey Breast & Ham	1	580	10	2	3	0	50	2420	93	11	40	6 starch, 2 lean meat
Veggie Delite	1	450	6	1	2	0	0	1000	88	11	18	6 starch, 1/2 fat
JARED SALADS W/ 6G OF FAT OR LESS												
✔Ham	1	120	3	2	1	0	25	840	14	4	12	1 starch, 1 lean meat
✔Oven Roasted Chicken Breast	1	140	3	2	0.5	0	50	390	11	4	19	1/2 starch, 1 lean meat
✔Roast Beef	1	120	3	2	1.5	0	20	480	12	4	13	1 starch, 2 lean meat
✔Subway Club	1	150	4	2	1.5	0	35	870	14	4	18	1 starch, 2 lean meat
✔Sweet Onion Chicken Teriyaki	1	210	3	1	1	0	50	780	26	4	20	1 1/2 starch, 2 lean meat

✔ = Healthiest Bets

(*Continued*)

JARED SALADS W/ 6G OF FAT OR LESS *(Continued)*	Amount	Cal.	Fat (g)	% Cal. Fat	Sat. Fat (g)	Trans Fat (g)	Chol. (mg)	Sod. (mg)	Carb. (g)	Fiber (g)	Pro. (g)	Choices/Exchanges
✔Turkey Breast	1	110	3	2	0.5	0	20	580	13	4	12	1 starch, 1 lean meat
✔Turkey Breast & Ham	1	120	3	2	0.5	0	25	790	14	4	14	1 starch, 2 lean meat
✔Veggie Delite	1	60	1	2	0	0	0	80	11	4	3	1/2 starch
SALAD DRESSING												
Fat Free Italian	2 oz.	35	0	0	0	0	0	720	7	0	1	Free
Ranch	2 oz.	320	35	10	6	0.5	30	560	3	0	0	7 fat
SANDWICH CONDIMENTS (AMOUNT ON 6" SUB)												
Bacon	2 strips	45	4	8	1.5	0	10	190	0	0	3	1 fat
Chipotle Southwest Sauce	1 oz.	96	10	9	2	0	8	215	1	0	0	2 fat
Honey Mustard Sauce, Fat Free	1 oz.	30	0	0	0	0	0	115	7	0	0	1/2 carb
✔Light Mayonnaise	1 T	50	5	9	1	0	5	100	<1	0	0	1 fat

Mayonnaise	1 T	110	12	10	2	0	10	80	0	0	0	2 1/2 fat
✔Mustard yellow or deli brown	2 tsp	5	0	0	0	0	0	115	<1	0	0	Free
Olive Oil Blend	1 tsp	45	5	10	0	0	0	0	0	0	0	1 fat
Ranch Dressing	1 oz.	120	13	10	2	0	10	210	1	0	0	2 1/2 fat
Red Wine Vinaigrette, Fat Free	1 oz.	29	0	0	0	0	1	340	6	0	0	Free
✔Sweet Onion Sauce, Fat Free	1 oz.	40	0	0	0	0	0	85	9	0	0	1/2 carb
SOUP												
Chicken and Dumpling	10 oz.	170	5	3	2	0	35	1390	23	2	8	1 1/2 starch, 1 fat
✔Chili con Carne	10 oz.	290	8	2	3.5	0	25	990	35	12	19	2 1/2 starch, 2 medium-fat meat
Cream of Broccoli	10 oz.	160	7	4	2.5	0	10	1010	18	5	6	1 starch, 1 1/2 fat

✔ = Healthiest Bets

(*Continued*)

SOUP *(Continued)*	Amount	Cal.	Fat (g)	% Cal. Fat	Sat. Fat (g)	Trans Fat (g)	Chol. (mg)	Sod. (mg)	Carb. (g)	Fiber (g)	Pro. (g)	Choices/Exchanges
Cream of Potato w/ Bacon	10 oz.	240	13	5	5	0	15	1050	26	3	5	1 1/2 starch, 2 1/2 fat
Golden Broccoli & Cheese	10 oz.	200	12	5	5	0	25	1180	17	3	5	1 starch, 2 1/2 fat
Minestrone	10 oz.	80	1	1	0.5	0	<5	1125	15	4	4	1 starch
✔New England Style Clam Chowder	10 oz.	150	5	3	1	0	10	990	20	4	6	1/2 starch, 1 milk, 1 fat
Roasted Chicken Noodle	10 oz.	80	2	2	0.5	0	15	1240	11	1	6	1/2 starch, 1 lean meat
Spanish Style Chicken w/ Rice	10 oz.	110	2	2	0.5	0	10	1300	17	1	6	1 starch, 1/2 fat
Tomato Garden Vegetable w/ Rotini	10 oz.	90	0	0	0	0	0	1140	20	2	3	1 starch, 1 veg
Vegetable Beef	10 oz.	100	2	2	0.5	0	10	1450	15	3	6	1 starch, 1/2 fat
Wild Rice w/ Chicken	10 oz.	210	11	5	4	0	25	1250	21	2	6	1 1/2 starch, 2 fat

VEGETABLES (AMOUNT ON 6" SUB)												
✔Banana Peppers	3 rings	0	0	0	0	0	0	20	0	0	0	Free
✔Cucumbers	3 slices	3	0	0	0	0	0	0	<1	0	0	Free
✔Jalapeno Peppers	3 rings	3	0	0	0	0	0	70	0	0	0	Free
✔Lettuce	1 srvg	3	0	0	0	0	0	0	0	0	0	Free
✔Olives	3 rings	3	0	0	0	0	0	25	0	0	0	Free
✔Onions	1 srvg	5	0	0	0	0	0	0	1	0	0	Free
✔Pickles	3 chips	0	0	0	0	0	0	115	0	0	0	Free
✔Tomatoes	3 wheels	5	0	0	0	0	0	0	2	0	0	Free

✔ = Healthiest Bets

Exclusive Web Content

Be sure to visit the following restaurants online at http://www.diabetes.org/healthyrestaurant

Carvel
Del Taco
El Pollo Loco
Frëshens
Godfather's
Jersey Mike's
Jimmy John's
Tim Hortons
Whataburger
Wienerschnitzel
Zaxby's

Chinese and Asian Fare

RESTAURANTS

Panda Express
P.F. Chang's China Bistro
Pei Wei Asian Diner

Note: When it comes to Chinese and Asian fare, most restaurants in the U.S. are independently owned, single-store operations. However, over the past few years three national chains have come on the scene, and they willingly provide at least some nutrition information. (P.F. Chang's and Pei Wei leave out the sodium, which, given that this is Asian food, is likely quite high. Because no sodium information is available for these two restaurants, there are no Healthiest Bets checked off.) Having this information is good news because eating Chinese and Asian foods can make blood glucose management difficult due to the hidden grams of carbohydrate that can raise blood glucose, including sugar, marinades, sauces, and corn starch (used to thicken dishes). Panda Express is typically found in food courts. P.F. Chang's China Bistro is a sit-down eatery, and Pei Wei Asian is its more casual cousin.

NUTRITION PROS

- Asian restaurant meals have the potential to be healthy if you choose soup, an entrée with lots of vegetables, no fried items, and eat your entrée with steamed rice (when available, go for brown rice). Oh yes, go ahead and enjoy the fortune cookie.

- If you order well, you can eat a bounty of vegetables.
- Eating family style is common and accepted. Order jointly and put the dishes in the middle for all to share. You can take advantage of this to control portions and get plenty of healthy items.
- It's reasonably easy to control the saturated fat and cholesterol count. Just stay away from shrimp and calamari (squid). Then get dishes filled with vegetables. Asian cooking uses little milk, cream, cheese, or eggs.
- Liquid peanut oil, which is mainly made of the healthy monounsaturated fats, is the main oil used in Asian stir-frying. It is not only healthy but also has a high smoking point and can withstand the high temperature of stir-frying.
- It's easy to fill up first on a low-calorie soup. Try hot and sour or sizzling rice with vegetables. These are especially helpful if your dining mates are choosing high-fat and high-calorie fried appetizers.

NUTRITION CONS

- Asian restaurant items tend to contain more carbohydrate than meets the eye. Sugar and sugar-containing ingredients can be in marinades and sauces. Cornstarch is commonly used to thicken sauces, especially in Chinese dishes.
- Asian dishes can contain more fat than you might think from the oil used to stir-fry and deep-fry. Read about the preparation in the menu descriptions to find out about the fat level.
- You might want to opt for soup and skip the appetizers. Most of them—egg rolls, spring rolls, fried dumplings, and spareribs—are fried or are high in fat.

- It's easy to eat a lot of carbohydrate from rice and noodles.
- Chinese food can be high in sodium due to the ingredients in marinades and sauces, such as soy sauce and MSG (monosodium glutamate).

Healthy Tips

- ★ To keep sodium levels low, don't dip appetizers in sauces. Go for the lighter white sauces. Choose steamed white or brown rice rather than fried rice. And request no MSG.
- ★ You'll be better able to control what you get if you choose a sit-down Asian restaurant rather than one in a food court or an all-you-can-eat buffet because you can customize your food order.
- ★ The hot mustard sauce or hot chili sauce can add some zing without adding too much sodium, sugar, or fat.
- ★ If you eat family style, order fewer dishes than the number of people at the table. This controls portions from the start. Order at least one dish that has only vegetables.
- ★ Use chopsticks. They will slow down your eating, particularly if you haven't mastered using them.

Get it Your Way

- ★ Order dishes with meats that aren't breaded and fried before they are stir-fried.
- ★ Ask to have one or two more vegetables added to a dish to fill it with vegetables. You might have to pay a bit more.
- ★ Because dishes are made to order in sit-down Asian restaurants, feel free to ask that one item be left out or another added in.
- ★ You may want to order a sauce on the side and use the dipping technique to limit the amount you eat. This will help decrease both your sodium and sugar intake. However, flavor and taste will likely be sacrificed.

Exclusive Web Content

Be sure to visit the following restaurants online at http://www.diabetes.org/healthyrestaurant

Carvel	**Godfather's**	**Whataburger**
Del Taco	**Jersey Mike's**	**Wienerschnitzel**
El Pollo Loco	**Jimmy John's**	**Zaxby's**
Frëshens	**Tim Hortons**	

Panda Express
(www.pandaexpress.com)

Light 'n Lean Choice

Veggie Spring Roll *(1)*
Beef with Broccoli *(1 serving)*
String Bean Chicken Breast *(1 serving)*
Steamed White Rice *(1/2 order, 4 oz)*

Calories	580	Cholesterol (mg)	50
Fat (g)	20	Sodium (mg)	1,345
% calories from fat	31	Carbohydrate (g)	73
Saturated fat (g)	4	Fiber (g)	12
Trans fat (g)	0	Protein (g)	30

Exchanges: 4 starch, 2 veg, 3 medium-fat meat, 1 1/2 fat

Healthy 'n Hearty Choice

Veggie Spring Roll *(1)*
Mushroom Chicken *(1 serving)*
Tangy Shrimp *(1 serving)*
Fried Rice *(1 serving)*

Calories	810	Cholesterol (mg)	235*
Fat (g)	29	Sodium (mg)	2,050
% calories from fat	32	Carbohydrate (g)	102
Saturated fat (g)	7	Fiber (g)	13
Trans fat (g)	0	Protein (g)	35

Exchanges: 6 starch, 2 veg, 2 lean meat, 4 1/2 fat

*shrimp raises the cholesterol level

(*Continued*)

Panda Express

	Amount	Cal.	Fat (g)	% Cal. Fat	Sat. Fat (g)	Trans Fat (g)	Chol. (mg)	Sod. (mg)	Carb. (g)	Fiber (g)	Pro. (g)	Choices/Exchanges
APPETIZERS												
Chicken Egg Roll	1 roll	170	8	4	1.5	0	25	410	17	2	8	1 starch, 1 1/2 fat
Chicken Potsticker	3 pcs	220	12	5	1.5	0	0	360	25	4	6	1 1/2 starch, 2 fat
Cream Cheese Rangoon	3 pcs	190	8	4	5	0	35	180	24	2	5	1 1/2 starch, 1 1/2 fat
✔Veggie Spring Roll	1 roll	80	4	5	1	0	0	270	11	2	2	1/2 starch, 1/2 fat
BEEF												
Beijing Beef	1 srvg	420	26	6	5	0	25	730	36	1	14	2 1/2 starch, 1 medium-fat meat, 3 1/2 fat
✔Broccoli Beef	1 srvg	150	7	4	1.5	0	25	510	11	4	11	1/2 starch, 1 medium-fat meat

✔Mongolian Beef	1 srvg	180	11	6	2	0	25	800	15	2	11	1 starch, 1 medium-fat meat, 1 fat
CHICKEN												
✔Black Pepper Chicken	1 srvg	200	12	5	2.5	0	80	820	11	2	13	1/2 starch, 2 lean meat, 1 1/2 fat
✔Kung Pao Chicken	1 srvg	240	15	6	3	0	65	540	12	5	16	1 starch, 2 lean meat, 2 fat
Mandarin Chicken	1 srvg	250	10	4	3	0	145	1150	8	0	31	1/2 starch, 4 lean meat
✔Mushroom Chicken	1 srvg	130	6	4	1.5	0	45	520	8	3	11	1/2 starch, 1 lean meat, 1/2 fat
Orange Chicken	1 srvg	500	27	5	5.5	1	100	810	42	3	23	3 starch, 2 lean meat, 4 fat
✔Potato Chicken	1 srvg	200	10	5	2	0	55	990	21	2	11	1 1/2 starch, 1 lean meat, 1 1/2 fat

✔ = Healthiest Bets

(*Continued*)

CHICKEN *(Continued)*	Amount	Cal.	Fat (g)	% Cal. Fat	Sat. Fat (g)	Trans Fat (g)	Chol. (mg)	Sod. (mg)	Carb. (g)	Fiber (g)	Pro. (g)	Choices/Exchanges
✔String Bean Chicken Breast	1 srvg	160	8	5	1.5	0	25	550	10	4	12	1/2 starch, 1 lean meat, 1/2 fat
✔Sweet & Sour Chicken	1 srvg	350	14	4	2.5	0	35	330	43	1	13	3 starch, 1 lean meat, 2 fat
COOKIES												
✔Fortune Cookies	1 cookie	32	0	0	0	0	0	8	7	0	1	1/2 carb
PORK												
BBQ Pork	1 srvg	440	23	5	9	0	140	1570	15	1	41	1 starch, 5 medium-fat meat
Sweet & Sour Pork	1 srvg	400	23	5	4.5	0	30	360	35	2	13	2 1/2 starch, 1 medium-fat meat, 3 1/2 fat
RICE & NOODLES												
Chow Mein	1 srvg	390	12	3	2	0	0	1020	59	7	11	4 starch, 2 fat

Fried Rice	1 srvg	450	14	3	3	0	105	710	67	6	13	4 1/2 starch, 3 fat
Steamed Rice	1 srvg	380	3	1	0.5	0	0	30	81	4	9	5 1/2 starch
SAUCES												
Mandarin Sauce	1.5 oz.	70	0	0	0	0	0	740	17	0	1	1 carb
Potsticker Sauce	1.5 oz.	35	0	0	0	0	0	970	8	0	1	1/2 carb
✔Sweet & Sour Sauce	1.5 oz.	80	0	0	0	0	0	135	19	0	0	1 carb
SHRIMP												
✔Crispy Shrimp	6 pcs	260	13	5	2.5	0	60	810	26	1	9	1 1/2 starch, 1 lean meat, 2 1/2 fat
✔Kung Pao Shrimp	1 srvg	240	14	5	2	0	95	640	14	4	16	1 starch, 2 lean meat, 1 1/2 fat
✔Tangy Shrimp	1 srvg	150	5	3	1	0	85	550	16	2	9	1 starch, 1 lean meat, 1/2 fat

✔ = Healthiest Bets

(*Continued*)

	Amount	Cal.	Fat (g)	% Cal. Fat	Sat. Fat (g)	Trans Fat (g)	Chol. (mg)	Sod. (mg)	Carb. (g)	Fiber (g)	Pro. (g)	Choices/Exchanges
SOUP												
✔Egg Flower Soup	12 oz.	88	2	2	0	0	55	895	16	0	2	1 starch, 1/2 fat
Hot & Sour Soup	12 oz.	110	4	3	1	0	85	1370	14	2	5	1 starch, 1/2 fat
VEGGIES												
✔Eggplant & Tofu	1 srvg	180	10	5	1.5	0	0	690	20	4	5	1 starch, 1 veg, 2 fat
✔Mixed Veggies	1 srvg	90	7	7	1	0	0	110	8	3	2	1 1/2 veg, 1 1/2 fat

✔ = Healthiest Bets

P.F. Chang's China Bistro

(www.pfchangs.com)

Light 'n Lean Choice

Hot and Sour Soup *(1 cup, 8 oz)*
Cantonese Shrimp *(1/2 dish)*
Buddha's Feast, stir-fried *(whole dish)*
Steamed Brown Rice *(1 cup)*

Calories	641	Cholesterol (mg)	na
Fat (g)	11	Sodium (mg)	na
% calories from fat	15	Carbohydrate (g)	104
Saturated fat (g)	1	Fiber (g)	20
Trans fat (g)	na	Protein (g)	35

Exchanges: 6 starch, 3 veg, 2 lean meat, 1 fat

Healthy 'n Hearty Choice

Bikini Shrimp Salad with
Watermelon Citrus Vinaigrette *(1/2 serving)*
Ginger Chicken with Broccoli *(1/3 dish)*
Vegetable Chow Fun *(1/3 dinner size)*

Calories	829	Cholesterol (mg)	na
Fat (g)	29	Sodium (mg)	na
% calories from fat	31	Carbohydrate (g)	109
Saturated fat (g)	3	Fiber (g)	15
Trans fat (g)	na	Protein (g)	36

Exchanges: 5 1/2 starch, 4 veg, 3 lean meat, 3 1/2 fat

(Continued)

P.F. Chang's China Bistro

	Amount	Cal.	Fat (g)	% Cal. Fat	Sat. Fat (g)	Trans Fat (g)	Chol. (mg)	Sod. (mg)	Carb. (g)	Fiber (g)	Pro. (g)	Choices/Exchanges
CHICKEN												
Chang's Spicy Chicken	entire dish	923	37	4	6	na	na	na	88	1	56	6 starch, 5 lean meat, 4 fat
Chicken w/ Black Bean Sauce	entire dish	678	23	3	4	na	na	na	33	1	76	2 starch, 10 lean meat
Dali Chicken	entire dish	1091	52	4	9	na	na	na	53	6	91	3 1/2 starch, 11 lean meat, 4 fat
Ginger Chicken w/ Broccoli	entire dish	656	26	4	3	na	na	na	45	7	60	3 starch, 7 lean meat, 1 fat
Ginger Chicken w/ Broccoli - Gluten Free	entire dish	677	30	4	5	na	na	na	43	7	61	3 starch, 7 lean meat, 1 fat

Ground Chicken & Eggplant	entire dish	792	40	5	7	na	na	na	73	9	33	5 starch, 3 lean meat, 6 fat
Kung Pao Chicken	entire dish	1228	79	6	12	na	na	na	58	8	74	4 starch, 9 lean meat, 10 fat
Mu Shu Chicken	entire dish	715	38	5	8	na	na	na	49	23	47	3 1/2 starch, 5 lean meat, 4 fat
Orange Peel Chicken	entire dish	1151	46	4	8	na	na	na	127	14	61	8 1/2 starch, 5 lean meat, 5 fat
Philip's Better Lemon Chicken	entire dish	1051	42	4	7	na	na	na	113	5	58	7 1/2 starch, 5 lean meat, 5 fat
Sweet & Sour Chicken	entire dish	764	20	2	4	na	na	na	107	3	40	7 starch, 3 lean meat, 2 fat
DESSERTS												
Apple Pie Mini Dessert	1	170	4	2	2	na	na	na	34	1	1	2 1/2 carb, 1 fat

✔ = Healthiest Bets; n/a = not available

(*Continued*)

DESSERTS *(Continued)*	Amount	Cal.	Fat (g)	% Cal. Fat	Sat. Fat (g)	Trans Fat (g)	Chol. (mg)	Sod. (mg)	Carb. (g)	Fiber (g)	Pro. (g)	Choices/Exchanges
Banana Split Mini Dessert	1	167	6	3	1	na	na	na	28	1	1	2 carb, 1 fat
Banana Spring Rolls	1 srvg	814	37	4	16	na	na	na	130	7	12	8 1/2 carb, 6 fat
Carrot Cake Mini Dessert	1	295	14	4	4	na	na	na	42	1	2	3 carb, 3 fat
Coconut - Pineapple Ice Cream	1 srvg	111	12	10	8	na	na	na	25	0	4	1 1/2 carb, 2 fat
Creamy Strawberry Cheesecake Mini Dessert	1	239	20	8	12	na	na	na	14	1	3	1 carb, 4 fat
Flourless Chocolate Dome	1 srvg	572	26	4	0	na	na	na	84	8	8	5 1/2 carb, 4 fat
Great Wall of Chocolate Cake	1 srvg	2237	90	4	21	na	na	na	376	13	20	25 carb, 15 fat
Great Wall of Chocolate Mini Dessert	1	336	26	7	4	na	na	na	24	2	1	1 1/2 carb, 5 fat
S'Mores Mini Dessert	1	323	12	3	7	na	na	na	50	1	3	3 1/2 carb, 2 1/2 fat

Tiramisu Mini Dessert	1	202	14	6	7	na	na	na	15	0	3	1 carb, 3 fat
Tres Leche Lemon Dream Mini Dessert	1	216	8	3	4	na	na	na	32	1	4	2 carb, 1 1/2 fat
THE GRILL												
Asian Marinated New York Strip	entire dish	1432	86	5	30	na	na	na	68	2	92	4 1/2 starch, 11 medium-fat meat, 6 fat
Citrus Soy Salmon - Served w/ Brown Rice	entire dish	1000	59	5	20	na	na	na	42	4	69	3 starch, 9 lean meat, 6 1/2 fat
Citrus Soy Salmon - Served w/ White Rice	entire dish	1025	58	5	20	na	na	na	49	2	70	3 1/2 starch, 9 lean meat, 6 1/2 fat
Lemongrass Prawns	entire dish	907	58	6	21	na	na	na	65	4	34	4 1/2 starch, 3 lean meat, 9 fat
Sichuan Chicken Flatbread	entire dish	1160	80	6	23	na	na	na	56	4	52	3 1/2 starch, 6 lean meat, 12 fat

✔ = Healthiest Bets; n/a = not available

(*Continued*)

	Amount	Cal.	Fat (g)	% Cal. Fat	Sat. Fat (g)	Trans Fat (g)	Chol. (mg)	Sod. (mg)	Carb. (g)	Fiber (g)	Pro. (g)	Choices/Exchanges
MEAT												
Beef a la Sichuan	entire dish	1172	64	5	17	na	na	na	56	5	86	3 1/2 starch, 11 medium-fat meat, 2 fat
Chengdu Spiced Lamb	entire dish	1056	75	6	19	na	na	na	34	5	62	2 1/2 starch, 8 medium-fat meat, 6 1/2 fat
Mongolian Beef	entire dish	1178	73	6	19	na	na	na	29	2	96	2 starch, 13 medium-fat meat, 1 fat
Mu Shu Pork	entire dish	871	50	5	13	na	na	na	50	25	57	3 1/2 starch, 7 medium-fat meat, 3 fat
Orange Peel Beef	entire dish	1568	85	5	20	na	na	na	115	14	88	7 1/2 starch, 9 medium-fat meat, 6 fat
Sweet & Sour Pork	entire dish	1095	46	4	14	na	na	na	106	3	61	7 starch, 6 medium-fat meat, 3 fat

Wok Charred Beef	entire dish	941	63	6	14	na	na	na	33	8	63	2 starch, 8 medium-fat meat, 4 fat
Wok Seared Lamb	entire dish	1081	80	7	28	na	na	na	29	8	62	2 starch, 8 medium-fat meat, 8 fat
NOODLES, MEINS, AND RICE												
Brown Rice	1 cup	254	2	1	0	na	na	na	53	4	5	4 starch, 1/2 fat
Cantonese Chow Fun w/ Beef	entire dish	1212	38	3	10	na	na	na	142	5	69	9 starch, 10 fat
Cantonese Chow Fun w/ Chicken	entire dish	1045	23	2	4	na	na	na	146	5	60	10 starch, 6 fat
Chow Mein Combo	entire dish	912	34	3	8	na	na	na	86	6	61	5 1/2 starch, 6 lean meat, 3 fat
Chow Mein w/ Beef	entire dish	793	26	3	7	na	na	na	84	7	54	5 1/2 starch, 5 medium-fat meat

✓ = Healthiest Bets; n/a = not available

(*Continued*)

NOODLES, MEINS, AND RICE *(Continued)*	Amount	Cal.	Fat (g)	% Cal. Fat	Sat. Fat (g)	Trans Fat (g)	Chol. (mg)	Sod. (mg)	Carb. (g)	Fiber (g)	Pro. (g)	Choices/Exchanges
Chow Mein w/ Chicken	entire dish	689	16	2	3	na	na	na	84	6	49	5 1/2 starch, 5 lean meat
Chow Mein w/ Pork	entire dish	898	34	3	10	na	na	na	83	6	61	5 1/2 starch, 6 medium-fat meat, 1/2 fat
Chow Mein w/ Shrimp	entire dish	625	13	2	2	na	na	na	84	6	41	5 1/2 starch, 3 lean meat
Dan Dan Noodles	entire dish	1087	30	2	6	na	na	na	145	7	51	10 starch, 6 fat
Double Pan-Fried Noodles Combo	entire dish	1384	69	4	13	na	na	na	118	7	68	8 starch, 16 fat
Double Pan-Fried Noodles w/ Beef	entire dish	1186	56	4	11	na	na	na	112	6	53	7 starch, 13 fat
Double Pan-Fried Noodles w/ Chicken	entire dish	1072	47	4	7	na	na	na	115	7	42	8 starch, 10 fat

Double Pan-Fried Noodles w/ Pork	entire dish	1208	60	4	12	na	na	na	114	7	50	8 starch, 13 1/2 fat
Double Pan-Fried Noodles w/ Shrimp	entire dish	1031	46	4	7	na	na	na	115	7	37	8 starch, 9 fat
Garlic Noodles	entire dish	612	11	2	2	na	na	na	111	6	18	7 starch, 1 fat
P.F. Chang's Fried Rice Combo	entire dish	1539	69	4	14	na	na	na	154	5	68	10 starch, 16 fat
P.F. Chang's Fried Rice w/ Beef	entire dish	1228	40	3	10	na	na	na	150	5	58	10 starch, 9 fat
P.F. Chang's Fried Rice w/ Chicken	entire dish	1208	44	3	8	na	na	na	151	5	47	10 starch, 9 fat
P.F. Chang's Fried Rice w/ Pork	entire dish	1360	57	4	13	na	na	na	150	5	55	10 starch, 12 fat
P.F. Chang's Fried Rice w/ Shrimp	entire dish	1154	41	3	7	na	na	na	149	4	40	10 starch, 8 fat

✔ = Healthiest Bets; n/a = not available

(*Continued*)

NOODLES, MEINS, AND RICE *(Continued)*	Amount	Cal.	Fat (g)	% Cal. Fat	Sat. Fat (g)	Trans Fat (g)	Chol. (mg)	Sod. (mg)	Carb. (g)	Fiber (g)	Pro. (g)	Choices/Exchanges
Singapore Street Noodles	entire dish	572	16	3	3	na	na	na	81	7	28	5 starch, 3 fat
Singapore Street Noodles - Gluten Free	entire dish	566	15	2	2	na	na	na	81	4	28	5 starch, 3 fat
Tam's Noodles	entire dish	1678	93	5	17	na	na	na	144	6	58	10 starch, 19 fat
White Rice	1 cup	295	1	0	0	na	na	na	64	1	6	4 starch
SALAD DRESSINGS												
Watermelon Citrus Vinaigrette	1 srvg	240	23	9	3	na	na	na	7	0	1	1/2 carb, 4 1/2 fat
Chang's Signature Ginger Dressing	1 srvg	483	48	9	7	na	na	na	9	0	1	1/2 carb, 9 1/2 fat
Creamy Wedge Dressing	1 srvg	443	43	9	7	na	na	na	8	1	3	1/2 carb, 9 fat

SALADS - NO DRESSING												
Bikini Shrimp Salad - no dressing	1 salad	192	6	3	0	na	na	na	30	4	8	1 starch, 3 veg, 1 lean meat, 1 fat
Chang's Wedge - no dressing	1 salad	244	19	7	5	na	na	na	12	5	8	3 veg, 1 lean meat, 3 fat
Chang's Wedge w/ Chicken - no dressing	1 salad	595	35	5	9	na	na	na	12	5	57	1 starch, 2 veg, 7 lean meat, 2 fat
Chicken Chopped Salad	1 salad	401	14	3	3	na	na	na	21	5	47	1 starch, 2 veg, 5 lean meat
SEAFOOD												
Cantonese Scallops	entire dish	408	16	4	3	na	na	na	26	4	39	1 1/2 starch, 5 lean meat, 1/2 fat
Cantonese Shrimp	entire dish	330	12	3	2	na	na	na	21	4	33	1 1/2 starch, 4 lean meat
Chang's Lemon Scallops	entire dish	952	28	3	4	na	na	na	100	3	69	6 1/2 starch, 7 lean meat, 1 fat

✓ = Healthiest Bets; n/a = not available

(*Continued*)

SEAFOOD *(Continued)*	Amount	Cal.	Fat (g)	% Cal. Fat	Sat. Fat (g)	Trans Fat (g)	Chol. (mg)	Sod. (mg)	Carb. (g)	Fiber (g)	Pro. (g)	Choices/Exchanges
Crispy Honey Shrimp	entire dish	1061	44	4	6	na	na	na	118	2	35	8 starch, 2 lean meat, 8 fat
Hot Fish	entire dish	1338	71	5	14	na	na	na	111	8	60	7 1/2 starch, 5 lean meat, 10 fat
Kung Pao Scallops	entire dish	1136	57	5	8	na	na	na	66	9	87	4 1/2 starch, 11 lean meat, 5 fat
Kung Pao Shrimp	entire dish	977	58	5	8	na	na	na	58	9	60	4 starch, 7 lean meat, 7 fat
Lemon Pepper Shrimp	entire dish	701	36	5	5	na	na	na	59	5	36	4 starch, 3 lean meat, 5 fat
Oolong Marinated Sea Bass	entire dish	521	12	2	3	na	na	na	40	3	64	2 1/2 starch, 7 lean meat
Orange Peel Shrimp	entire dish	1010	41	4	6	na	na	na	118	14	47	8 starch, 3 lean meat, 5 fat

Salt & Pepper Prawns	entire dish	844	50	5	7	na	na	na	55	5	45	3 1/2 starch, 5 lean meat, 7 fat
Shrimp w/ Candied Walnuts	entire dish	1225	80	6	12	na	na	na	74	2	60	5 starch, 6 lean meat, 11 fat
Sichuan from the Sea Calamari	entire dish	1078	36	3	6	na	na	na	118	4	69	8 starch, 6 lean meat, 3 fat
Sichuan from the Sea Scallops	entire dish	1030	36	3	5	na	na	na	98	3	70	6 1/2 starch, 7 lean meat, 3 fat
Sichuan from the Sea Shrimp	entire dish	728	37	5	5	na	na	na	55	3	44	3 1/2 starch, 5 lean meat, 4 fat
Wild Alaskan Sockeye Salmon Steamed w/ Ginger	entire dish	646	36	5	6	na	na	na	23	5	60	1 1/2 starch, 8 lean meat, 2 fat
Wild Alaskan Sockeye Salmon Steamed w/ Ginger - Gluten Free	entire dish	672	36	5	6	na	na	na	30	6	60	2 starch, 8 lean meat, 2 fat

✔ = Healthiest Bets; n/a = not available

(*Continued*)

	Amount	Cal.	Fat (g)	% Cal. Fat	Sat. Fat (g)	Trans Fat (g)	Chol. (mg)	Sod. (mg)	Carb. (g)	Fiber (g)	Pro. (g)	Choices/Exchanges
SIDES												
Asian Slaw	entire dish	585	57	9	8	na	na	na	19	5	5	4 veg, 11 1/2 fat
Garlic Snap Peas	sm	129	7	5	1	na	na	na	13	4	4	3 veg, 1 1/2 fat
Garlic Snap Peas	lg	205	10	4	1	na	na	na	23	7	7	5 veg, 2 fat
Shanghai Cucumbers	entire dish	124	6	4	1	na	na	na	8	4	10	2 veg, 1 fat
Sichuan-Style Asparagus	sm	97	3	3	0	na	na	na	16	3	6	3 veg, 1/2 fat
Sichuan-Style Asparagus	lg	204	6	3	1	na	na	na	34	6	11	7 veg, 1 fat
Spicy Green Beans	sm	234	13	5	3	na	na	na	23	6	7	5 veg, 2 1/2 fat
Spicy Green Beans	lg	602	40	6	7	na	na	na	48	13	14	9 veg, 8 fat
Spinach Stir-Fried w/ Garlic	lg	140	6	4	1	na	na	na	16	11	12	3 veg, 1 fat

Spinach Stir-Fried w/ Garlic	sm	77	3	4	0	na	na	na	9	6	7	2 veg, 1/2 fat
SOUPS												
Chang's Chicken Noodle Soup	1 bowl	512	13	2	3	na	na	na	30	2	64	2 starch, 8 lean meat
Egg Drop Soup	1 cup	48	2	4	0	na	na	na	7	0	1	1/2 starch, 1/2 fat
Egg Drop Soup	1 bowl	367	14	3	3	na	na	na	51	1	7	3 starch, 3 fat
Hot and Sour Soup	1 cup	85	2	2	0	na	na	na	11	4	5	1 starch, 1/2 fat
Hot and Sour Soup	1 bowl	652	18	2	4	na	na	na	82	34	37	5 1/2 starch, 3 lean meat
Wonton Soup	1 bowl	354	10	3	2	na	na	na	44	3	21	3 starch, 2 medium-fat meat
STARTERS												
Chang's Chicken Lettuce Wraps	1 wrap	377	12	3	3	na	na	na	35	5	28	2 starch, 1 veg, 3 lean meat, 1/2 fat

✓ = Healthiest Bets; n/a = not available

(*Continued*)

STARTERS *(Continued)*	Amount	Cal.	Fat (g)	% Cal. Fat	Sat. Fat (g)	Trans Fat (g)	Chol. (mg)	Sod. (mg)	Carb. (g)	Fiber (g)	Pro. (g)	Choices/Exchanges
Chang's Chicken Lettuce Wraps - Gluten Free	1 wrap	477	12	2	3	na	na	na	63	5	31	3 1/2 starch, 2 veg, 3 lean meat
Chang's Spare Ribs	entire dish	1356	89	6	24	na	na	na	43	1	93	3 starch, 12 medium-fat meat, 5 fat
Chang's Vegetarian Lettuce Wraps	1 wrap	281	4	1	0	na	na	na	37	7	25	1 1/2 starch, 3 veg, 2 lean meat
Crab Wontons	entire dish	440	26	5	9	na	na	na	32	2	19	2 starch, 2 lean meat, 4 fat
Crispy Green Beans	entire dish	507	28	5	4	na	na	na	59	8	8	Free
Harvest Spring Rolls	1 roll	287	15	5	2	na	na	na	30	2	6	2 starch, 3 fat
Northern Style Spare Ribs	entire dish	720	54	7	14	na	na	na	6	0	49	1/2 starch, 7 medium-fat meat, 4 fat

Peking Dumplings - Pan Fried	entire dish	367	23	6	7	na	na	na	21	1	18	1 1/2 starch, 2 medium-fat meat, 2 fat
Peking Dumplings - Steamed	entire dish	327	18	5	6	na	na	na	21	1	18	1 1/2 starch, 2 medium-fat meat, 1 1/2 fat
Salt and Pepper Calamari	entire dish	720	11	1	3	na	na	na	118	3	33	8 starch, 1 lean meat, 1 fat
Seared Ahi Tuna	entire dish	210	9	4	1	na	na	na	9	1	26	1/2 starch, 3 lean meat
Shrimp Dumplings - Pan Fried	entire dish	305	13	4	2	na	na	na	25	1	21	1 1/2 starch, 2 lean meat, 1 fat
Shrimp Dumplings - Steamed	entire dish	265	8	3	1	na	na	na	25	1	21	1 1/2 starch, 2 lean meat
Vegetable Dumplings - Pan Fried	entire dish	307	11	3	2	na	na	na	43	2	9	2 1/2 starch, 1 veg, 2 fat
Vegetable Dumplings - Steamed	entire dish	267	7	2	1	na	na	na	43	2	9	3 starch, 1 veg, 1 fat

✔ = Healthiest Bets; n/a = not available

(*Continued*)

	Amount	Cal.	Fat (g)	% Cal. Fat	Sat. Fat (g)	Trans Fat (g)	Chol. (mg)	Sod. (mg)	Carb. (g)	Fiber (g)	Pro. (g)	Choices/Exchanges
STARTERS ADDS												
Chili Bean Sauce	1 srvg	81	1	1	0	na	na	na	12	0	3	1 carb
Crispy Green Bean Sauce	1 srvg	451	48	10	6	na	na	na	5	0	0	1 veg, 9 1/2 fat
Mustard Vinaigrette	1 srvg	66	2	3	0	na	na	na	7	0	4	1/2 carb, 1/2 fat
Potsticker Sauce	1 srvg	36	1	3	0	na	na	na	6	0	2	1/2 starch
Rice Sticks	1 srvg	135	0	0	0	na	na	na	33	0	0	2 starch
Shrimp Dumpling Sauce	1 srvg	24	0	0	0	na	na	na	1	0	3	Free
Special Sauce	1 srvg	55	1	2	0	na	na	na	9	0	2	1/2 starch
Spicy Plum Sauce	1 srvg	110	0	0	0	na	na	na	28	0	0	2 carb
Sweet & Sour Sauce	1 srvg	57	0	0	0	na	na	na	15	0	0	1 carb

TRADITIONAL LUNCH BOWLS

Almond & Cashew Chicken Lunch Bowl - Served w/ Brown Rice	entire dish	909	27	3	4	na	na	na	101	9	62	6 1/2 starch, 6 lean meat, 2 fat
Almond & Cashew Chicken Lunch Bowl - Served w/ White Rice	entire dish	955	26	2	4	na	na	na	112	5	63	7 1/2 starch, 6 lean meat, 1 fat
Beef w/ Broccoli Lunch Bowl - Served w/ Brown Rice	entire dish	844	27	3	18	na	na	na	87	8	58	6 starch, 1 veg, 6 medium-fat meat
Beef w/ Broccoli Lunch Bowl - Served w/ White Rice	entire dish	890	26	3	8	na	na	na	99	5	59	6 starch, 1 veg, 6 medium-fat meat
Buddha's Feast Lunch Bowl - Served w/ Brown Rice	entire dish	541	8	1	1	na	na	na	101	11	23	6 1/2 starch, 1 fat

✔ = Healthiest Bets; n/a = not available

(Continued)

TRADITIONAL, LUNCH BOWLS *(Continued)*	Amount	Cal.	Fat (g)	% Cal. Fat	Sat. Fat (g)	Trans Fat (g)	Chol. (mg)	Sod. (mg)	Carb. (g)	Fiber (g)	Pro. (g)	Choices/Exchanges
Buddha's Feast Lunch Bowl - Served w/ White Rice	entire dish	587	6	1	1	na	na	na	113	7	24	7 1/2 starch, 1 fat
Citrus Soy Salmon Lunch Bowl - Served w/ Brown Rice	entire dish	1047	63	5	20	na	na	na	67	6	48	4 1/2 starch, 5 lean meat, 9 1/2 fat
Citrus Soy Salmon Lunch Bowl - Served w/ White Rice	entire dish	1093	62	5	20	na	na	na	79	2	49	5 1/2 starch, 5 lean meat, 9 1/2 fat
Crispy Honey Chicken Lunch Bowl - Served w/ Brown Rice	entire dish	943	13	1	3	na	na	na	126	6	61	8 1/2 starch, 5 lean meat
Crispy Honey Chicken Lunch Bowl - Served w/ White Rice	entire dish	989	12	1	3	na	na	na	138	2	62	9 starch, 5 lean meat

Moo Goo Gai Pan Lunch Bowl - Served w/ Brown Rice	entire dish	545	8	1	2	na	na	na	76	7	40	5 starch, 4 lean meat
Moo Goo Gai Pan Lunch Bowl - Served w/ White Rice	entire dish	591	6	1	1	na	na	na	88	3	41	6 starch, 3 lean meat
Pepper Steak Lunch Bowl Served w/ Brown Rice	entire dish	820	28	3	8	na	na	na	82	7	54	5 1/2 starch, 5 medium-fat meat
Pepper Steak Lunch Bowl Served w/ White Rice	entire dish	968	39	4	10	na	na	na	94	3	55	6 1/2 starch, 5 medium-fat meat, 2 fat
Shrimp w/ Lobster Sauce Lunch Bowl - Served w/ Brown Rice	entire dish	686	25	3	5	na	na	na	75	6	37	5 starch, 3 lean meat, 3 fat
Shrimp w/ Lobster Sauce Lunch Bowl - Served w/ White Rice	entire dish	732	23	3	4	na	na	na	87	2	38	6 starch, 3 lean meat, 3 fat

✓ = Healthiest Bets

(*Continued*)

	Amount	Cal.	Fat (g)	% Cal. Fat	Sat. Fat (g)	Trans Fat (g)	Chol. (mg)	Sod. (mg)	Carb. (g)	Fiber (g)	Pro. (g)	Choices/Exchanges
TRADITIONS												
Almond & Cashew Chicken	entire dish	815	30	3	5	na	na	na	63	5	81	4 starch, 9 lean meat
Beef w/ Broccoli	entire dish	1118	65	5	17	na	na	na	38	7	93	2 1/2 starch, 12 medium-fat meat, 1 fat
Crispy Honey Chicken	entire dish	867	11	1	3	na	na	na	121	3	53	8 starch, 4 lean meat
Lo Mein Combo	entire dish	1409	83	5	16	na	na	na	98	8	66	6 1/2 starch, 7 lean meat, 12 fat
Lo Mein w/ Beef	entire dish	1374	80	5	16	na	na	na	94	8	67	6 1/2 starch, 7 medium-fat meat, 9 fat
Lo Mein w/ Chicken	entire dish	1198	67	5	11	na	na	na	97	8	51	6 1/2 starch, 5 lean meat, 10 fat

Lo Mein w/ Pork	entire dish	1400	54	3	17	na	na	na	95	8	63	6 1/2 starch, 6 medium-fat meat, 7 fat
Lo Mein w/ Shrimp	entire dish	1134	64	5	10	na	na	na	97	8	43	6 1/2 starch, 3 lean meat, 11 fat
Moo Goo Gai Pan	entire dish	661	34	5	5	na	na	na	32	4	54	2 starch, 7 lean meat, 2 1/2 fat
Pepper Steak	entire dish	971	48	4	15	na	na	na	32	4	95	2 starch, 12 medium-fat meat
Shrimp w/ Lobster Sauce	entire dish	480	22	4	3	na	na	na	24	1	42	1 1/2 starch, 5 lean meat, 1 fat
VEGETARIAN PLATES												
Buddha's Feast - Steamed	entire dish	137	1	1	0	na	na	na	29	10	8	6 veg
Buddha's Feast - Stir Fried	entire dish	367	5	1	0	na	na	na	66	10	25	2 starch, 7 veg, 1 fat

✔ = Healthiest Bets

(Continued)

VEGETARIAN, PLATES *(Continued)*	Amount	Cal.	Fat (g)	% Cal. Fat	Sat. Fat (g)	Trans Fat (g)	Chol. (mg)	Sod. (mg)	Carb. (g)	Fiber (g)	Pro. (g)	Choices/Exchanges
Coconut Curry Vegetables	entire dish	686	46	6	25	na	na	na	48	12	30	3 starch, 1 veg, 9 fat
Stir-Fried Eggplant	entire dish	590	34	5	5	na	na	na	64	10	10	3 1/2 starch, 2 veg, 6 fat
Vegetable Chow Fun	entire dish	878	8	1	1	na	na	na	181	26	22	10 starch, 3 veg, 1 fat
Vegetarian Ma Po Tofu	entire dish	537	19	3	1	na	na	na	51	6	40	3 starch, 2 veg, 6 fat

✔ = Healthiest Bets

Pei Wei Asian Diner

(www.peiwei.com)

Light 'n Lean Choice

Pei Wei Spring Rolls *(2)*
Mongolian Shrimp *(1 serving)*
Brown Rice *(1 serving)*
Fortune Cookie *(1)*

Calories	500	Cholesterol (mg)	na
Fat (g)	13	Sodium (mg)	na
% calories from fat	23	Carbohydrate (g)	67
Saturated fat (g)	na	Fiber (g)	5
Trans fat (g)	na	Protein (g)	27

Exchanges: 4 starch, 1/2 carb, 1 veg, 2 1/2 lean meat, 1 1/2 fat

Healthy 'n Hearty Choice

Crispy Potstickers *(1/2 order, 3 pieces)*
Ginger Broccoli with Beef *(1 serving)*
Beef Fried Rice *(1/2)*
Fortune Cookie *(1)*

Calories	645	Cholesterol (mg)	na
Fat (g)	26	Sodium (mg)	na
% calories from fat	36	Carbohydrate (g)	56
Saturated fat (g)	na	Fiber (g)	3
Trans fat (g)	na	Protein (g)	41

Exchanges: 3 starch, 1/2 carb, 1 veg, 4 medium-fat meat, 1 1/2 fat

(Continued)

Pei Wei Asian Diner

	Amount	Cal.	Fat (g)	% Cal. Fat	Sat. Fat (g)	Trans Fat (g)	Chol. (mg)	Sod. (mg)	Carb. (g)	Fiber (g)	Pro. (g)	Choices/Exchanges
FIRST TASTES												
Crab Wontons (4)	2 srvgs	190	13	6	na	na	na	na	9	0	8	1/2 starch, 1 lean meat, 2 fat
Crab Wontons (6)	2 srvgs	230	16	6	na	na	na	na	9	0	11	1/2 starch, 1 lean meat, 2 1/2 fat
Crispy Potstickers (4)	2 srvgs	130	7	5	na	na	na	na	10	0	6	1/2 starch, 2 fat
Crispy Potstickers (6)	2 srvgs	150	8	5	na	na	na	na	10	0	8	1/2 starch, 2 fat
Edamame	2 srvgs	156	8	5	na	na	na	na	12	5	14	1 starch, 2 lean meat
Hot & Sour Soup	bowl	500	28	5	na	na	na	na	37	6	24	2 1/2 starch, 2 lean meat, 4 fat
Hot & Sour Soup	cup	150	9	5	na	na	na	na	11	2	6	1/2 starch, 1 lean meat, 1 1/2 fat

Minced Chicken w/ Cool Lettuce Wrap	2 srvgs	250	4	1	na	na	na	na	31	3	22	2 starch, 2 lean meat
Pei Wei Spring Rolls	2 srvgs	90	5	5	na	na	na	na	11	1	2	1/2 starch, 1 fat
KID'S WEI												
Chicken Teriyaki	1 srvg	240	5	2	na	na	na	na	20	0	23	1 1/2 starch, 3 lean meat
Chicken Wei Lo Mein	1 srvg	180	7	4	na	na	na	na	7	0	20	1/2 starch, 3 lean meat
Honey Seared Chicken	1 srvg	290	17	5	na	na	na	na	19	0	16	1 1/2 starch, 2 lean meat, 2 1/2 fat
NOODLE & RICE BOWLS (2 SERVINGS/DISH)												
Beef Fried Rice	1 srvg	630	21	3	na	na	na	na	68	3	37	4 1/2 starch, 3 medium-fat meat, 1 fat
Chicken Fried Rice	1 srvg	525	11	2	na	na	na	na	68	3	32	4 1/2 starch, 2 lean meat

✓ = Healthiest Bets; na = not available

(*Continued*)

NOODLE & RICE BOWLS (2 SERVINGS/DISH) *(Continued)*	Amount	Cal.	Fat (g)	% Cal. Fat	Sat. Fat (g)	Trans Fat (g)	Chol. (mg)	Sod. (mg)	Carb. (g)	Fiber (g)	Pro. (g)	Choices/Exchanges
Dan Dan Noodles - Chicken	1 srvg	390	7	2	na	na	na	na	54	3	26	3 1/2 starch, 1 lean meat, 2 fat
Japanese Teriyaki bowl - Beef & Brown Rice	1 srvg	580	17	3	na	na	na	na	66	4	33	4 1/2 starch, 3 medium-fat meat, 1/2 fat
Japanese Teriyaki bowl - Beef & White Rice	1 srvg	560	16	3	na	na	na	na	62	3	32	4 starch, 3 medium-fat meat, 1/2 fat
Japanese Teriyaki bowl - Chicken & Brown Rice	1 srvg	460	7	1	na	na	na	na	64	4	28	4 1/2 starch, 2 lean meat
Japanese Teriyaki bowl - Chicken & White Rice	1 srvg	440	6	1	na	na	na	na	60	3	28	4 starch, 2 lean meat
Japanese Teriyaki bowl - Shrimp & Brown Rice	1 srvg	410	5	1	na	na	na	na	64	4	20	4 1/2 starch, 1 lean meat, 1/2 fat
Japanese Teriyaki bowl - Shrimp & White Rice	1 srvg	390	5	1	na	na	na	na	61	3	20	4 starch, 1 lean meat, 1/2 fat

Japanese Teriyaki bowl - Vegetables, Tofu & Brown Rice	1 srvg	410	6	1	na	na	na	na	71	7	13	3 starch, 3 veg, 2 fat
Japanese Teriyaki bowl - Vegetables, Tofu & White Rice	1 srvg	390	5	1	na	na	na	na	68	5	13	3 starch, 3 veg, 2 fat
Lo Mein Noodles - Beef	1 srvg	570	21	3	na	na	na	na	61	5	36	4 starch, 3 medium-fat meat, 1 fat
Lo Mein Noodles - Chicken	1 srvg	460	11	2	na	na	na	na	61	5	31	4 starch, 3 lean meat, 1/2 fat
Lo Mein Noodles - Shrimp	1 srvg	400	8	2	na	na	na	na	60	5	23	4 starch, 2 lean meat, 1/2 fat
Lo Mein Noodles - Vegetables & Tofu	1 srvg	400	8	2	na	na	na	na	66	7	16	3 starch, 3 veg, 2 fat
Pad Thai - Beef	1 srvg	670	30	4	na	na	na	na	63	2	40	4 starch, 4 medium-fat meat, 1 fat
Pad Thai - Chicken	1 srvg	560	20	3	na	na	na	na	61	2	35	4 starch, 3 lean meat, 2 fat

✔ = Healthiest Bets; na = not available

(*Continued*)

NOODLE & RICE BOWLS (2 SERVINGS/DISH) *(Continued)*	Amount	Cal.	Fat (g)	% Cal. Fat	Sat. Fat (g)	Trans Fat (g)	Chol. (mg)	Sod. (mg)	Carb. (g)	Fiber (g)	Pro. (g)	Choices/Exchanges
Pad Thai - Shrimp	1 srvg	490	17	3	na	na	na	na	60	2	27	4 starch, 2 lean meat, 2 fat
Pad Thai - Vegetables & Tofu	1 srvg	470	17	3	na	na	na	na	66	4	18	3 starch, 3 veg, 1 lean meat, 2 fat
Shrimp Fried Rice	1 srvg	475	10	2	na	na	na	na	67	3	24	4 1/2 starch, 2 lean meat, 1 fat
Thai Blazing Noodles - Beef	1 srvg	630	32	5	na	na	na	na	55	4	28	3 1/2 starch, 2 medium-fat meat, 4 fat
Thai Blazing Noodles - Chicken	1 srvg	520	22	4	na	na	na	na	55	4	24	3 1/2 starch, 2 lean meat, 3 1/2 fat
Thai Blazing Noodles - Shrimp	1 srvg	485	22	4	na	na	na	na	55	4	16	3 1/2 starch, 1 lean meat, 4 fat
Thai Blazing Noodles - Vegetables & Tofu	1 srvg	430	18	4	na	na	na	na	59	6	10	3 starch, 3 veg, 3 fat

Vegetables & Tofu Fried Rice	1 srvg	440	7	1	na	na	na	na	73	5	17	4 starch, 3 veg, 1 fat
RICE & NOODLES (2 SERVINGS/DISH)												
Brown Rice	1 srvg	170	2	1	na	na	na	na	37	3	4	2 1/2 starch, 1/2 fat
Egg Noodles	1 srvg	210	3	1	na	na	na	na	39	2	7	2 1/2 starch, 1/2 fat
Rice Noodles	1 srvg	130	0	0	na	na	na	na	32	0	0	2 starch
White Rice	1 srvg	200	0	0	na	na	na	na	44	1	4	3 starch
SALADS												
Asian Chopped Chicken Salad - no dressing	2 srvgs	200	8	4	na	na	na	na	10	2	23	2 veg, 3 lean meat
Asian Chopped Chicken Salad w/ dressing	2 srvgs	280	15	5	na	na	na	na	13	2	24	2 1/2 veg, 3 lean meat, 1 fat
Pei Wei Spicy Chicken Salad - no dressing	2 srvgs	210	3	1	na	na	na	na	23	2	22	1/2 starch, 3 veg, 3 lean meat

✔ = Healthiest Bets; na = not available

(Continued)

SALADS *(Continued)*	Amount	Cal.	Fat (g)	% Cal. Fat	Sat. Fat (g)	Trans Fat (g)	Chol. (mg)	Sod. (mg)	Carb. (g)	Fiber (g)	Pro. (g)	Choices/Exchanges
Pei Wei Spicy Chicken Salad w/ dressing	2 srvgs	350	16	4	na	na	na	na	28	2	22	1 starch, 3 veg, 3 lean meat, 1 1/2 fat
Vietnamese Chicken Salad Rolls	3 srvgs	53	3	5	na	na	na	na	5	1	3	1/2 starch, 1/2 fat
SAUCES AND SIDES												
Chocolate Chip Cookie	1	342	14	4	na	na	na	na	53	2	5	3 1/2 carb, 2 1/2 fat
Fortune Cookie	1	30	0	0	na	na	na	na	7	0	0	1/2 carb
Lettuce Wrap Sauce, 2 oz	1 srvg	70	5	6	na	na	na	na	2	0	4	1/2 carb, 1 fat
Lime Vinaigrette, 2 oz	1 srvg	230	20	8	na	na	na	na	13	0	0	1 carb, 3 1/2 fat
Rice Sticks	1 srvg	130	0	0	na	na	na	na	33	0	0	2 starch
Sesame Ginger Dressing, 2 oz	1 srvg	170	16	8	na	na	na	na	5	0	1	1/2 carb, 3 fat
Sweet Chile Sauce, 2 oz	1 srvg	140	0	0	na	na	na	na	34	2	0	2 carb
Thai Peanut Sauce, 2 oz	1 srvg	168	11	6	na	na	na	na	15	1	5	1 carb, 2 fat

SIGNATURE DISHES (2 SERVINGS/DISH)												
Ginger Broccoli - Beef	1 srvg	450	22	4	na	na	na	na	19	2	37	1 1/2 starch, 5 medium-fat meat
Ginger Broccoli - Chicken	1 srvg	300	9	3	na	na	na	na	19	2	31	1 1/2 starch, 4 lean meat
Ginger Broccoli - Shrimp	1 srvg	230	7	3	na	na	na	na	18	2	22	1 starch, 3 lean meat
Ginger Broccoli - Vegetables & Tofu	1 srvg	170	4	2	na	na	na	na	23	4	10	1/2 starch, 3 veg, 1 lean meat
Honey Seared - Chicken	1 srvg	420	15	3	na	na	na	na	45	1	21	3 starch, 2 lean meat, 2 fat
Honey Seared - Shrimp	1 srvg	370	14	3	na	na	na	na	43	0	14	3 starch, 1 lean meat, 2 1/2 fat
Lemon Pepper - Beef	1 srvg	550	31	5	na	na	na	na	32	2	38	2 starch, 5 medium-fat meat, 1 1/2 fat

✔ = Healthiest Bets; na = not available

(*Continued*)

SIGNATURE DISHES (2 SERVINGS/DISH) *(Continued)*	Amount	Cal.	Fat (g)	% Cal. Fat	Sat. Fat (g)	Trans Fat (g)	Chol. (mg)	Sod. (mg)	Carb. (g)	Fiber (g)	Pro. (g)	Choices/Exchanges
Lemon Pepper - Chicken	1 srvg	440	20	4	na	na	na	na	34	2	31	2 1/2 starch, 3 lean meat, 2 fat
Lemon Pepper - Shrimp	1 srvg	380	18	4	na	na	na	na	34	2	22	2 1/2 starch, 2 lean meat, 2 1/2 fat
Lemon Pepper - Vegetables & Tofu	1 srvg	230	10	4	na	na	na	na	29	4	10	1 starch, 3 veg, 2 fat
Mandarin Kung Pao - Beef	1 srvg	610	34	5	na	na	na	na	31	3	10	2 starch, 1 medium-fat meat, 8 fat
Mandarin Kung Pao - Chicken	1 srvg	450	21	4	na	na	na	na	28	3	10	2 starch, 1 lean meat, 5 fat
Mandarin Kung Pao - Shrimp	1 srvg	400	19	4	na	na	na	na	28	3	10	2 starch, 1 lean meat, 4 fat
Mandarin Kung Pao - Vegetables & Tofu	1 srvg	290	15	5	na	na	na	na	23	4	10	1/2 starch, 3 veg, 1 lean meat, 2 1/2 fat

Mongolian - Beef	1 srvg	420	22	5	na	na	na	na	14	1	36	1 starch, 5 medium-fat meat
Mongolian - Chicken	1 srvg	280	9	3	na	na	na	na	14	1	30	1 starch, 4 lean meat
Mongolian - Shrimp	1 srvg	210	6	3	na	na	na	na	12	1	21	1 starch, 3 lean meat
Mongolian - Vegetables & Tofu	1 srvg	180	6	3	na	na	na	na	19	3	10	1 starch, 3 veg, 1 fat
Orange Peel - Beef	1 srvg	660	31	4	na	na	na	na	52	3	33	3 1/2 starch, 3 medium-fat meat, 3 fat
Orange Peel - Chicken	1 srvg	520	18	3	na	na	na	na	52	3	33	3 1/2 starch, 3 lean meat, 1 1/2 fat
Orange Peel - Shrimp	1 srvg	460	16	3	na	na	na	na	51	3	33	3 1/2 starch, 3 lean meat, 1/2 fat
Orange Peel - Vegetables & Tofu	1 srvg	330	10	3	na	na	na	na	46	4	33	2 starch, 3 veg, 2 lean meat

✓ = Healthiest Bets; na = not available

(*Continued*)

SIGNATURE DISHES (2 SERVINGS/DISH) *(Continued)*	Amount	Cal.	Fat (g)	% Cal. Fat	Sat. Fat (g)	Trans Fat (g)	Chol. (mg)	Sod. (mg)	Carb. (g)	Fiber (g)	Pro. (g)	Choices/Exchanges
Pei Wei Spicy - Beef	1 srvg	480	26	5	na	na	na	na	25	2	34	1 1/2 starch, 4 medium-fat meat, 1 fat
Pei Wei Spicy - Chicken	1 srvg	330	13	4	na	na	na	na	25	2	28	1 1/2 starch, 3 lean meat, 1/2 fat
Pei Wei Spicy - Shrimp	1 srvg	300	11	3	na	na	na	na	29	2	19	2 starch, 2 lean meat, 1 fat
Pei Wei Spicy - Vegetables & Tofu	1 srvg	250	16	6	na	na	na	na	21	3	6	1/2 starch, 3 veg, 3 fat
Spicy Korean - Beef	1 srvg	490	24	4	na	na	na	na	26	3	41	1 1/2 starch, 5 medium-fat meat
Spicy Korean - Chicken	1 srvg	350	11	3	na	na	na	na	26	3	35	1 1/2 starch, 4 lean meat
Spicy Korean - Shrimp	1 srvg	280	9	3	na	na	na	na	24	3	26	1 1/2 starch, 3 lean meat

Spicy Korean - Vegetables & Tofu	1 srvg	240	9	3	na	na	na	na	27	4	15	1 starch, 3 veg, 2 fat
Sweet & Sour - Chicken	1 srvg	440	13	3	na	na	na	na	61	2	21	4 starch, 1 lean meat, 1 fat
Sweet & Sour - Shrimp	1 srvg	390	11	3	na	na	na	na	59	2	14	4 starch, 2 fat
Thai Coconut Curry - Beef	1 srvg	550	37	6	na	na	na	na	20	2	36	1 1/2 starch, 5 medium-fat meat, 3 fat
Thai Coconut Curry - Chicken	1 srvg	380	19	5	na	na	na	na	23	2	30	1 1/2 starch, 4 lean meat, 1 1/2 fat
Thai Coconut Curry - Shrimp	1 srvg	300	17	5	na	na	na	na	18	2	21	1 starch, 2 lean meat, 2 fat
Thai Coconut Curry - Vegetables & Tofu	1 srvg	220	14	6	na	na	na	na	19	2	8	1/2 starch, 3 veg, 3 fat
Thai Dynamite - Chicken	1 srvg	390	19	4	na	na	na	na	20	2	33	1 1/2 starch, 4 lean meat, 1 1/2 fat

✔ = Healthiest Bets; na = not available

(*Continued*)

SIGNATURE DISHES (2 SERVINGS/DISH) *(Continued)*	Amount	Cal.	Fat (g)	% Cal. Fat	Sat. Fat (g)	Trans Fat (g)	Chol. (mg)	Sod. (mg)	Carb. (g)	Fiber (g)	Pro. (g)	Choices/Exchanges
Thai Dynamite - Shrimp	1 srvg	280	16	5	na	na	na	na	20	2	15	1 1/2 starch, 2 lean meat, 2 1/2 fat
Thai Dynamite - Vegetables & Tofu	1 srvg	220	16	7	na	na	na	na	15	3	6	3 veg, 3 fat

✓ = Healthiest Bets; na = not available

Exclusive Web Content

Be sure to visit the following restaurants online at http://www.diabetes.org/healthyrestaurant

Carvel
Del Taco
El Pollo Loco
Frëshens
Godfather's
Jersey Mike's
Jimmy John's
Tim Hortons
Whataburger
Wienerschnitzel
Zaxby's

Pizza, Pasta, and All Else Italian

RESTAURANTS

CiCi's Pizza
Domino's Pizza
Fazoli's
Little Caesars
Papa John's Pizza
Papa Murphy's Take 'N' Bake
Pizza Hut

EXCLUSIVE WEB CONTENT

Godfather's Pizza
(http://www.diabetes.org/healthyrestaurant)

Note: The criteria for the Healthiest Bets for pizza are based on two slices, although the nutrition information provided in the table is generally for one slice. Read page 55 for more details about selecting Healthiest Bets.

NUTRITION PROS

- Surprisingly, pizza and pasta—as long as you top them wisely and control the portions—can be healthy restaurant choices.
- Pizza and pasta can hold the line on fat and calories better than some meals with a burger and French fries.
- Pizza and pasta meals can match today's diabetes nutrition goals: low in fat and moderate in protein and carbohydrate.

- You can eat vegetables, both raw and cooked, in most pizza and pasta restaurants. That's an accomplishment in a fast-food restaurant. Raw vegetables come as salads. Cooked vegetables come as pizza sauce and toppings or as tomato-based sauces and toppings on pasta.
- Splitting and sharing is the way to go in most pizza restaurants.
- You can design your own pizza with healthier toppings (see list on the next page). Pizza parlors are used to made-for-you orders.
- Most pizza chains offer a veggie combination pizza. Order it and skip the high-fat meats!
- Pizza chains are slowly but surely divulging their nutrition information, so you can pick and choose with nutrition facts in hand.
- Several pizza chains have gone uptown. That's good news for health-focused pizza lovers. They bake their pizzas in brick ovens, and they offer novel and healthy toppings. Pineapple, spinach, feta cheese, roasted red peppers, and grilled chicken are just a few.
- Taking home leftovers is a snap. Boxes are ready.

NUTRITION CONS

- It's hard to eat just two or three slices. There's always just one more piece of pizza begging you to eat it.
- High-fat pizza toppings—extra cheese, pepperoni, and sausage—can quickly add fat and calories.
- High-fat toppings also add more sodium.
- Some pizza chains now promote more toppings, extra cheese, and bigger pizzas. This all adds up to more fat and calories.

- Restaurant combination pizzas often add high-fat and high-calorie toppers.
- Pasta with high-fat and high-calorie toppings—cream sauce, creamy cheese sauce, butter sauce—is too easy to find.
- Pasta portions are often heavy-handed.
- Breadsticks and garlic bread sound healthy, but they are often drenched in fat. Check their nutrition numbers.

HEALTHY PIZZA TOPPINGS

part-skim cheese	sliced tomatoes	chicken
green peppers	spinach	ham
onions	broccoli	Canadian bacon
mushrooms	pineapple	

NOT-SO-HEALTHY PIZZA TOPPINGS

extra cheese	pepperoni	anchovies
several types of cheese	sausage	bacon
hamburger meat		

Get It Your Way

- ★ Ask your pizza maker to go light on the cheese and heavy on the veggies.
- ★ Request a half-order (may be called "appetizer size") of pasta if you don't have someone with whom to split it.
- ★ Remember to order your salad dressing on the side.

Healthy Tips

- ★ If you count calories carefully, stick with the thin crust and load up on the veggies.
- ★ If your favorite chain does not publish nutrition information, check the nutrition information for similar items from two other pizza chains. This will give you ballpark figures on which to base your choice.
- ★ If your dining partner wants not-so-healthy pizza toppings, order healthier toppings on one half and let your partner handle the other.
- ★ If you count grams of carbohydrate, make sure the slices you eat are average. If they are bigger or smaller, change your carbohydrate estimate based on the carbohydrate information. Your eyes will tell the tale.
- ★ Order just enough for everyone at the table to avoid that just-one-more-slice syndrome.
- ★ If you know extra pieces will be left over, package them up before you take your first bite.
- ★ Try an appetizer-size portion of pasta, split an order with your dining partner, or stash a portion in a take-home container before you lift your fork to your mouth.
- ★ Along with pizza or pasta, crunch on a healthy garden salad to fill you up and not out.
- ★ The red pepper flakes you'll probably find sitting right on your table (or in your spice cabinet for take-home pizza) add zip to your pizza, pasta, or salad without adding calories.

CiCi's Pizza

(www.cicispizza.com)

Light 'n Lean Choice

12" Buffet Pizzas with Ham and Pineapple *(3 slices)*

Calories	423	Cholesterol (mg)	31
Fat (g)	13	Sodium (mg)	956
% calories from fat	28	Carbohydrate (g)	56
Saturated fat (g)	8	Fiber (g)	4
Trans fat (g)	0	Protein (g)	21

Exchanges: 4 starch, 2 1/2 fat

Healthy 'n Hearty Choice

15" To-Go Pizzas, Ole *(4 slices)*

Calories	677	Cholesterol (mg)	3
Fat (g)	16	Sodium (mg)	1,401
% calories from fat	21	Carbohydrate (g)	106
Saturated fat (g)	9	Fiber (g)	13
Trans fat (g)	0	Protein (g)	28

Exchanges: 7 starch, 3 fat

(Continued)

CiCi's Pizza

	Amount	Cal.	Fat (g)	% Cal. Fat	Sat. Fat (g)	Trans Fat (g)	Chol. (mg)	Sod. (mg)	Carb. (g)	Fiber (g)	Pro. (g)	Choices/Exchanges
12" BUFFET PIZZAS												
✔Alfredo	1 slice	139	5	3	3	0	10	199	18	1	6	1 starch, 1 fat
✔Bacon Cheddar	1 slice	145	5	3	2	0	13	312	18	3	6	1 starch, 1 fat
✔Bar-B-Que	1 slice	172	6	3	4	0.5	12	311	21	2	8	1 1/2 starch, 1 1/2 fat
✔Beef	1 slice	170	7	4	3.5	0	20	281	18	1	9	1 starch, 1 medium-fat meat, 1/2 fat
✔Cheese	1 slice	152	5	3	3	0	9	305	20	1	7	1 1/2 starch, 1 fat
✔Ham & Pineapple	1 slice	141	4	3	3	0	10	319	19	1	7	1 1/2 starch, 1 fat
✔Olé	1 slice	108	4	3	2	0	1	261	13	2	5	1 starch, 1/2 fat
✔Pepperoni	1 slice	175	7	4	4	0	13	384	21	2	8	1 1/2 starch, 1 medium-fat meat, 1 fat

✔Pepperoni & Jalapeño	1 slice	163	6	3	3.5	0	11	394	20	2	8	1 1/2 starch, 1 medium-fat meat, 1/2 fat
✔Sausage	1 slice	197	7	3	4	0	11	358	19	1	8	1 1/2 starch, 1 medium-fat meat, 1 fat
✔Spinach Alfredo	1 slice	151	5	3	3.5	0	11	215	20	2	7	1 1/2 starch, 1 fat
✔Zesty Ham & Cheddar	1 slice	153	6	4	3	0.5	9	271	18	1	6	1 starch, 1 fat
✔Zesty Pepperoni	1 slice	157	7	4	2.5	1	7	302	18	1	6	1 starch, 1 1/2 fat
✔Zesty Tomato Alfredo	1 slice	136	5	3	3	0	10	202	18	2	6	1 starch, 1 fat
✔Zesty Veggie	1 slice	124	4	3	2	0.5	4	224	17	1	5	1 starch, 1 fat
15" TO-GO PIZZAS												
✔Alfredo	1 slice	216	8	3	5.5	0.5	12	366	27	2	8	2 starch, 1 1/2 fat
Bacon Cheddar	1 slice	257	8	3	3.5	0	16	495	36	4	10	2 1/2 starch, 1 1/2 fat
Bar-B-Que	1 slice	289	10	3	6.5	0.5	17	446	36	2	13	2 1/2 starch, 1 medium-fat meat, 1 1/2 fat

✔ = Healthiest Bets

(*Continued*)

15" TO-GO PIZZAS *(Continued)*	Amount	Cal.	Fat (g)	% Cal. Fat	Sat. Fat (g)	Trans Fat (g)	Chol. (mg)	Sod. (mg)	Carb. (g)	Fiber (g)	Pro. (g)	Choices/Exchanges
Beef	1 slice	260	10	3	6.5	0	30	436	28	3	14	2 starch, 1 medium-fat meat, 1 fat
✔Cheese	1 slice	223	8	3	5.5	0	17	428	28	3	11	2 starch, 1 medium-fat meat, 1 fat
✔Ham & Pineapple	1 slice	225	8	3	5.5	0	21	394	27	2	11	2 starch, 1 medium-fat meat, 1 fat
✔Olé	1 slice	169	4	2	2	0	1	350	26	3	7	2 starch, 1 fat
Pepperoni	1 slice	240	10	4	6	0	21	504	27	3	11	2 starch, 1 medium-fat meat, 1 fat
✔Pepperoni & Jalapeño	1 slice	221	9	4	5.5	0	18	535	25	3	10	1 1/2 starch, 1 medium-fat meat, 1 fat
Sausage	1 slice	290	10	3	6.5	0	20	517	28	3	12	2 starch, 1 medium-fat meat, 1 fat

✔Spinach Alfredo	1 slice	243	8	3	5.5	0	18	347	32	3	11	2 starch, 1 medium-fat meat, 1 fat
Zesty Ham & Cheddar	1 slice	229	11	4	5	1.5	15	450	24	2	11	1 1/2 starch, 1 medium-fat meat, 1 1/2 fat
Zesty Pepperoni	1 slice	246	12	4	4.5	1.5	11	475	26	2	10	1 1/2 starch, 1 medium-fat meat, 1 1/2 fat
✔Zesty Tomato Alfredo	1 slice	217	8	3	5.5	0.5	12	379	27	2	8	2 starch, 1 1/2 fat
✔Zesty Veggie	1 slice	213	9	4	3.5	1.5	7	394	25	2	9	1 1/2 starch, 2 fat
EXTRAS & DESSERT												
✔Apple Pizza	1 slice	149	4	2	1	0.5	0	193	26	1	3	1 1/2 starch, 1/2 fat
Brownies	1 brownie	143	6	4	1	1	0	96	22	1	1	1 1/2 carb, 1 fat
✔Cinnamon Rolls	1 roll	139	6	4	1	0.5	0	99	20	1	2	1 1/2 starch, 1 fat
✔Garlic Bread	1 slice	99	5	5	1.5	0	5	120	10	0	4	1/2 starch, 1 fat

✔ = Healthiest Bets

Domino's Pizza

(www.dominos.com)

Light 'n Lean Choice

14" Large Crunchy Thin-Crust Pizza with Green Peppers *(3 slices)*

Calories	540	Cholesterol (mg)	15
Fat (g)	29	Sodium (mg)	1,020
% calories from fat	48	Carbohydrate (g)	63
Saturated fat (g)	9	Fiber (g)	6
Trans fat (g)	0	Protein (g)	21

Exchanges: 4 starch, 1 veg, 2 medium-fat meat, 2 fat

Healthy 'n Hearty Choice

12" Medium Feast, Classic Hand-Tossed Crust Pizza, Vegi Feast *(3 slices)*

Calories	885	Cholesterol (mg)	25
Fat (g)	42	Sodium (mg)	2,025
% calories from fat	43	Carbohydrate (g)	102
Saturated fat (g)	18	Fiber (g)	6
Trans fat (g)	0	Protein (g)	42

Exchanges: 6 starch, 2 veg, 3 medium-fat meat, 5 fat

Domino's Pizza

	Amount	Cal.	Fat (g)	% Cal. Fat	Sat. Fat (g)	Trans Fat (g)	Chol. (mg)	Sod. (mg)	Carb. (g)	Fiber (g)	Pro. (g)	Choices/Exchanges
12" MEDIUM FEAST PIZZAS: OPTIONAL TOPPING												
✔Extra Cheese	1 slice	250	2	1	1	0	4	85	1	0	2	1/2 fat
12" MEDIUM FEAST, CLASSIC HAND-TOSSED CRUST PIZZAS												
America's Favorite Feast	1 slice	345	18	5	7	0	30	785	34	2	15	2 1/2 starch, 1 medium-fat meat, 2 1/2 fat
Bacon Cheeseburger Feast	1 slice	355	19	5	8	0	40	725	33	2	18	2 starch, 2 medium-fat meat, 2 fat
Barbecue Feast	1 slice	345	16	4	7	0	30	695	38	1	16	2 1/2 starch, 1 medium-fat meat, 2 fat
Deluxe Feast	1 slice	315	16	5	6.5	0	25	715	34	2	14	2 1/2 starch, 1 medium-fat meat, 2 fat

✔ = Healthiest Bets

(*Continued*)

12" MEDIUM FEAST, CLASSIC HAND-TOSSED CRUST PIZZAS *(Continued)*	Amount	Cal.	Fat (g)	% Cal. Fat	Sat. Fat (g)	Trans Fat (g)	Chol. (mg)	Sod. (mg)	Carb. (g)	Fiber (g)	Pro. (g)	Choices/Exchanges
ExtravaganZZa	1 slice	375	20	5	8	0	40	925	35	2	18	2 1/2 starch, 2 medium-fat meat, 2 1/2 fat
Hawaiian Feast	1 slice	305	14	4	6	0	25	725	35	2	15	2 1/2 starch, 1 medium-fat meat, 1 1/2 fat
MeatZZa Feast	1 slice	365	19	5	8	0	40	895	34	2	17	2 1/2 starch, 1 medium-fat meat, 2 1/2 fat
Pepperoni Feast	1 slice	345	19	5	8	0	35	865	34	2	16	2 1/2 starch, 1 medium-fat meat, 2 1/2 fat
Philly Cheese Steak Feast	1 slice	315	15	4	7.5	0	30	695	31	1	16	2 starch, 1 medium-fat meat, 1 1/2 fat
Vegi Feast	1 slice	295	14	4	6	0	25	675	34	2	14	2 1/2 starch, 1 medium-fat meat, 2 fat
12" MEDIUM FEAST, CRUNCHY THIN CRUST PIZZAS												
America's Favorite Feast	1 slice	265	19	6	6.5	0	30	690	18	2	11	1 starch, 1 medium-fat meat, 2 1/2 fat

Bacon Cheeseburger Feast	1 slice	275	20	7	7.5	0	40	630	17	2	14	1 starch, 2 medium-fat meat, 2 1/2 fat
Barbecue Feast	1 slice	265	17	6	6.5	0	30	600	22	1	12	1 1/2 starch, 1 medium-fat meat, 2 fat
Deluxe Feast	1 slice	235	17	7	6	0	25	620	18	2	10	1 starch, 1 medium-fat meat, 2 1/2 fat
ExtravaganZZa	1 slice	295	21	6	7.5	0	40	830	19	2	14	1 1/2 starch, 1 medium-fat meat, 2 1/2 fat
Hawaiian Feast	1 slice	225	14	6	5.5	0	25	630	19	2	11	1 1/2 starch, 1 medium-fat meat, 2 fat
MeatZZa Feast	1 slice	285	20	6	7.5	0	40	800	18	2	13	1 starch, 1 medium-fat meat, 2 1/2 fat
Pepperoni Feast	1 slice	265	20	7	7.5	0	35	770	18	2	12	1 starch, 1 medium-fat meat, 2 1/2 fat
Philly Cheese Steak Feast	1 slice	235	16	6	7	0	30	600	15	1	12	1 starch, 1 medium-fat meat, 2 fat

✓ = Healthiest Bets

(*Continued*)

12" MEDIUM FEAST, CRUNCHY THIN CRUST PIZZAS *(Continued)*	Amount	Cal.	Fat (g)	% Cal. Fat	Sat. Fat (g)	Trans Fat (g)	Chol. (mg)	Sod. (mg)	Carb. (g)	Fiber (g)	Pro. (g)	Choices/Exchanges
Vegi Feast	1 slice	215	15	6	5.5	0	25	580	18	2	10	1 starch, 1 medium-fat meat, 2 fat
12" MEDIUM FEAST, ULTIMATE DEEP DISH PIZZAS												
America's Favorite Feast	1 slice	360	22	6	7.5	0	30	975	31	4	14	2 starch, 1 medium-fat meat, 3 1/2 fat
Bacon Cheeseburger Feast	1 slice	370	23	6	8.5	0	40	915	30	4	17	2 starch, 2 medium-fat meat, 3 fat
Barbecue Feast	1 slice	360	20	5	7.5	0	30	885	35	3	15	2 1/2 starch, 1 medium-fat meat, 3 fat
Deluxe Feast	1 slice	330	20	5	7	0	25	905	31	4	13	2 starch, 1 medium-fat meat, 3 fat
ExtravaganZZa	1 slice	390	24	6	8.5	0	40	1115	32	4	17	2 starch, 2 medium-fat meat, 3 1/2 fat
Hawaiian Feast	1 slice	320	18	5	6.5	0	25	915	32	4	14	2 starch, 1 medium-fat meat, 2 1/2 fat

MeatZZa Feast	1 slice	380	23	5	8.5	0	40	1085	31	4	16	2 starch, 1 medium-fat meat, 3 fat
Pepperoni Feast	1 slice	360	23	6	8.5	0	35	1055	31	4	15	2 starch, 1 medium-fat meat, 3 1/2 fat
Philly Cheese Steak Feast	1 slice	330	19	5	8	0	30	885	28	3	15	2 starch, 1 medium-fat meat, 2 1/2 fat
Vegi Feast	1 slice	310	18	5	6.5	0	25	865	31	4	13	2 starch, 1 medium-fat meat, 2 1/2 fat
12" MEDIUM, 1 TOPPING, CLASSIC HAND-TOSSED PIZZAS												
✔Beef	1 slice	210	9	4	3.5	0	20	420	24	1	9	1 1/2 starch, 1 medium-fat meat, 1 fat
✔Black Olives	1 slice	180	7	4	2	0	10	415	25	1	7	1 1/2 starch, 1 1/2 fat
✔Extra Cheese	1 slice	195	8	4	3	0	15	435	25	1	9	1 1/2 starch, 1 medium-fat meat, 1 fat
✔Green Peppers	1 slice	170	6	3	2	0	10	350	24	1	7	1 1/2 starch, 1 fat

✔ = Healthiest Bets

(*Continued*)

12" MEDIUM, 1 TOPPING, CLASSIC HAND-TOSSED PIZZAS *(Continued)*	Amount	Cal.	Fat (g)	% Cal. Fat	Sat. Fat (g)	Trans Fat (g)	Chol. (mg)	Sod. (mg)	Carb. (g)	Fiber (g)	Pro. (g)	Choices/Exchanges
✔Ham	1 slice	180	6	3	2	0	15	450	24	1	9	1 1/2 starch, 1 medium-fat meat, 1/2 fat
✔Mushrooms	1 slice	170	6	3	2	0	10	350	24	1	7	1 1/2 starch, 1 fat
✔Onions	1 slice	170	6	3	2	0	10	350	25	1	7	1 1/2 starch, 1 fat
✔Pepperoni	1 slice	210	9	4	3	0	15	490	24	1	9	1 1/2 starch, 1 medium-fat meat, 1 fat
✔Pineapple	1 slice	180	6	3	2	0	10	350	26	1	7	1 1/2 starch, 1 fat
✔Sausage	1 slice	215	9	4	3.5	0	15	480	25	1	9	1 1/2 starch, 1 medium-fat meat, 1 fat
12" MEDIUM, 1 TOPPING, CRUNCHY THIN CRUST PIZZAS												
Beef	1 slice	170	11	6	4	0	20	310	14	1	7	1 starch, 1 medium-fat meat, 1 1/2 fat
✔Black Olives	1 slice	140	9	6	2.5	0	10	305	15	1	5	1 starch, 1 1/2 fat

✔Extra Cheese	1 slice	155	10	6	3.5	0	15	325	15	1	7	1 starch, 1 medium-fat meat, 1 1/2 fat
✔Green Peppers	1 slice	130	8	6	2.5	0	10	240	14	1	5	1 starch, 1 1/2 fat
✔Ham	1 slice	140	8	5	2.5	0	15	340	14	1	7	1 starch, 1 medium-fat meat, 1 fat
✔Mushrooms	1 slice	130	8	6	2.5	0	10	240	14	1	5	1 starch, 1 1/2 fat
✔Onions	1 slice	130	8	6	2.5	0	10	240	15	1	5	1 starch, 1 1/2 fat
Pepperoni	1 slice	170	11	6	3.5	0	15	380	14	1	7	1 starch, 1 medium-fat meat, 1 1/2 fat
✔Pineapple	1 slice	140	8	5	2.5	0	10	240	16	1	5	1 starch, 1 1/2 fat
Sausage	1 slice	175	11	6	4	0	15	370	15	1	7	1 starch, 1 medium-fat meat, 1 1/2 fat
12" MEDIUM, 1 TOPPING, OPTIONAL TOPPINGS												
American Cheese	1 slice	40	3	7	2	0	10	190	0	0	2	1 fat
✔Anchovies	1 slice	0	0	0	0	0	0	35	0	0	0	Free

✔ = Healthiest Bets

(*Continued*)

12" MEDIUM, 1 TOPPING, OPTIONAL TOPPINGS *(Continued)*	Amount	Cal.	Fat (g)	% Cal. Fat	Sat. Fat (g)	Trans Fat (g)	Chol. (mg)	Sod. (mg)	Carb. (g)	Fiber (g)	Pro. (g)	Choices/Exchanges
Bacon	1 slice	40	3	7	1	0	10	115	0	0	4	1 medium-fat meat
✔Banana Peppers	1 slice	0	0	0	0	0	0	130	0	0	0	Free
Cheddar Cheese	1 slice	30	3	9	1.5	0	5	45	0	0	2	1 fat
✔Chicken Grilled	1 slice	15	0	0	0	0	5	90	0	0	2	Free
✔Garlic	1 slice	10	0	0	0	0	0	0	1	0	0	Free
✔Green Chile Peppers	1 slice	0	0	0	0	0	0	0	0	0	0	Free
✔Green Olive	1 slice	15	2	12	0	0	0	95	0	0	0	Free
✔Jalapeno	1 slice	0	0	0	0	0	0	100	0	0	0	Free
✔Philly Meat	1 slice	10	0	0	0	0	5	60	0	0	2	Free
Provolone Cheese	1 slice	45	4	8	0	0	10	110	0	0	3	1 fat
✔Tomatoes	1 slice	5	0	0	0	0	0	20	1	0	0	Free

12" MEDIUM, 1 TOPPING, ULTIMATE DEEP-DISH PIZZAS

Beef	1 slice	265	14	5	5	0	20	595	27	3	10	2 starch, 1 medium-fat meat, 2 fat
Black Olives	1 slice	235	12	5	3.5	0	10	590	28	3	8	2 starch, 2 1/2 fat
Extra Cheese	1 slice	250	13	5	4.5	0	15	610	28	3	10	2 starch, 1 medium-fat meat, 2 fat
Green Peppers	1 slice	225	11	4	3.5	0	10	525	27	3	8	2 starch, 2 fat
Ham	1 slice	235	11	4	3.5	0	15	625	27	3	10	2 starch, 1 medium-fat meat, 1 1/2 fat
Mushrooms	1 slice	225	11	4	3.5	0	10	525	27	3	8	2 starch, 2 fat
Onions	1 slice	225	11	4	3.5	0	10	525	28	3	8	2 starch, 2 fat
Pepperoni	1 slice	265	15	5	4.5	0	15	665	27	3	10	2 starch, 1 medium-fat meat, 2 fat
Pineapple	1 slice	235	11	4	3.5	0	10	525	29	3	8	2 starch, 2 fat

✓ = Healthiest Bets

(*Continued*)

12" MEDIUM, 1 TOPPING, ULTIMATE DEEP-DISH PIZZAS *(Continued)*	Amount	Cal.	Fat (g)	% Cal. Fat	Sat. Fat (g)	Trans Fat (g)	Chol. (mg)	Sod. (mg)	Carb. (g)	Fiber (g)	Pro. (g)	Choices/Exchanges
Sausage	1 slice	270	15	5	5	0	15	655	28	3	10	2 starch, 1 medium-fat meat, 2 1/2 fat
14" BROOKLYN STYLE PIZZA												
Pepperoni	1 slice	330	8	2	4	0.5	35	750	30	2	16	2 starch, 1 medium-fat meat, 2 fat
Sausage	1 slice	350	8	2	4	0.5	35	740	31	2	16	2 starch, 1 medium-fat meat, 2 fat
14" LARGE FEAST PIZZAS: OPTIONAL TOPPING												
Extra Cheese	1 slice	30	2.5	8	1.5	0	5	120	1	0	2	1 fat
14" LARGE FEAST, CLASSIC HAND-TOSSED PIZZAS												
America's Favorite Feast	1 slice	460	23	5	9.5	0	35	1110	48	4	21	3 starch, 2 medium-fat meat, 2 1/2 fat
Bacon Cheeseburger Feast	1 slice	490	24	4	10.5	0	45	1020	46	4	24	3 starch, 2 medium-fat meat, 2 1/2 fat

Barbecue Feast	1 slice	460	20	4	8.5	0	35	970	53	3	21	3 1/2 starch, 1 medium-fat meat, 2 fat
Deluxe Feast	1 slice	420	19	4	8.5	0	25	970	47	4	19	3 starch, 1 medium-fat meat, 2 fat
ExtravaganZZa	1 slice	490	25	5	10.5	0	45	1250	49	4	24	3 1/2 starch, 2 medium-fat meat, 3 fat
Hawaiian Feast	1 slice	420	17	4	7.5	0	30	1020	49	4	20	3 1/2 starch, 1 medium-fat meat, 2 fat
MeatZZa Feast	1 slice	500	26	5	11.5	0	45	1280	48	4	24	3 starch, 2 medium-fat meat, 2 1/2 fat
Pepperoni Feast	1 slice	470	24	5	10.5	0	40	1200	47	4	22	3 starch, 2 medium-fat meat, 2 1/2 fat
Philly Cheese Steak Feast	1 slice	420	18	4	9.5	0	35	940	44	3	21	3 starch, 2 medium-fat meat, 2 fat
Vegi Feast	1 slice	410	17	4	7.5	0	25	950	48	4	19	3 starch, 1 medium-fat meat, 2 fat

✔ = Healthiest Bets

(Continued)

	Amount	Cal.	Fat (g)	% Cal. Fat	Sat. Fat (g)	Trans Fat (g)	Chol. (mg)	Sod. (mg)	Carb. (g)	Fiber (g)	Pro. (g)	Choices/Exchanges
14" LARGE FEAST, CRUNCHY THIN CRUST PIZZAS												
America's Favorite Feast	1 slice	350	24	6	9	0	35	980	26	3	16	1 1/2 starch, 2 medium-fat meat, 2 1/2 fat
Bacon Cheeseburger Feast	1 slice	380	25	6	10	0	45	890	24	3	19	1 1/2 starch, 2 medium-fat meat, 3 fat
Barbecue Feast	1 slice	350	21	5	8	0	35	840	31	2	16	2 starch, 1 medium-fat meat, 2 fat
Deluxe Feast	1 slice	310	20	6	8	0	25	840	25	3	14	1 1/2 starch, 1 medium-fat meat, 2 fat
ExtravaganZZa	1 slice	380	26	6	10	0	45	1120	27	3	19	2 starch, 2 medium-fat meat, 2 1/2 fat
Hawaiian Feast	1 slice	310	18	5	7	0	30	890	27	3	15	2 starch, 1 medium-fat meat, 2 fat

MeatZZa Feast	1 slice	390	27	6	11	0	45	1150	26	3	19	1 1/2 starch, 2 medium-fat meat, 3 fat
Pepperoni Feast	1 slice	360	25	6	10	0	40	1070	25	3	17	1 1/2 starch, 2 medium-fat meat, 2 1/2 fat
Philly Cheese Steak Feast	1 slice	310	19	6	9	0	35	810	22	2	16	1 1/2 starch, 2 medium-fat meat, 2 fat
Vegi Feast	1 slice	300	18	5	7	0	25	820	26	3	14	1 1/2 starch, 1 medium-fat meat, 2 fat
14" LARGE FEAST, ULTIMATE DEEP DISH PIZZAS												
America's Favorite Feast	1 slice	490	28	5	11	0	45	1380	46	6	20	3 starch, 2 medium-fat meat, 3 fat
Bacon Cheeseburger Feast	1 slice	520	29	5	12	0	55	1290	44	6	23	3 starch, 2 medium-fat meat, 3 fat
Barbecue Feast	1 slice	490	25	5	10	0	45	1240	51	5	20	3 1/2 starch, 1 medium-fat meat, 3 fat

✔ = Healthiest Bets

(*Continued*)

14" LARGE FEAST, ULTIMATE DEEP-DISH PIZZAS *(Continued)*	Amount	Cal.	Fat (g)	% Cal. Fat	Sat. Fat (g)	Trans Fat (g)	Chol. (mg)	Sod. (mg)	Carb. (g)	Fiber (g)	Pro. (g)	Choices/Exchanges
Deluxe Feast	1 slice	450	24	5	10	0	35	1240	45	6	18	3 starch, 1 medium-fat meat, 3 fat
ExtravaganZZa	1 slice	520	30	5	12	0	55	1520	47	6	23	3 starch, 2 medium-fat meat, 3 fat
Hawaiian Feast	1 slice	450	22	4	9	0	40	1290	47	6	19	3 starch, 1 medium-fat meat, 3 fat
MeatZZa Feast	1 slice	530	31	5	13	0	55	1550	46	6	23	3 starch, 2 medium-fat meat, 3 1/2 fat
Pepperoni Feast	1 slice	500	29	5	12	0	50	1470	45	6	21	3 starch, 2 medium-fat meat, 3 fat
Philly Cheese Steak Feast	1 slice	450	23	5	11	0	45	1210	42	5	20	3 starch, 2 medium-fat meat, 2 1/2 fat
Vegi Feast	1 slice	440	22	5	9	0	35	1220	46	6	18	3 starch, 1 medium-fat meat, 3 fat

14" LARGE, 1 TOPPING, CLASSIC HAND-TOSSED PIZZAS												
Beef	1 slice	280	12	4	4.5	0	15	590	34	2	13	2 1/2 starch, 1 medium-fat meat, 1 1/2 fat
Black Olives	1 slice	240	8	3	2.5	0	5	550	35	2	10	2 1/2 starch, 1 1/2 fat
Extra Cheese	1 slice	260	10	3	4	0	10	610	35	2	12	2 1/2 starch, 1 medium-fat meat, 1 1/2 fat
Green Peppers	1 slice	230	8	3	2.5	0	5	490	35	2	10	2 1/2 starch, 1 1/2 fat
Ham	1 slice	245	8	3	2.5	0	10	630	34	2	12	2 1/2 starch, 1 medium-fat meat, 1 fat
Mushrooms	1 slice	230	8	3	2.5	0	5	490	35	2	10	2 1/2 starch, 1 1/2 fat
Onions	1 slice	230	7	3	2.5	0	5	490	35	2	10	2 1/2 starch, 1 1/2 fat
Pepperoni	1 slice	280	12	4	4	0	15	680	34	2	12	2 1/2 starch, 1 medium-fat meat, 1 1/2 fat
Pineapple	1 slice	245	8	3	2.5	0	5	490	37	2	10	2 1/2 starch, 1 1/2 fat

✓ = Healthiest Bets

(*Continued*)

14" LARGE, 1 TOPPING, CLASSIC HAND-TOSSED PIZZAS *(Continued)*	Amount	Cal.	Fat (g)	% Cal. Fat	Sat. Fat (g)	Trans Fat (g)	Chol. (mg)	Sod. (mg)	Carb. (g)	Fiber (g)	Pro. (g)	Choices/Exchanges
Sausage	1 slice	290	13	4	4.5	0	15	680	36	3	12	2 1/2 starch, 1 medium-fat meat, 2 fat
14" LARGE, 1 TOPPING CRUNCHY THIN CRUST PIZZAS												
Beef	1 slice	230	14	5	5	0	15	440	20	2	10	1 1/2 starch, 1 medium-fat meat, 2 fat
✔Black Olives	1 slice	190	10	5	3	0	5	400	21	2	7	1 1/2 starch, 2 fat
Extra Cheese	1 slice	210	12	5	4.5	0	10	460	21	2	9	1 1/2 starch, 1 medium-fat meat, 1 1/2 fat
✔Green Peppers	1 slice	180	10	5	3	0	5	340	21	2	7	1 1/2 starch, 2 fat
✔Ham	1 slice	195	10	5	3	0	10	480	20	2	9	1 1/2 starch, 1 medium-fat meat, 1 1/2 fat
✔Mushrooms	1 slice	180	10	5	3	0	5	340	21	2	7	1 1/2 starch, 2 fat
Onions	1 slice	180	10	5	3	0	5	340	21	2	7	1 1/2 starch, 2 fat

Pepperoni	1 slice	230	14	5	4.5	0	15	530	20	2	9	1 1/2 starch, 1 medium-fat meat, 2 fat
✔Pineapple	1 slice	195	10	5	3	0	5	340	23	2	7	1 1/2 starch, 2 fat
Sausage	1 slice	240	15	6	5	0	15	530	22	3	9	1 1/2 starch, 1 medium-fat meat, 2 1/2 fat
14" LARGE, 1 TOPPING, OPTIONAL TOPPINGS												
American Cheese	1 slice	45	4	8	2.5	0	10	220	0	0	2	1 fat
✔Anchovies	1 slice	0	0	0	0	0	0	35	0	0	0	Free
Bacon	1 slice	60	4	6	1.5	0	15	170	0	0	6	1 medium-fat meat
✔Banana Peppers	1 slice	0	0	0	0	0	0	180	1	0	0	Free
Cheddar Cheese	1 slice	35	3	8	2	0	10	55	0	0	2	1 fat
✔Chicken Grilled	1 slice	20	1	5	0	0	10	130	0	0	3	1/2 fat
✔Garlic	1 slice	15	0	0	0	0	0	0	1	0	0	Free
✔Green Chile Peppers	1 slice	0	0	0	0	0	0	0	0	0	0	Free

✔ = Healthiest Bets

(*Continued*)

14" LARGE, 1 TOPPING, OPTIONAL TOPPINGS *(Continued)*	Amount	Cal.	Fat (g)	% Cal. Fat	Sat. Fat (g)	Trans Fat (g)	Chol. (mg)	Sod. (mg)	Carb. (g)	Fiber (g)	Pro. (g)	Choices/Exchanges
✔Green Olive	1 slice	20	2	9	0	0	0	125	1	0	0	1/2 fat
✔Jalapeno	1 slice	0	0	0	0	0	0	135	0	0	0	Free
✔Philly Meat	1 slice	15	1	6	0	0	5	85	0	0	2	Free
Provolone Cheese	1 slice	60	5	8	3	0	10	160	0	0	5	1 medium-fat meat
✔Tomatoes	1 slice	0	0	0	0	0	0	25	1	0	0	Free
14" LARGE, 1 TOPPING, ULTIMATE DEEP DISH PIZZAS												
Beef	1 slice	370	19	5	7	0	25	840	40	5	14	2 1/2 starch, 1 medium-fat meat, 3 fat
Black Olives	1 slice	330	15	4	5	0	15	800	41	5	11	2 1/2 starch, 3 fat
Extra Cheese	1 slice	350	17	4	6.5	0	20	860	41	5	13	2 1/2 starch, 1 medium-fat meat, 2 1/2 fat
Green Peppers	1 slice	320	14	4	5	0	15	740	41	5	11	2 1/2 starch, 3 fat

Ham	1 slice	335	15	4	5	0	20	880	40	5	13	2 1/2 starch, 1 medium-fat meat, 2 fat
Mushrooms	1 slice	320	14	4	5	0	15	740	41	5	11	2 1/2 starch, 3 fat
Onions	1 slice	320	14	4	5	0	15	740	41	5	11	2 1/2 starch, 3 fat
Pepperoni	1 slice	370	19	5	6.5	0	25	930	40	5	13	2 1/2 starch, 1 medium-fat meat, 3 fat
Pineapple	1 slice	335	14	4	5	0	15	740	43	5	11	3 starch, 3 fat
Sausage	1 slice	380	20	5	7	0	25	930	42	6	13	3 starch, 1 medium-fat meat, 3 fat
16" BROOKLYN STYLE PIZZA												
Pepperoni	1 slice	460	11	2	5	1	45	990	43	3	22	3 starch, 2 medium-fat meat, 2 fat
Sausage	1 slice	480	11	2	6	0.5	45	1000	44	3	22	3 starch, 2 medium-fat meat, 2 1/2 fat

✔ = Healthiest Bets

(Continued)

	Amount	Cal.	Fat (g)	% Cal. Fat	Sat. Fat (g)	Trans Fat (g)	Chol. (mg)	Sod. (mg)	Carb. (g)	Fiber (g)	Pro. (g)	Choices/Exchanges
SIDE ITEMS: BREAD												
Breadsticks	1 stick	110	6	5	1.5	0	0	100	11	0	2	1/2 starch, 1 fat
Cheesy Bread	1 stick	120	6	5	2	0	5	150	11	0	4	1/2 starch, 1 fat
Cinna Stix	1 stick	120	6	5	1	0	0	85	14	1	2	1 starch, 1 fat
SIDE ITEMS: BREAD DIPPING SAUCES												
Garlic Dipping Sauce	2 oz.	440	49	10	10	7	0	390	0	0	0	10 fat
✔Marinara Dipping Sauce	2 oz.	25	0	0	0	0	0	260	5	1	1	1/2 carb
Sweet Icing Dipper Cup	2.5 oz.	250	3	1	2.5	0	0	0	57	0	0	4 carb
SIDE ITEMS: CHICKEN												
Barbeque Buffalo Wings	2 pieces	230	14	5	3.5	0	50	410	6	0	17	1/2 starch, 2 lean meat, 1 1/2 fat
✔Buffalo Chicken Kickers	2 pieces	90	3	3	0.5	0	20	90	6	1	9	1/2 starch, 1 lean meat

Hot Buffalo Wings	2 pieces	210	14	6	3.5	0	50	440	5	0	16	1/2 starch, 2 lean meat, 1 1/2 fat
SIDE ITEMS: CHICKEN DIPPING SAUCES												
Blue Cheese Dipping Cup	1.5 oz.	210	22	9	4	0	20	390	2	0	1	4 1/2 fat
Hot Dipping Cup	1.5 oz.	120	12	9	2	0	0	790	3	0	0	3 fat
Ranch Dipping Cup	1.5 oz.	190	21	10	3	0	10	390	2	0	1	4 fat
SIDE ITEMS: SALAD DRESSINGS												
Blue Cheese Dressing	1.5 oz.	230	24	9	5	0	30	450	2	0	2	5 fat
Buttermilk Ranch Dressing	1.5 oz.	220	24	10	4	0	10	420	2	0	1	5 fat
Creamy Caesar Dressing	1.5 oz.	210	22	9	3.5	0	10	510	2	0	1	4 1/2 fat
✔Golden Italian Dressing	1.5 oz.	220	23	9	3.5	0	0	370	2	0	0	4 1/2 fat
✔Light Italian Dressing	1.5 oz.	20	1	5	0	0	0	780	2	0	0	Free

✔ = Healthiest Bets

(Continued)

	Amount	Cal.	Fat (g)	% Cal. Fat	Sat. Fat (g)	Trans Fat (g)	Chol. (mg)	Sod. (mg)	Carb. (g)	Fiber (g)	Pro. (g)	Choices/Exchanges
SIDE ITEMS: SALADS												
✔Garden Fresh Salad	1 salad	70	4	5	2.5	0	10	80	5	2	4	1 veg, 1 fat
✔Grilled Chicken Caesar Salad	1 salad	100	5	5	2	0	20	310	6	2	10	1 veg, 1 lean meat

✔ = Healthiest Bets

Exclusive Web Content

Be sure to visit the following restaurants online at http://www.diabetes.org/healthyrestaurant

Carvel
Del Taco
El Pollo Loco
Frëshens
Godfather's
Jersey Mike's
Jimmy John's
Tim Hortons
Whataburger
Wienerschnitzel
Zaxby's

Fazoli's

(www.fazolis.com)

Light 'n Lean Choice

Penne with Marinara *(small)*
Garden Salad with
Fat-Free Italian Dressing *(1.5 oz, 3 Tbsp)*

Calories	500	Cholesterol (mg)	0
Fat (g)	3	Sodium (mg)	1,190
% calories from fat	5	Carbohydrate (g)	98
Saturated fat (g)	0	Fiber (g)	10
Trans fat (g)	0	Protein (g)	17

Exchanges: 6 starch, 1 veg

Healthy 'n Hearty Choice

Ravioli with Marinara Sauce *(1 regular serving)*
Caesar Salad with
Caesar Dressing *(1/2 serving, 1 1/2 Tbsp)*

Calories	645	Cholesterol (mg)	108
Fat (g)	30	Sodium (mg)	1,455
% calories from fat	42	Carbohydrate (g)	74
Saturated fat (g)	11	Fiber (g)	9
Trans fat (g)	0	Protein (g)	27

Exchanges: 4 1/2 starch, 1 veg, 6 fat

(Continued)

Fazoli's

	Amount	Cal.	Fat (g)	% Cal. Fat	Sat. Fat (g)	Trans Fat (g)	Chol. (mg)	Sod. (mg)	Carb. (g)	Fiber (g)	Pro. (g)	Choices/Exchanges
DESSERTS												
Chocolate Chunk Cookie	1 cookie	510	26	5	15	0	75	350	68	3	5	4 1/2 carb, 4 fat
Chocolate Overload Torte	1 srvg	490	28	5	20	1	15	380	55	3	5	3 1/2 carb, 5 fat
New York Style Cheesecake	1 pc	600	39	6	21	0	115	370	53	1	5	3 1/2 carb, 8 fat
Oatmeal Raisin Cookie	1 cookie	450	16	3	8	0	20	380	70	3	7	4 1/2 carb, 2 fat
Turtle Cheesecake	1 pc	590	37	6	17	0	95	330	56	2	7	3 1/2 carb, 7 fat
DRINKS												
Original Lemon Ice	reg	170	0	0	0	0	0	15	46	0	0	3 carb
Original Lemon Ice	lg	250	0	0	0	0	0	20	65	0	0	4 1/2 carb
Peach Lemon Ice	20.9 oz.	360	0	0	0	0	0	20	90	0	0	6 carb

Pomegranate Lemon Ice	20.9 oz.	360	0	0	0	0	0	20	90	0	0	6 carb
Strawberry Lemon Ice	20.9 oz.	320	0	0	0	0	0	60	81	0	0	5 1/2 carb
Triple Berry Lemon Ice	20.9 oz.	360	0	0	0	0	0	20	91	0	0	6 carb
EXTRAS												
✔Breadstick, Dry	1	100	2	2	0	0	0	160	20	0	3	1 starch, 1/2 fat
Garlic Breadstick	1	150	7	4	1.5	0	0	290	20	1	3	1 starch, 1 1/2 fat
KIDS MEALS												
Cheese Pizza	1 slice	270	11	4	4	0.5	25	700	31	2	13	2 starch, 1 medium-fat meat, 1 fat
✔Fettuccine Alfredo	1 srvg	290	5	2	1.5	0	5	420	50	2	9	3 starch, 1 fat
✔Meat Lasagna	1 srvg	260	13	5	6	0	35	920	21	2	14	1 1/2 starch, 1 medium-fat meat, 1 fat
Pepperoni Pizza	1 slice	310	14	4	5	0.5	30	850	31	2	14	2 starch, 1 medium-fat meat, 1 1/2 fat

✔ = Healthiest Bets

(*Continued*)

KIDS MEALS *(Continued)*	Amount	Cal.	Fat (g)	% Cal. Fat	Sat. Fat (g)	Trans Fat (g)	Chol. (mg)	Sod. (mg)	Carb. (g)	Fiber (g)	Pro. (g)	Choices/Exchanges
✔Ravioli w/ Marinara Sauce	1 srvg	290	7	2	3.5	0	30	580	43	3	13	3 starch, 1 1/2 fat
✔Ravioli w/ Meat Sauce	1 srvg	320	9	3	4	0	35	840	44	4	16	3 starch, 1 medium-fat meat, 1 fat
✔Side of Mandarin Oranges	1 srvg	25	0	0	0	0	0	0	7	1	1	Free
✔Spaghetti w/ Marinara	1 srvg	270	2	1	0	0	0	390	53	4	9	4 starch, 1/2 fat
✔Spaghetti w/ Meat Sauce	1 srvg	300	5	2	1	0	5	570	52	4	12	3 1/2 starch, 1 fat
✔Spaghetti w/ Meatballs	1 srvg	350	7	2	2.5	0	20	620	55	4	14	3 1/2 starch, 1 1/2 fat
✔Ziti w/ Meat Sauce	1 srvg	180	6	3	2.5	0	15	680	23	3	9	1 1/2 starch, 1 medium-fat meat, 1/2 fat
OVEN-BAKED PASTAS												
Baked Spaghetti	1 srvg	680	22	3	9	0.5	65	1480	90	7	32	6 starch, 4 1/2 fat
Baked Spaghetti w/ Meatballs	1 srvg	940	40	4	17	1	120	2370	100	9	46	6 1/2 starch, 4 medium-fat meat, 4 fat

Chicken Broccoli Penne Bake	1 srvg	810	33	4	14	1	145	2630	75	6	58	5 starch, 6 lean meat, 2 fat
Chicken Parmesan	1 srvg	1030	39	3	12	1	115	2700	115	9	55	7 1/2 starch, 5 lean meat, 4 fat
Meat Lasagna	1 srvg	520	26	5	12	0	70	1840	42	5	29	3 starch, 3 medium-fat meat, 2 1/2 fat
Rigatoni Romano	1 srvg	1110	56	5	21	1	140	3360	100	11	54	7 starch, 11 fat
PANINI												
Chicken Parmesan	1 srvg	650	24	3	6	0	65	1770	75	4	36	5 starch, 3 lean meat, 2 1/2 fat
Four Cheese & Tomato	1 srvg	510	22	4	12	0.5	60	960	53	3	28	3 1/2 starch, 2 medium-fat meat, 2 fat
Grilled Chicken	1 srvg	480	14	3	3.5	0	80	1470	55	3	40	3 1/2 starch, 4 lean meat
Smoked Turkey	1 srvg	550	24	4	9	0	85	2150	55	3	35	3 1/2 starch, 3 lean meat, 2 fat

✓ = Healthiest Bets

(*Continued*)

	Amount	Cal.	Fat (g)	% Cal. Fat	Sat. Fat (g)	Trans Fat (g)	Chol. (mg)	Sod. (mg)	Carb. (g)	Fiber (g)	Pro. (g)	Choices/Exchanges
PASTA BOWLS												
Fettuccine w/ Alfredo	sm	520	12	2	4	0	15	1060	83	4	16	6 starch, 2 fat
Fettuccine w/ Alfredo	reg	780	18	2	6	0	20	1600	125	5	24	8 starch, 3 fat
Fettuccine w/ Marinara	sm	450	3	1	0	0	0	770	88	7	15	6 starch, 1/2 fat
Fettuccine w/ Marinara	reg	670	4	1	0	0	0	1160	132	10	23	9 starch, 1/2 fat
Fettuccine w/ Meat Sauce	sm	510	8	1	2	0	15	1150	87	7	21	6 starch, 1 medium-fat meat, 1 fat
Fettuccine w/ Meat Sauce	reg	770	12	1	3.5	0	20	1730	130	10	32	8 1/2 starch, 1 medium-fat meat, 1 fat
Penne w/ Alfredo	sm	520	12	2	4	0	15	1060	83	4	16	6 starch, 2 fat
Penne w/ Alfredo	reg	780	18	2	6	0	25	1600	125	5	24	8 starch, 3 fat
Penne w/ Marinara	sm	450	3	1	0	0	0	770	88	7	15	6 starch
Penne w/ Marinara	reg	670	4	1	0	0	0	1160	132	10	23	9 starch, 1/2 fat

Penne w/ Meat Sauce	sm	510	8	1	2	0	15	1150	87	7	21	6 starch, 1 medium-fat meat, 1 fat
Penne w/ Meat Sauce	reg	770	12	1	3.5	0	20	1730	130	10	32	8 1/2 starch, 1 medium-fat meat, 1 fat
Ravioli w/ Marinara Sauce	1 srvg	490	15	3	8	0	80	1210	69	7	22	5 starch, 3 fat
Ravioli w/ Meat Sauce	1 srvg	570	21	3	10	0	95	1590	70	7	28	4 1/2 starch, 2 medium-fat meat, 1 1/2 fat
Spaghetti w/ Alfredo	sm	520	12	2	4	0	15	1060	83	4	16	6 starch, 2 fat
Spaghetti w/ Alfredo	reg	780	18	2	6	0	25	1600	125	5	24	8 starch, 3 fat
Spaghetti w/ Marinara	sm	450	3	1	0	0	0	770	88	7	15	6 starch
Spaghetti w/ Marinara	reg	670	4	1	0	0	0	1160	132	10	23	9 starch, 1/2 fat
Spaghetti w/ Meat Sauce	sm	510	8	1	2	0	15	1150	87	7	21	6 starch, 1 medium-fat meat, 1 fat
Spaghetti w/ Meat Sauce	reg	770	12	1	3.5	0	20	1730	130	10	32	8 1/2 starch, 1 medium-fat meat, 1 fat

✔ = Healthiest Bets

(*Continued*)

PASTA BOWLS *(Continued)*	Amount	Cal.	Fat (g)	% Cal. Fat	Sat. Fat (g)	Trans Fat (g)	Chol. (mg)	Sod. (mg)	Carb. (g)	Fiber (g)	Pro. (g)	Choices/Exchanges
Ziti w/ Meat Sauce	sm	480	16	3	6	0.5	45	1470	63	6	23	4 starch, 1 medium-fat meat, 1 fat
Ziti w/ Meat Sauce	reg	700	23	3	9	1	65	2240	91	9	35	6 starch, 2 medium-fat meat, 2 fat
PIZZA												
Cheese	1 slice	270	11	4	4	0.5	25	700	31	2	13	2 starch, 1 medium-fat meat, 1 fat
Pepperoni	1 slice	310	14	4	5	0.5	30	850	31	2	14	2 starch, 1 medium-fat meat, 1 1/2 fat
SALAD DRESSINGS & CROUTONS												
Caesar	1.5 oz.	230	25	10	4	0	45	350	1	0	1	5 fat
✔Croutons	1 pkg	70	3	4	0	0	0	100	8	0	2	1 starch, 1/2 fat
✔Fat Free Honey Mustard	1.5 oz.	60	0	0	0	0	0	350	15	1	0	1 carb
✔Fat Free Italian	1.5 oz.	25	0	0	0	0	0	390	6	0	0	1/2 carb

Honey French	1.5 oz.	220	18	7	3	0	0	310	14	0	0	1 carb, 3 1/2 fat
✔Italian	1.5 oz.	160	14	8	2	0	0	760	7	0	0	1/2 carb, 3 fat
✔Lite Ranch	1.5 oz.	120	12	9	2	0	5	350	2	0	1	2 1/2 fat
Ranch	1.5 oz.	220	24	10	4	0	10	420	2	0	1	5 fat
SALADS												
✔Caesar Side	1 srvg	40	2	5	1	0	5	70	4	2	4	1 veg, 1/2 fat
Crispy Chicken & Fruit	1 srvg	450	18	4	3	0	55	1080	49	5	24	1 starch, 2 veg, 3 lean meat, 3 fat
Crispy Chicken & Pasta Caesar	1 srvg	620	30	4	7	0	65	1660	57	5	32	4 starch, 3 lean meat, 4 fat
Crispy Chicken Club	1 srvg	550	32	5	9	0	95	1680	33	4	37	2 starch, 4 lean meat, 4 fat
✔Garden Side	1 srvg	25	0	0	0	0	0	30	4	3	2	1 veg
✔Grilled Chicken & Fruit	1 srvg	220	2	1	0	0	65	780	26	4	27	2 veg, 4 lean meat

✔ = Healthiest Bets

(*Continued*)

SALADS *(Continued)*	Amount	Cal.	Fat (g)	% Cal. Fat	Sat. Fat (g)	Trans Fat (g)	Chol. (mg)	Sod. (mg)	Carb. (g)	Fiber (g)	Pro. (g)	Choices/Exchanges
Grilled Chicken & Pasta Caesar	1 srvg	390	14	3	4	0	75	1370	35	4	34	1 starch, 3 veg, 4 lean meat
Grilled Chicken Club	1 srvg	320	16	5	6	0	105	1380	11	3	40	1/2 starch, 5 lean meat
Pasta Side	1 srvg	250	11	4	2.5	0	5	590	32	1	6	2 starch, 2 fat
SAMPLER PLATTERS												
Classic Sampler	1 srvg	810	25	3	10	0	55	2220	108	8	35	7 starch, 2 medium-fat meat, 3 fat
Ultimate Sampler	1 srvg	990	31	3	12	0.5	70	2900	132	11	44	9 starch, 3 medium-fat meat, 3 fat
SUBMARINOS												
Club	1 srvg	670	29	4	9	0	65	2910	65	3	37	4 1/2 starch, 3 medium-fat meat, 2 fat

Ham n Swiss	1 srvg	620	25	4	7	0	50	2480	65	3	34	4 1/2 starch, 3 lean meat, 2 1/2 fat
Italian Beef	1 srvg	660	24	3	9	0	90	2320	68	3	46	4 1/2 starch, 5 medium-fat meat
Original	1 srvg	880	53	5	16	0	85	3080	68	4	36	4 1/2 starch, 3 medium-fat meat, 7 fat
TOPPINGS												
✔Broccoli	1 srvg	25	0	0	0	0	0	10	5	3	3	1 veg
✔Broccoli & Tomatoes	1 srvg	30	0	0	0	0	0	10	6	3	3	1 veg
✔Garlic Shrimp	1 srvg	160	12	7	2.5	0	45	440	3	1	10	1 lean meat, 1 1/2 fat
Italian Sausage	1 srvg	240	21	8	7	0	45	770	3	1	10	1 medium-fat meat, 3 fat
✔Meatballs	1 srvg	250	18	6	8	0	55	700	6	1	13	1/2 starch, 2 medium-fat meat, 2 fat
✔Peppery Chicken	1 srvg	80	3	3	0.5	0	35	370	1	0	13	2 lean meat

✔ = Healthiest Bets

Little Caesars

(www.littlecaesars.com)

Light 'n Lean Choice

Vegetarian *(2 slices)*

Calories	440	Cholesterol (mg)	30
Fat (g)	18	Sodium (mg)	1,020
% calories from fat	37	Carbohydrate (g)	54
Saturated fat (g)	8	Fiber (g)	4
Trans fat (g)	0	Protein (g)	22

Exchanges: 3 1/2 starch, 1 1/2 medium-fat meat, 2 fat

Healthy 'n Hearty Choice

14" Round Hot-n-Ready Cheese Pizza *(3 slices)*

Calories	600	Cholesterol (mg)	45
Fat (g)	21	Sodium (mg)	1,020
% calories from fat	32	Carbohydrate (g)	75
Saturated fat (g)	10.5	Fiber (g)	3
Trans fat (g)	0	Protein (g)	30

Exchanges: 5 starch, 2 medium-fat meat, 2 fat

Little Caesars

	Amount	Cal.	Fat (g)	% Cal. Fat	Sat. Fat (g)	Trans Fat (g)	Chol. (mg)	Sod. (mg)	Carb. (g)	Fiber (g)	Pro. (g)	Choices/Exchanges
BREADS												
✔Crazy Bread	1 stick	100	3	3	0.5	0	0	150	15	1	3	1 starch, 1/2 fat
✔Italian Cheese Bread	1 pc	130	7	5	2.5	0	10	230	13	0	6	1 starch, 1 1/2 fat
✔Pepperoni Cheese Bread - 10 pcs	1 pc	150	8	5	3	0	15	280	13	0	7	1 starch, 1 medium-fat meat, 1 fat
✔Pepperoni Cheese Bread - 16 pcs	1 pc	160	8	5	3	0	15	280	16	1	7	1 starch, 1 medium-fat meat, 1 fat
CAESAR DIPS												
Buffalo	1	140	14	9	2	0	0	940	4	0	0	1/2 carb, 3 fat
Buffalo Ranch	1	230	24	9	3.5	0	15	520	3	0	0	5 fat

✔ = Healthiest Bets

(*Continued*)

CAESAR DIPS (*Continued*)	Amount	Cal.	Fat (g)	% Cal. Fat	Sat. Fat (g)	Trans Fat (g)	Chol. (mg)	Sod. (mg)	Carb. (g)	Fiber (g)	Pro. (g)	Choices/Exchanges
Buttery Garlic	1	380	42	10	9	0	0	420	0	0	0	8 1/2 fat
Cheezy	1	210	21	9	4	0	15	450	3	0	1	4 fat
Chipotle	1	220	24	10	3.5	0	15	560	2	0	0	5 fat
Ranch	1	250	26	9	4	0	15	380	3	0	0	5 fat
CHURROS												
✔Churros	1 stick	150	4	2	0.5	1.5	0	95	25	1	2	1 1/2 starch, 1/2 fat
CHURROS SAUCE												
✔Chocolate	1	90	3	3	1	0.5	0	60	16	0	0	1 carb, 1/2 fat
✔Dulce De Leche	1	90	3	3	0.5	0.5	0	90	16	0	0	1 carb, 1/2 fat
CRAZY SAUCE												
✔Crazy Sauce	1	45	0	0	0	0	0	260	10	1	2	1/2 carb

PIZZAS

✔14" Round Hot-n-Ready Cheese	1 slice	200	7	3	3.5	0	15	340	25	1	10	1 1/2 starch, 1 medium-fat meat, 1/2 fat
✔14" Round Hot-n-Ready Pepperoni	1 slice	230	9	4	4.5	0	20	420	25	1	11	1 1/2 starch, 1 medium-fat meat, 1 fat
3 Meat Treat	1 slice	280	14	5	6	0	30	590	25	1	14	1 1/2 starch, 1 medium-fat meat, 1 fat
Baby Pan!Pan! Cheese & Pepperoni	1 pan	360	18	5	7	0	35	610	33	1	16	2 starch, 1 medium-fat meat, 2 1/2 fat
Baby Pan!Pan! Just Cheese	1 pan	320	15	4	6	0	25	500	33	1	14	2 starch, 1 medium-fat meat, 2 fat
Deep Dish Just Cheese	1 slice	320	13	4	5	0	25	490	38	1	14	2 1/2 starch, 1 medium-fat meat, 1 fat
Deep Dish Pepperoni	1 slice	360	16	4	6	0	30	610	38	1	16	2 1/2 starch, 1 medium-fat meat, 2 fat

✔ = Healthiest Bets

(*Continued*)

PIZZAS (*Continued*)	Amount	Cal.	Fat (g)	% Cal. Fat	Sat. Fat (g)	Trans Fat (g)	Chol. (mg)	Sod. (mg)	Carb. (g)	Fiber (g)	Pro. (g)	Choices/Exchanges
✔Hula Hawaiian	1 slice	230	8	3	3.5	0	25	500	28	1	12	2 starch, 1 medium-fat meat, 1/2 fat
Ultimate Supreme	1 slice	260	11	4	5	0	25	520	26	1	12	1 1/2 starch, 1 medium-fat meat, 1 fat
✔Vegetarian	1 slice	220	9	4	4	0	15	510	27	2	11	2 starch, 1 medium-fat meat, 1 fat
WINGS												
Barbecue	1 wing	70	4	5	1	0	20	220	3	0	4	1 lean meat, 1 fat
Hot	1 wing	60	5	8	1	0	20	430	1	0	4	1 lean meat, 1/2 fat
Mild	1 wing	60	4	6	1	0	20	290	1	0	4	1 lean meat, 1 fat
Oven Roasted	1 wing	50	4	7	1	0	20	150	0	0	4	1 lean meat, 1/2 fat

✔ = Healthiest Bets

Papa John's Pizza

(www.papajohns.com)

Light 'n Lean Choice

14" Original-Crust Garden Fresh Pizza *(2 slices)*

Calories	560	Cholesterol (mg)	30
Fat (g)	18	Sodium (mg)	1,360
% calories from fat	29	Carbohydrate (g)	78
Saturated fat (g)	5	Fiber (g)	4
Trans fat (g)	0	Protein (g)	22

Exchanges: 5 starch, 3 1/2 fat

Healthy 'n Hearty Choice

14" Original Crust Spinach Alfredo Chicken Tomato Pizza *(3 slices)*

Calories	600	Cholesterol (mg)	50
Fat (g)	22	Sodium (mg)	1,400
% calories from fat	33	Carbohydrate (g)	74
Saturated fat (g)	9	Fiber (g)	4
Trans fat (g)	0	Protein (g)	28

Exchanges: 5 starch, 1 veg, 2 medium-fat meat, 2 fat

(Continued)

Papa John's Pizza

	Amount	Cal.	Fat (g)	% Cal. Fat	Sat. Fat (g)	Trans Fat (g)	Chol. (mg)	Sod. (mg)	Carb. (g)	Fiber (g)	Pro. (g)	Choices/Exchanges
10" ORIGINAL CRUST PIZZAS												
BBQ Chicken & Bacon Pizza	1 slice	220	8	3	2.5	0	20	640	30	1	10	2 starch, 1 medium-fat meat, 1 fat
✔Cheese	1 slice	180	6	3	1.5	0	10	430	25	1	7	1 1/2 starch, 1 fat
✔Chicken Bacon Ranch	1 slice	220	10	4	2.5	0	20	470	26	1	10	1 1/2 starch, 1 medium-fat meat, 1 fat
✔Garden Fresh	1 slice	180	6	3	1.5	0	10	460	26	1	8	1 1/2 starch, 1 fat
Hawaiian BBQ Chicken	1 slice	230	8	3	2.5	0	20	640	31	1	10	2 starch, 1 medium-fat meat, 1 fat
Italian Meats Trio	1 slice	170	6	3	3	0	15	510	19	1	8	1 1/2 starch, 1 medium-fat meat, 1/2 fat

The Meats	1 slice	230	11	4	3.5	0	20	620	25	1	10	1 1/2 starch, 1 medium-fat meat, 1 1/2 fat
✔Papa's White	1 slice	190	7	3	2.5	0	15	490	25	1	8	1 1/2 starch, 1 1/2 fat
Pepperoni	1 slice	210	9	4	2.5	0	15	540	25	1	9	1 1/2 starch, 1 medium-fat meat, 1 fat
Sausage	1 slice	220	10	4	3	0	15	540	25	2	8	1 1/2 starch, 2 fat
Sicilian Classic Pizza	1 slice	240	9	3	4.5	0	20	700	26	2	10	1 1/2 starch, 1 medium-fat meat, 1 fat
Smokehouse Bacon & Ham	1 slice	220	9	4	2.5	0	20	590	26	1	10	1 1/2 starch, 1 medium-fat meat, 1 fat
Spicy Italian	1 slice	230	7	3	5	0	20	600	26	2	9	1 1/2 starch, 1 medium-fat meat, 1 fat
✔Spinach Alfredo	1 slice	190	7	3	3	0	15	420	24	1	8	1 1/2 starch, 1 1/2 fat
✔Spinach Alfredo Chicken Tomato	1 slice	200	8	4	3	0	20	470	25	1	9	1 1/2 starch, 1 medium-fat meat, 1 fat

✔ = Healthiest Bets

(Continued)

10" ORIGINAL CRUST PIZZAS *(Continued)*	Amount	Cal.	Fat (g)	% Cal. Fat	Sat. Fat (g)	Trans Fat (g)	Chol. (mg)	Sod. (mg)	Carb. (g)	Fiber (g)	Pro. (g)	Choices/Exchanges
Tuscan Six Cheese	1 slice	210	8	3	3	0	15	530	26	1	10	1 1/2 starch, 1 medium-fat meat, 1 fat
The Works	1 slice	220	8	3	4	0	15	610	26	2	9	1 1/2 starch, 1 medium-fat meat, 1 fat
12" ORIGINAL CRUST PIZZAS												
BBQ Chicken & Bacon Pizza	1 slice	240	8	3	2.5	0	20	690	32	1	11	2 starch, 1 medium-fat meat, 1 fat
Cheese	1 slice	210	8	3	2.5	0	15	510	27	1	9	2 starch, 1 medium-fat meat, 1 fat
✔Chicken Bacon Ranch	1 slice	240	10	4	2.5	0	20	500	27	1	11	2 starch, 1 medium-fat meat, 1 fat
✔Garden Fresh	1 slice	200	7	3	2	0	10	490	28	2	8	2 starch, 1 1/2 fat
Hawaiian BBQ Chicken	1 slice	240	8	3	2.5	0	20	690	33	1	11	2 starch, 1 medium-fat meat, 1 fat

Italian Meats Trio	1 slice	250	8	3	5	0	25	740	27	2	12	2 starch, 1 medium-fat meat, 1/2 fat
The Meats	1 slice	240	11	4	3.5	0	20	640	26	1	11	1 1/2 starch, 1 medium-fat meat, 1 1/2 fat
Papa's White	1 slice	200	8	4	2.5	0	15	520	26	1	8	1 1/2 starch, 1 1/2 fat
Pepperoni	1 slice	220	9	4	3	0	15	580	26	1	9	1 1/2 starch, 1 medium-fat meat, 1 1/2 fat
Sausage	1 slice	240	11	4	3.5	0	15	580	26	2	9	1 1/2 starch, 1 medium-fat meat, 1 1/2 fat
Sicilian Classic Pizza	1 slice	260	10	3	5	0	25	770	27	2	12	2 starch, 1 medium-fat meat, 1 fat
Smokehouse Bacon & Ham	1 slice	240	9	3	3	0	20	640	27	1	11	2 starch, 1 medium-fat meat, 1 fat
Spicy Italian	1 slice	260	8	3	7	0	20	680	27	2	11	2 starch, 1 medium-fat meat, 1 fat

✓ = Healthiest Bets

(Continued)

12" ORIGINAL CRUST PIZZAS *(Continued)*	Amount	Cal.	Fat (g)	% Cal. Fat	Sat. Fat (g)	Trans Fat (g)	Chol. (mg)	Sod. (mg)	Carb. (g)	Fiber (g)	Pro. (g)	Choices/Exchanges
✔Spinach Alfredo	1 slice	210	8	3	3	0	15	450	26	1	8	1 1/2 starch, 1 1/2 fat
✔Spinach Alfredo Chicken Tomato	1 slice	220	8	3	3.5	0	20	500	26	1	10	1 1/2 starch, 1 medium-fat meat, 1 fat
Tuscan Six Cheese	1 slice	230	9	4	3.5	0	20	570	27	1	11	2 starch, 1 medium-fat meat, 1 fat
The Works	1 slice	230	8	3	3.5	0	15	610	28	2	10	2 starch, 1 medium-fat meat, 1 fat
12" PAN CRUST PIZZAS												
BBQ Chicken & Bacon Pizza	1 slice	430	22	5	7	0	30	940	43	1	15	3 starch, 1 medium-fat meat, 3 fat
Cheese	1 slice	410	23	5	7	0	20	750	38	1	13	2 1/2 starch, 1 medium-fat meat, 4 fat
Chicken Bacon Ranch	1 slice	430	25	5	7	0	25	680	37	1	15	2 1/2 starch, 1 medium-fat meat, 4 fat

Garden Fresh	1 slice	370	19	5	6	0	15	660	39	2	11	2 1/2 starch, 4 fat
Hawaiian BBQ Chicken	1 slice	440	22	5	7	0	30	940	45	1	15	3 starch, 1 medium-fat meat, 3 fat
Italian Meats Trio	1 slice	440	21	4	11	0	30	1040	38	2	16	2 1/2 starch, 1 medium-fat meat, 3 fat
The Meats	1 slice	440	26	5	8	0	30	890	37	1	15	2 1/2 starch, 1 medium-fat meat, 4 fat
Papa's White	1 slice	370	21	5	7	0	20	700	35	1	11	2 1/2 starch, 1 medium-fat meat, 3 fat
Pepperoni	1 slice	410	24	5	8	0	20	820	37	1	13	2 1/2 starch, 1 medium-fat meat, 4 fat
Sausage	1 slice	420	25	5	8	0	20	790	37	2	12	2 1/2 starch, 1 medium-fat meat, 4 fat
Sicilian Classic Pizza	1 slice	450	23	5	11	0	35	1040	37	2	16	2 1/2 starch, 1 medium-fat meat, 3 1/2 fat

✔ = Healthiest Bets

(*Continued*)

12" PAN CRUST PIZZAS *(Continued)*	Amount	Cal.	Fat (g)	% Cal. Fat	Sat. Fat (g)	Trans Fat (g)	Chol. (mg)	Sod. (mg)	Carb. (g)	Fiber (g)	Pro. (g)	Choices/Exchanges
Smokehouse Bacon & Ham	1 slice	420	23	5	7	0	30	870	38	1	15	2 1/2 starch, 1 medium-fat meat, 3 fat
Spicy Italian	1 slice	470	21	4	14	0	30	950	38	3	15	2 1/2 starch, 1 medium-fat meat, 4 fat
Spinach Alfredo	1 slice	380	22	5	8	0	20	610	35	1	12	2 1/2 starch, 1 medium-fat meat, 3 fat
Spinach Alfredo Chicken Tomato	1 slice	390	22	5	8	0	25	660	36	2	13	2 1/2 starch, 1 medium-fat meat, 3 fat
Tuscan Six Cheese	1 slice	410	23	5	8	0	25	760	37	1	15	2 1/2 starch, 1 medium-fat meat, 3 fat
The Works	1 slice	420	21	5	9	0	25	860	38	2	14	2 1/2 starch, 1 medium-fat meat, 3 1/2 fat

14" ORIGINAL CRUST PIZZAS												
BBQ Chicken & Bacon Pizza	1 slice	340	11	3	3.5	0	30	960	44	2	15	3 starch, 1 medium-fat meat, 1 fat
Cheese	1 slice	300	11	3	3.5	0	20	750	39	2	13	2 1/2 starch, 1 medium-fat meat, 1 1/2 fat
Chicken Bacon Ranch	1 slice	340	14	4	3.5	0	25	700	38	2	15	2 1/2 starch, 1 medium-fat meat, 1 1/2 fat
Garden Fresh	1 slice	280	9	3	2.5	0	15	680	39	2	11	2 1/2 starch, 2 fat
Hawaiian BBQ Chicken	1 slice	340	11	3	3.5	0	30	960	46	2	16	3 starch, 1 medium-fat meat, 1 fat
Italian Meats Trio	1 slice	340	11	3	7	0	30	1030	38	2	16	2 1/2 starch, 1 medium-fat meat, 1 fat
The Meats	1 slice	350	16	4	5	0	30	930	38	2	15	2 1/2 starch, 1 medium-fat meat, 2 fat

✔ = Healthiest Bets

(*Continued*)

14" ORIGINAL CRUST PIZZAS *(Continued)*	Amount	Cal.	Fat (g)	% Cal. Fat	Sat. Fat (g)	Trans Fat (g)	Chol. (mg)	Sod. (mg)	Carb. (g)	Fiber (g)	Pro. (g)	Choices/Exchanges
Papa's White	1 slice	280	10	3	3.5	0	20	720	37	1	12	2 1/2 starch, 1 medium-fat meat, 1 fat
Pepperoni	1 slice	310	13	4	4	0	20	810	38	2	13	2 1/2 starch, 1 medium-fat meat, 2 fat
Sausage	1 slice	330	15	4	4.5	0	20	810	37	3	13	2 1/2 starch, 1 medium-fat meat, 2 fat
Sicilian Classic Pizza	1 slice	360	13	3	7	0	35	1060	38	3	16	2 1/2 starch, 1 medium-fat meat, 1 1/2 fat
Smokehouse Bacon & Ham	1 slice	330	13	4	3.5	0	30	890	39	2	16	2 1/2 starch, 1 medium-fat meat, 1 fat
Spicy Italian	1 slice	370	11	3	10	0	30	960	38	4	15	2 1/2 starch, 1 medium-fat meat, 1 fat
Spinach Alfredo	1 slice	280	11	4	4.5	0	20	630	36	2	11	2 1/2 starch, 1 medium-fat meat, 1 fat

Spinach Alfredo Chicken Tomato	1 slice	300	11	3	4.5	0	25	700	37	2	14	2 1/2 starch, 1 medium-fat meat, 1 fat
Tuscan Six Cheese	1 slice	320	13	4	4.5	0	25	780	38	2	15	2 1/2 starch, 1 medium-fat meat, 1 fat
The Works	1 slice	330	11	3	6	0	25	890	39	3	14	2 1/2 starch, 1 medium-fat meat, 1 1/2 fat
14" THIN CRUST PIZZAS												
BBQ Chicken & Bacon Pizza	1 slice	290	14	4	3.5	0	30	740	29	< 1	13	2 starch, 1 medium-fat meat, 2 fat
Cheese	1 slice	240	13	5	3.5	0	20	500	22	1	10	1 1/2 starch, 1 medium-fat meat, 2 fat
Chicken Bacon Ranch	1 slice	270	16	5	4	0	25	490	21	1	12	1 1/2 starch, 1 medium-fat meat, 2 fat
✔Garden Fresh	1 slice	210	11	5	2.5	0	15	430	23	2	8	1 1/2 starch, 2 fat
Hawaiian BBQ Chicken	1 slice	290	14	4	3.5	0	30	740	31	1	13	2 starch, 1 medium-fat meat, 2 fat

✔ = Healthiest Bets

(*Continued*)

14" THIN CRUST PIZZAS *(Continued)*	Amount	Cal.	Fat (g)	% Cal. Fat	Sat. Fat (g)	Trans Fat (g)	Chol. (mg)	Sod. (mg)	Carb. (g)	Fiber (g)	Pro. (g)	Choices/Exchanges
Italian Meats Trio	1 slice	280	12	4	7	0	30	820	22	2	13	1 1/2 starch, 1 medium-fat meat, 1 1/2 fat
The Meats	1 slice	300	18	5	5	0	30	700	23	2	13	1 1/2 starch, 1 medium-fat meat, 2 fat
Papa's White	1 slice	220	12	5	4	0	20	510	20	1	9	1 1/2 starch, 1 medium-fat meat, 1 1/2 fat
Pepperoni	1 slice	260	15	5	4.5	0	20	580	23	1	10	1 1/2 starch, 1 medium-fat meat, 2 fat
Sausage	1 slice	280	17	5	5	0	20	590	22	2	10	1 1/2 starch, 1 medium-fat meat, 2 1/2 fat
Sicilian Classic Pizza	1 slice	290	14	4	8	0	35	850	21	2	13	1 1/2 starch, 1 medium-fat meat, 2 fat
Smokehouse Bacon & Ham	1 slice	260	14	5	4	0	30	680	22	1	12	1 1/2 starch, 1 medium-fat meat, 1 1/2 fat

Spicy Italian	1 slice	320	14	4	11	0	30	740	24	3	12	1 1/2 starch, 1 medium-fat meat, 2 fat
Spinach Alfredo	1 slice	220	13	5	4.5	0	20	370	19	1	8	1 1/2 starch, 1 medium-fat meat, 2 fat
Spinach Alfredo Chicken Tomato	1 slice	230	13	5	4.5	0	25	430	21	1	10	1 1/2 starch, 1 medium-fat meat, 2 fat
Tuscan Six Cheese	1 slice	250	14	5	5	0	25	570	21	1	12	1 1/2 starch, 1 medium-fat meat, 1 fat
The Works	1 slice	280	14	5	6	0	25	670	24	2	12	1 1/2 starch, 1 medium-fat meat, 2 fat
16" ORIGINAL CRUST PIZZAS												
BBQ Chicken & Bacon Pizza	1 slice	370	13	3	4	0	30	1050	48	2	17	3 starch, 1 medium-fat meat, 1 fat
Cheese	1 slice	310	11	3	3.5	0	20	760	41	2	13	2 1/2 starch, 1 medium-fat meat, 1 fat

✓ = Healthiest Bets

(*Continued*)

16" ORIGINAL CRUST PIZZAS *(Continued)*	Amount	Cal.	Fat (g)	% Cal. Fat	Sat. Fat (g)	Trans Fat (g)	Chol. (mg)	Sod. (mg)	Carb. (g)	Fiber (g)	Pro. (g)	Choices/Exchanges
Chicken Bacon Ranch	1 slice	370	16	4	4.5	0	30	790	41	2	17	2 1/2 starch, 1 medium-fat meat, 2 fat
Garden Fresh	1 slice	310	10	3	3	0	15	760	43	2	13	3 starch, 1 medium-fat meat, 1 fat
Hawaiian BBQ Chicken	1 slice	370	13	3	4	0	30	1010	48	2	17	3 starch, 1 medium-fat meat, 1 fat
Italian Meats Trio	1 slice	380	12	3	8	0	35	1160	41	3	18	2 1/2 starch, 1 medium-fat meat, 1 1/2 fat
The Meats	1 slice	390	18	4	6	0	35	1040	41	2	17	2 1/2 starch, 1 medium-fat meat, 2 fat
Papa's White	1 slice	310	12	3	4	0	25	810	40	1	13	2 1/2 starch, 1 medium-fat meat, 1 fat
Pepperoni	1 slice	350	15	4	5	0	25	910	41	2	15	2 1/2 starch, 1 medium-fat meat, 2 fat

Sausage	1 slice	370	18	4	5	0	25	910	41	3	14	2 1/2 starch, 1 medium-fat meat, 3 fat
Sicilian Classic Pizza	1 slice	400	15	3	8	0	40	1190	41	3	18	2 1/2 starch, 1 medium-fat meat, 1 1/2 fat
Smokehouse Bacon & Ham	1 slice	370	15	4	4.5	0	35	1010	42	2	18	3 starch, 1 medium-fat meat, 1 fat
Spicy Italian	1 slice	410	13	3	11	0	35	1070	42	4	17	3 starch, 1 medium-fat meat, 2 fat
Spinach Alfredo	1 slice	320	13	4	5	0	25	710	39	2	13	2 1/2 starch, 1 medium-fat meat, 2 fat
Spinach Alfredo Chicken Tomato	1 slice	340	13	3	5	0	30	790	41	2	16	2 1/2 starch, 1 medium-fat meat, 1 1/2 fat
Tuscan Six Cheese	1 slice	340	13	3	5	0	25	820	41	2	16	2 1/2 starch, 1 medium-fat meat, 1 1/2 fat
The Works	1 slice	370	13	3	7	0	30	1000	42	3	16	3 starch, 1 medium-fat meat, 1 1/2 fat

✔ = Healthiest Bets

(Continued)

	Amount	Cal.	Fat (g)	% Cal. Fat	Sat. Fat (g)	Trans Fat (g)	Chol. (mg)	Sod. (mg)	Carb. (g)	Fiber (g)	Pro. (g)	Choices/Exchanges
BREADSTICKS												
Garlic Parmesan	2 sticks	330	10	3	1.5	0	0	720	54	2	10	3 1/2 starch, 2 fat
Plain	2 sticks	290	5	2	0.5	0	0	540	53	2	9	3 1/2 starch, 1 fat
Whole Wheat	2 sticks	270	5	2	0.5	0	0	500	53	8	8	3 1/2 starch, 1 fat
DESSERTS												
Apple Twist Sweetreat	2 slices	380	16	4	4	0	0	530	54	1	5	3 1/2 carb, 2 fat
Chocolate Pastry Delights	1 pastry	180	11	6	6	0	5	140	18	1	2	1 carb, 2 fat
Cinna Swirl Sweetreat	2 slices	420	21	5	5	0	0	570	53	1	5	3 1/2 carb, 3 fat
Cinnamon Sweetsticks	4 sticks	570	15	2	3	0	0	750	98	3	12	6 1/2 carb, 2 fat
DIPPING SAUCES												
✔Barbeque Sauce	1 cup	40	0	0	0	0	0	240	11	0	0	1/2 carb
Blue Cheese	1 cup	170	18	10	3.5	0	20	240	1	0	1	3 1/2 fat

Buffalo Sauce	1 cup	15	0.5	3	0	0	0	890	2	0	0	Free
Cheese Sauce	1 cup	70	6	8	1.5	0	0	150	1	0	1	1 1/2 fat
Honey Mustard	1 cup	150	15	9	2	0	10	120	5	0	0	1/2 carb, 3 fat
✔Pizza Sauce	1 cup	20	0	0	0	0	0	140	3	0	0	Free
Ranch Sauce	1 cup	110	11	9	2	0	10	250	1	0	1	2 fat
Special Garlic	1 cup	150	17	10	3	0	0	310	0	0	0	3 1/2 fat
SEASONINGS												
✔Crushed Red Pepper	1 pkt	5	0	0	0	n/a	n/a	0	1	0	0	Free
✔Parmesan Cheese	1 pkt	15	1	6	0.5	n/a	5	45	0	0	n/a	Free
✔Special Seasonings	1 pkt	5	0	0	0	n/a	0	410	1	0	0	Free
SIDES												
BBQ Wings	2 wings	200	12	5	3.5	0	105	700	6	0	17	1/2 starch, 2 lean meat, 1 fat

✔ = Healthiest Bets

(*Continued*)

SIDES *(Continued)*	Amount	Cal.	Fat (g)	% Cal. Fat	Sat. Fat (g)	Trans Fat (g)	Chol. (mg)	Sod. (mg)	Carb. (g)	Fiber (g)	Pro. (g)	Choices/Exchanges
Buffalo Wings	2 wings	200	14	6	4	0	110	840	1	1	18	3 lean meat, 1 1/2 fat
Cheesesticks	4 sticks	370	16	4	4.5	0	25	830	42	2	15	3 starch, 1 medium-fat meat, 2 fat
Chickenstrips	2 strips	160	8	5	2	0	25	350	10	0	10	1/2 starch, 1 lean meat, 1 fat

✔ = Healthiest Bets

Exclusive Web Content

Be sure to visit the following restaurants online at http://www.diabetes.org/healthyrestaurant

Carvel
Del Taco
El Pollo Loco
Frëshens
Godfather's
Jersey Mike's
Jimmy John's
Tim Hortons
Whataburger
Wienerschnitzel
Zaxby's

Papa Murphy's Take 'N' Bake

(www.papamurphys.com)

Light 'n Lean Choice

Lasagna *(1 serving)*
Garden Salad
(1 serving, no dressing info included)

Calories	355	Cholesterol (mg)	46
Fat (g)	20	Sodium (mg)	941
% calories from fat	50	Carbohydrate (g)	25
Saturated fat (g)	10	Fiber (g)	6
Trans fat (g)	1	Protein (g)	20

Exchanges: 1 starch, 2 veg, 2 medium-fat meat, 2 fat

Healthy 'n Hearty Choice

Large (14") Original Crust Pizza,
Vegetarian Combo *(3 slices)*

Calories	780	Cholesterol (mg)	78
Fat (g)	33	Sodium (mg)	2,025
% calories from fat	38	Carbohydrate (g)	87
Saturated fat (g)	15	Fiber (g)	3
Trans fat (g)	0	Protein (g)	36

Exchanges: 6 starch, 1 veg, 2 1/2 medium-fat meat, 3 fat

(Continued)

Papa Murphy's Take 'n' Bake

	Amount	Cal.	Fat (g)	% Cal. Fat	Sat. Fat (g)	Trans Fat (g)	Chol. (mg)	Sod. (mg)	Carb. (g)	Fiber (g)	Pro. (g)	Choices/Exchanges
BREADS												
Cheesy Bread	2 slices	220	8	3	3	0	7	489	31	1	7	2 starch, 1 1/2 fat
DESSERT PIZZAS W/O ICING												
Apple	1 slice	245	5	2	1.5	1	1	335	46	2	4	3 carb, 1 fat
Cherry	1 slice	235	5	2	1.5	1	1	335	44	1	5	3 carb, 1 fat
DESSERTS												
Chocolate Chip Cookies	1 srvg	245	11	4	3.5	2	9	225	34	1	3	2 1/2 carb, 2 fat
Cinnamon Rolls w/o icing	1 roll	344	10	3	3.8	0	0	577	58	1	6	4 carb, 2 fat
Cinnamon Wheel w/o frosting	2 slices	250	7	3	2.2	0	0	415	42	1	5	3 carb, 1 1/2 fat

FAMILY SIZE (16") ORIGINAL CRUST PIZZAS

Barbecue Chicken	1 slice	334	12	3	6	0	46	785	36	1	19	2 1/2 starch, 2 medium-fat meat, 1 fat
Cheese	1 slice	260	10	3	5.5	0	28	625	29	1	12	2 starch, 1 medium-fat meat, 1 fat
Cowboy	1 slice	340	17	5	8	0	37	965	31	1	17	2 starch, 2 medium-fat meat, 2 fat
Gourmet Chicken Garlic	1 slice	320	14	4	6.5	0	44	687	30	1	18	2 starch, 2 medium-fat meat, 1 fat
Gourmet Classic Italian	1 slice	352	18	5	8	0	38	850	31	1	17	2 starch, 1 medium-fat meat, 2 fat
Gourmet Vegetarian	1 slice	302	13	4	6	0	31	692	31	1	14	2 starch, 1 medium-fat meat, 1 1/2 fat
Hawaiian	1 slice	285	11	3	6	0	35	735	33	1	14	2 starch, 1 medium-fat meat, 1 fat
Herb Chicken Mediterranean	1 slice	338	15	4	6	0	37	737	35	2	17	2 1/2 starch, 1 medium-fat meat, 1 fat

✔ = Healthiest Bets

(*Continued*)

FAMILY SIZE (16") ORIGINAL CRUST PIZZAS *(Continued)*	Amount	Cal.	Fat (g)	% Cal. Fat	Sat. Fat (g)	Trans Fat (g)	Chol. (mg)	Sod. (mg)	Carb. (g)	Fiber (g)	Pro. (g)	Choices/Exchanges
Murphy's Combination	1 slice	355	18	5	8	0	40	1010	31	1	17	2 starch, 2 medium-fat meat, 2 fat
Papa-Roni Signature	1 slice	340	17	5	8	0	47	885	29	1	16	2 starch, 1 medium-fat meat, 2 fat
Papa's All Meat	1 slice	350	17	4	8	0	50	1000	30	1	18	2 starch, 2 medium-fat meat, 1 1/2 fat
Papa's Favorite	1 slice	355	18	5	8	0	40	1005	31	1	17	2 starch, 2 medium-fat meat, 2 fat
Pepperoni	1 slice	310	15	4	7	0	40	785	29	1	14	2 starch, 1 medium-fat meat, 2 fat
Rancher	1 slice	325	15	4	7	0	44	890	30	1	17	2 starch, 2 medium-fat meat, 1 fat
Specialty of the House	1 slice	310	14	4	7	0	30	870	31	1	15	2 starch, 1 medium-fat meat, 1 1/2 fat

Vegetarian Combo	1 slice	285	12	4	6	0	28	740	32	1	13	2 starch, 1 medium-fat meat, 1 fat
Veggie Mediterranean	1 slice	320	14	4	6	0	27	705	34	2	13	2 1/2 starch, 1 medium-fat meat, 2 fat
FAMILY SIZE CALZONES												
Chicken Florentine	1 srvg	457	19	4	8	0	56	1042	46	1	25	3 starch, 2 medium-fat meat, 1 fat
Combo	1 srvg	434	19	4	9.5	0	50	1020	45	1	21	3 starch, 2 medium-fat meat, 2 fat
Italian	1 srvg	449	20	4	9	0	37	1180	46	1	22	3 starch, 2 medium-fat meat, 1 1/2 fat
Veggie	1 srvg	390	16	4	7.5	0	35	965	45	2	18	3 starch, 1 medium-fat meat, 2 fat
FAMILY SIZE STUFFED PIZZAS												
5-Meat	1 slice	365	16	4	7.2	0	40	984	38	1	18	2 1/2 starch, 1 medium-fat meat, 1 fat

✓ = Healthiest Bets

(*Continued*)

FAMILY SIZE STUFFED PIZZAS *(Continued)*	Amount	Cal.	Fat (g)	% Cal. Fat	Sat. Fat (g)	Trans Fat (g)	Chol. (mg)	Sod. (mg)	Carb. (g)	Fiber (g)	Pro. (g)	Choices/Exchanges
Big Murphy	1 slice	360	16	4	7	0	32	960	40	1	17	2 1/2 starch, 1 medium-fat meat, 2 fat
Chicago-Style	1 slice	365	16	4	7	0	37	935	38	1	17	2 1/2 starch, 1 medium-fat meat, 2 fat
Chicken & Bacon	1 slice	373	15	4	6.5	0	47	875	38	1	20	2 1/2 starch, 2 medium-fat meat, 1 1/2 fat
LARGE (14") ORIGINAL CRUST PIZZAS												
Barbecue Chicken	1 slice	308	11	3	5.5	0	42	734	35	1	17	2 1/2 starch, 1 medium-fat meat, 1 fat
Cheese	1 slice	240	10	4	5	0	26	565	26	1	11	1 1/2 starch, 1 medium-fat meat, 1 fat
Cowboy	1 slice	310	16	5	7	0	34	880	28	1	15	2 starch, 1 medium-fat meat, 1 1/2 fat

Gourmet Chicken Garlic	1 slice	291	12	4	5.7	0	40	626	27	1	16	2 starch, 2 medium-fat meat, 1 fat
Gourmet Classic Italian	1 slice	315	16	5	7	0	34	760	27	1	15	2 starch, 1 medium-fat meat, 2 fat
Gourmet Vegetarian	1 slice	273	12	4	5.5	0	28	625	28	1	13	2 starch, 1 medium-fat meat, 1 1/2 fat
Hawaiian	1 slice	255	10	4	5	0	30	665	29	1	13	2 starch, 1 medium-fat meat, 1 fat
Herb Chicken Mediterranean	1 slice	300	13	4	5.5	0	33	662	31	2	15	2 starch, 1 medium-fat meat, 1 1/2 fat
Murphy's Combination	1 slice	320	16	5	7.5	0	37	915	28	1	16	2 starch, 1 medium-fat meat, 2 fat
Papa's All Meat	1 slice	315	16	5	7.5	0	42	880	27	1	17	2 starch, 2 medium-fat meat, 1 1/2 fat
Papa's Favorite	1 slice	320	16	5	7	0	35	910	28	1	16	2 starch, 1 medium-fat meat, 1 1/2 fat

✓ = Healthiest Bets

(*Continued*)

LARGE (14") ORIGINAL CRUST PIZZAS *(Continued)*	Amount	Cal.	Fat (g)	% Cal. Fat	Sat. Fat (g)	Trans Fat (g)	Chol. (mg)	Sod. (mg)	Carb. (g)	Fiber (g)	Pro. (g)	Choices/Exchanges
Pepperoni	1 slice	280	14	5	6.5	0	37	710	26	1	13	1 1/2 starch, 1 medium-fat meat, 1 1/2 fat
Rancher	1 slice	290	14	4	6.5	0	40	795	27	1	15	2 starch, 1 medium-fat meat, 1 1/2 fat
Specialty of the House	1 slice	290	14	4	6.5	0	27	800	28	1	15	2 starch, 1 medium-fat meat, 1 fat
Vegetarian Combo	1 slice	260	11	4	5	0	26	675	29	1	12	2 starch, 1 medium-fat meat, 1 fat
Veggie Mediterranean	1 slice	285	13	4	5.5	0	25	640	31	2	12	2 starch, 1 medium-fat meat, 1 fat
LARGE (14") THIN CRUST DELITE PIZZAS												
✔Barbecue Chicken	1 slice	181	8	4	4	0	30	379	17	1	11	1 starch, 1 medium-fat meat, 1/2 fat
✔Cheese	1 slice	140	7	5	3.5	0	20	270	13	1	8	1 starch, 1 medium-fat meat, 1/2 fat

Cowboy	1 slice	190	11	5	5	0	24	510	13	1	11	1 starch, 1 medium-fat meat, 1 fat
✔Gourmet Chicken Bacon Artichoke	1 slice	181	9	4	4	0	30	400	13	1	12	1 starch, 1 medium-fat meat, 1/2 fat
✔Gourmet Chicken Garlic	1 slice	172	9	5	4	0	28	315	13	1	11	1 starch, 1 medium-fat meat, 1/2 fat
✔Gourmet Classic Italian	1 slice	180	10	5	5	0	24	430	13	1	10	1 starch, 1 medium-fat meat, 1 fat
✔Gourmet Vegetarian	1 slice	161	8	4	4	0	21	313	13	1	8	1 starch, 1 medium-fat meat, 1 fat
✔Hawaiian	1 slice	150	7	4	3.5	0	22	335	15	1	9	1 starch, 1 medium-fat meat, 1/2 fat
✔Herb Chicken Mediterranean	1 slice	180	9	5	4	0	24	341	16	2	10	1 starch, 1 medium-fat meat, 1 fat
Meat	1 slice	190	11	5	5	0	27	465	13	1	11	1 starch, 1 medium-fat meat, 1 fat

✔ = Healthiest Bets

(*Continued*)

LARGE (14") THIN CRUST DELITE PIZZAS *(Continued)*	Amount	Cal.	Fat (g)	% Cal. Fat	Sat. Fat (g)	Trans Fat (g)	Chol. (mg)	Sod. (mg)	Carb. (g)	Fiber (g)	Pro. (g)	Choices/Exchanges
Murphy's Combination	1 slice	195	12	6	5	0	27	535	14	1	11	1 starch, 1 medium-fat meat, 1 fat
Papa's All Meat	1 slice	187	11	5	5	0	30	485	13	1	11	1 starch, 1 medium-fat meat, 1 fat
Papa's Favorite	1 slice	195	11	5	5	0	25	520	14	1	11	1 starch, 1 medium-fat meat, 1 fat
✔Pepperoni	1 slice	165	9	5	4.5	0	26	365	13	1	9	1 starch, 1 medium-fat meat, 1 fat
✔Rancher	1 slice	175	9	5	4.5	0	29	440	13	1	10	1 starch, 1 medium-fat meat, 1/2 fat
✔Specialty of the House	1 slice	170	9	5	4.5	0	20	450	13	1	10	1 starch, 1 medium-fat meat, 1 fat
✔Vegetarian Combo	1 slice	150	8	5	3.5	0	20	360	14	1	8	1 starch, 1 medium-fat meat, 1 fat

✔Veggie	1 slice	152	8	5	4	0	20	275	13	1	8	1 starch, 1 medium-fat meat, 1 fat
✔Veggie Mediterranean	1 slice	165	9	5	4	0	20	325	15	2	8	1 starch, 1 medium-fat meat, 1 fat
LARGE SIZE CALZONES												
Chicken Florentine	1 srvg	455	19	4	9	0	60	1008	45	1	25	3 starch, 2 medium-fat meat, 1 fat
Combo	1 srvg	440	20	4	10	0	55	995	44	1	20	3 starch, 2 medium-fat meat, 2 fat
Italian	1 srvg	440	20	4	9.5	0	41	1080	45	1	21	3 starch, 2 medium-fat meat, 2 fat
✔Veggie	1 srvg	390	16	4	8	0	38	890	44	2	18	3 starch, 1 medium-fat meat, 2 fat
LARGE SIZE STUFFED PIZZAS												
5-Meat	1 slice	361	15	4	7	0	40	975	37	1	18	2 1/2 starch, 1 medium-fat meat, 1 1/2 fat

✔ = Healthiest Bets

(*Continued*)

LARGE SIZE STUFFED PIZZAS *(Continued)*	Amount	Cal.	Fat (g)	% Cal. Fat	Sat. Fat (g)	Trans Fat (g)	Chol. (mg)	Sod. (mg)	Carb. (g)	Fiber (g)	Pro. (g)	Choices/Exchanges
Big Murphy	1 slice	355	15	4	7	0	32	935	38	1	17	2 1/2 starch, 1 medium-fat meat, 1 fat
Chicago-Style	1 slice	356	15	4	7	0	37	915	38	1	17	2 1/2 starch, 1 medium-fat meat, 1 fat
Chicken & Bacon	1 slice	366	15	4	6.5	0	45	850	38	1	19	2 1/2 starch, 2 medium-fat meat, 1 fat
MEDIUM (12") ORIGINAL CRUST PIZZAS												
Barbecue Chicken	1 slice	273	10	3	5	0	37	643	30	1	15	2 starch, 1 medium-fat meat, 1/2 fat
Cheese	1 slice	215	9	4	4.5	0	25	520	24	1	10	1 1/2 starch, 1 medium-fat meat, 1 fat
Cowboy	1 slice	280	14	5	6.5	0	30	805	25	1	14	1 1/2 starch, 1 medium-fat meat, 1 1/2 fat

Gourmet Chicken Garlic	1 slice	263	12	4	5.5	0	36	563	24	1	15	1 1/2 starch, 1 medium-fat meat, 1 fat
Gourmet Classic Italian	1 slice	271	13	4	6.5	0	30	706	25	1	14	1 1/2 starch, 1 medium-fat meat, 1 1/2 fat
Gourmet Vegetarian	1 slice	248	11	4	5	0	26	562	25	1	11	1 1/2 starch, 1 medium-fat meat, 1 1/2 fat
✔Hawaiian	1 slice	190	7	3	4	0	22	470	22	1	10	1 1/2 starch, 1 medium-fat meat, 1/2 fat
Herb Chicken Mediterranean	1 slice	272	12	4	5	0	30	596	28	2	14	2 starch, 1 medium-fat meat, 1 fat
Murphy's Combination	1 slice	290	15	5	7	0	33	840	26	1	14	1 1/2 starch, 1 medium-fat meat, 1 1/2 fat
Papa's All Meat	1 slice	280	14	5	6.5	0	37	780	24	1	15	1 1/2 starch, 1 medium-fat meat, 1 1/2 fat
Papa's Favorite	1 slice	290	15	5	6.5	0	32	820	26	1	14	1 1/2 starch, 1 medium-fat meat, 1 1/2 fat

✔ = Healthiest Bets

(*Continued*)

MEDIUM (12") ORIGINAL CRUST PIZZAS *(Continued)*	Amount	Cal.	Fat (g)	% Cal. Fat	Sat. Fat (g)	Trans Fat (g)	Chol. (mg)	Sod. (mg)	Carb. (g)	Fiber (g)	Pro. (g)	Choices/Exchanges
Pepperoni	1 slice	250	12	4	6	0	33	640	24	1	12	1 1/2 starch, 1 medium-fat meat, 1 1/2 fat
Rancher	1 slice	265	12	4	6	0	36	720	25	1	14	1 1/2 starch, 1 medium-fat meat, 1 fat
Specialty of the House	1 slice	210	10	4	4.5	0	20	585	20	1	10	1 1/2 starch, 1 medium-fat meat, 1 fat
Vegetarian Combo	1 slice	235	10	4	5	0	24	620	26	1	11	1 1/2 starch, 1 medium-fat meat, 1/2 fat
Veggie Mediterranean	1 slice	255	12	4	5	0	23	575	28	2	11	2 starch, 1 medium-fat meat, 1 fat
PASTA												
✔Lasagna	1 portion	255	14	5	7	0.5	35	681	17	2	14	1 starch, 2 medium-fat meat, 1 1/2 fat

SALADS W/O DRESSINGS OR CROUTONS

✔Caesar	1 salad	47	2	4	1.1	0	5	122	4	3	4	1 veg, 1/2 fat
✔Chicken Caesar	1 salad	108	3	3	1.5	0	35	215	5	3	15	1 veg, 2 lean meat
✔Club	1 salad	145	9	6	4.2	0	33	490	6	3	12	1 veg, 1 lean meat, 1 fat
✔Garden	1 salad	100	6	5	3	0	12	260	8	4	6	2 veg, 1 fat
Italian	1 salad	136	10	7	4.5	0	22	400	7	3	7	2 veg, 2 fat

✔ = Healthiest Bets

Exclusive Web Content

Be sure to visit the following restaurants online at http://www.diabetes.org/healthyrestaurant

Carvel
Del Taco
El Pollo Loco
Fröshens
Godfather's
Jersey Mike's
Jimmy John's
Tim Hortons
Whataburger
Wienerschnitzel
Zaxby's

Pizza Hut

(www.pizzahut.com)

Light 'n Lean Choice

12" Fit 'N' Delicious Pizza, Diced Chicken, Mushroom, and Jalapeño *(3 slices)*

Calories	480	Cholesterol (mg)	45
Fat (g)	15	Sodium (mg)	2,190
% calories from fat	28	Carbohydrate (g)	66
Saturated fat (g)	6	Fiber (g)	3
Trans fat (g)	0	Protein (g)	27

Exchanges: 4 1/2 starch, 1 veg, 2 medium-fat meat

Healthy 'n Hearty Choice

14" Fit 'N' Delicious Pizza, Ham, Pineapple, and Diced Red Tomato *(3 slices)*

Calories	690	Cholesterol (mg)	60
Fat (g)	18	Sodium (mg)	2,490
% calories from fat	23	Carbohydrate (g)	96
Saturated fat (g)	7.5	Fiber (g)	3
Trans fat (g)	0	Protein (g)	33

Exchanges: 6 1/2 starch, 1 veg, 2 medium-fat meat, 1 1/2 fat

Pizza Hut

	Amount	Cal.	Fat (g)	% Cal. Fat	Sat. Fat (g)	Trans Fat (g)	Chol. (mg)	Sod. (mg)	Carb. (g)	Fiber (g)	Pro. (g)	Choices/Exchanges
12" FIT N' DELICIOUS PIZZA												
Diced Chicken, Mushroom, & Jalapeno	1 slice	160	5	3	2	0	15	730	22	1	9	1 1/2 starch, 1 medium-fat meat
Diced Chicken, Red Onion & Green Pepper	1 slice	170	5	3	2	0	15	520	23	1	9	1 1/2 starch, 1 medium-fat meat, 1/2 fat
Diced Red Tomato, Mushroom & Jalapeno	1 slice	150	4	2	1.5	0	10	630	22	1	6	1 1/2 starch, 1 fat
✔Green Pepper, & Diced Red Tomato	1 slice	150	4	2	1.5	0	10	420	23	1	6	1 1/2 starch, 1 medium-fat meat
Ham, Pineapple, & Diced Red Tomato	1 slice	160	5	3	2	0	15	580	13	1	8	1 starch, 1 medium-fat meat, 1 fat

✔ = Healthiest Bets

(Continued)

12" FIT N' DELICIOUS PIZZA (*Continued*)	Amount	Cal.	Fat (g)	% Cal. Fat	Sat. Fat (g)	Trans Fat (g)	Chol. (mg)	Sod. (mg)	Carb. (g)	Fiber (g)	Pro. (g)	Choices/Exchanges
Ham, Red Onion, & Mushroom	1 slice	160	5	3	2	0	15	580	23	1	8	1 1/2 starch, 1 medium-fat meat
12" MEDIUM HAND-TOSSED STYLE PIZZA												
Cheese Only	1 slice	230	10	4	4.5	1	25	620	25	1	12	1 1/2 starch, 1 medium-fat meat, 1 fat
Italian Sausage & Red Onion	1 slice	260	12	4	5	1	30	670	26	1	12	1 1/2 starch, 1 medium-fat meat, 1 1/2 fat
Meat Lovers	1 slice	340	19	5	7	1	45	1040	25	1	17	1 1/2 starch, 2 medium-fat meat, 2 fat
Pepperoni	1 slice	240	11	4	4.5	1	25	690	24	1	12	1 1/2 starch, 1 medium-fat meat, 1 fat
Pepperoni & Mushroom	1 slice	230	9	4	4	1	20	610	25	1	11	1 1/2 starch, 1 medium-fat meat, 1 fat

Quartered Ham & Pineapple	1 slice	220	8	3	3.5	1	20	620	26	1	10	1 1/2 starch, 1 medium-fat meat, 1 fat
Supreme	1 slice	270	13	4	5	1	30	780	26	2	13	1 1/2 starch, 1 medium-fat meat, 1 fat
Veggie Lovers	1 slice	210	8	3	3.5	1	15	580	26	2	10	1 1/2 starch, 1 medium-fat meat, 1 fat
12" MEDIUM PAN PIZZA												
Cheese Only	1 slice	270	13	4	5	0	25	570	27	1	11	2 starch, 1 medium-fat meat, 2 fat
Italian Sausage & Red Onion	1 slice	300	15	5	5	0	30	610	38	1	12	2 1/2 starch, 1 medium-fat meat, 2 fat
Meat Lovers	1 slice	370	22	5	8	0	45	990	28	2	17	2 starch, 2 medium-fat meat, 3 fat
Pepperoni	1 slice	260	14	5	5	0	25	640	27	1	12	2 starch, 1 medium-fat meat, 2 fat

✔ = Healthiest Bets

(*Continued*)

12" MEDIUM PAN PIZZA (*Continued*)	Amount	Cal.	Fat (g)	% Cal. Fat	Sat. Fat (g)	Trans Fat (g)	Chol. (mg)	Sod. (mg)	Carb. (g)	Fiber (g)	Pro. (g)	Choices/Exchanges
Pepperoni & Mushroom	1 slice	260	13	5	4.85	0	20	560	27	1	11	2 starch, 1 medium-fat meat, 2 fat
Quartered Ham & Pineapple	1 slice	250	11	4	4	0	20	560	28	1	10	2 starch, 1 medium-fat meat, 1 1/2 fat
Supreme	1 slice	310	16	5	6	0	30	720	28	2	13	2 starch, 1 medium-fat meat, 2 fat
Veggie Lovers	1 slice	250	11	4	4	0	15	530	28	2	10	2 starch, 1 medium-fat meat, 1 1/2 fat
12" MEDIUM THIN N' CRISPY PIZZA												
Cheese Only	1 slice	200	8	4	4.5	0	25	570	21	1	10	1 1/2 starch, 1 medium-fat meat, 1 fat
Italian Sausage & Red Onion	1 slice	230	11	4	4.5	0	30	620	23	1	10	1 1/2 starch, 1 medium-fat meat, 1 1/2 fat

Meat Lovers	1 slice	310	18	5	7	0.5	45	1010	22	1	15	1 1/2 starch, 2 medium-fat meat, 2 fat
Pepperoni	1 slice	210	10	4	4.5	0	25	640	21	1	10	1 1/2 starch, 1 medium-fat meat, 1 fat
Pepperoni & Mushroom	1 slice	190	8	4	3.5	0	20	560	21	1	9	1 1/2 starch, 1 medium-fat meat, 1 fat
Quartered Ham & Pineapple	1 slice	180	6	3	3	0	20	570	23	1	9	1 1/2 starch, 1 medium-fat meat, 1/2 fat
Supreme	1 slice	230	11	4	5	0	30	730	22	1	11	1 1/2 starch, 1 medium-fat meat, 1 1/2 fat
Veggie Lovers	1 slice	180	7	4	3	0	15	550	23	1	8	1 1/2 starch, 1 1/2 fat
14" LARGE HAND-TOSSED STYLE PIZZA												
Cheese Only	1 slice	340	14	4	7	1.5	35	900	36	2	17	2 1/2 starch, 1 medium-fat meat, 1 fat

✔ = Healthiest Bets

(*Continued*)

14" LARGE HAND-TOSSED STYLE PIZZA (*Continued*)	Amount	Cal.	Fat (g)	% Cal. Fat	Sat. Fat (g)	Trans Fat (g)	Chol. (mg)	Sod. (mg)	Carb. (g)	Fiber (g)	Pro. (g)	Choices/Exchanges
Italian Sausage & Red Onion	1 slice	370	17	4	7	1.5	40	960	38	2	17	2 1/2 starch, 1 medium-fat meat, 2 fat
Meat Lovers	1 slice	490	27	5	11	1.5	65	1510	37	2	24	2 1/2 starch, 2 medium-fat meat, 3 fat
Pepperoni	1 slice	380	15	4	7	1.5	40	1010	35	2	17	2 1/2 starch, 1 medium-fat meat, 2 fat
Pepperoni & Mushroom	1 slice	330	14	4	6	1.5	30	890	36	2	16	2 1/2 starch, 1 medium-fat meat, 1 fat
Quartered Ham & Pineapple	1 slice	310	11	3	5	1.5	30	900	38	2	15	2 1/2 starch, 1 medium-fat meat, 1 fat
Supreme	1 slice	390	18	4	8	1.5	40	1130	37	2	19	2 1/2 starch, 2 medium-fat meat, 2 fat
Veggie Lovers	1 slice	310	12	3	5	1.5	25	840	37	2	14	2 1/2 starch, 1 medium-fat meat, 1 fat

14" FIT N' DELICIOUS PIZZA												
Diced Chicken, Mushroom, & Jalapeno	1 slice	230	6	2	2.5	0	25	1010	43	2	13	3 starch, 1 medium-fat meat
Diced Chicken, Red Onion & Green Pepper	1 slice	230	8	3	2.5	0	25	730	32	2	13	2 starch, 1 medium-fat meat
Diced Red Tomato, Mushroom & Jalapeno	1 slice	210	6	3	2.5	0	10	870	31	2	9	2 starch, 1 fat
Green Pepper, & Diced Red Tomato	1 slice	210	6	3	2.5	0	10	580	32	2	8	2 starch, 1 fat
Ham, Pineapple, & Diced Red Tomato	1 slice	230	6	2	2.5	0	20	830	32	1	11	2 starch, 1 medium-fat meat, 1/2 fat
Ham, Red Onion, & Mushroom	1 slice	230	7	3	205	0	20	820	31	2	11	2 starch, 1 medium-fat meat, 1/2 fat
14" LARGE PAN PIZZA												
Cheese Only	1 slice	390	19	4	7	0	35	800	38	2	18	2 1/2 starch, 1 medium-fat meat, 2 fat

✔ = Healthiest Bets

(*Continued*)

14" LARGE PAN PIZZA (*Continued*)	Amount	Cal.	Fat (g)	% Cal. Fat	Sat. Fat (g)	Trans Fat (g)	Chol. (mg)	Sod. (mg)	Carb. (g)	Fiber (g)	Pro. (g)	Choices/Exchanges
Italian Sausage & Red Onion	1 slice	420	22	5	8	0	40	860	39	2	17	2 1/2 starch, 1 medium-fat meat, 3 fat
Meat Lovers	1 slice	530	31	5	11	0.5	65	1400	39	2	23	2 1/2 starch, 2 medium-fat meat, 4 fat
Pepperoni	1 slice	400	21	5	7	0	40	900	37	2	18	2 1/2 starch, 2 medium-fat meat, 2 fat
Pepperoni & Mushroom	1 slice	380	18	4	6	0	30	790	37	2	15	2 1/2 starch, 1 medium-fat meat, 2 1/2 fat
Quartered Ham & Pineapple	1 slice	360	16	4	6	0	30	790	39	2	15	2 1/2 starch, 1 medium-fat meat, 2 fat
Supreme	1 slice	440	23	5	7	0.5	40	1020	30	2	18	2 starch, 2 medium-fat meat, 3 fat
Veggie Lovers	1 slice	350	16	4	6	0	25	730	39	2	14	2 1/2 starch, 1 medium-fat meat, 2 fat

14" LARGE STUFFED CRUST PIZZA

Cheese Only	1 slice	360	16	4	5	1.5	40	1050	37	2	18	2 1/2 starch, 2 medium-fat meat, 1 fat
Italian Sausage & Red Onion	1 slice	410	20	4	9	1.5	50	1190	39	2	19	2 1/2 starch, 2 medium-fat meat, 2 fat
Meat Lovers	1 slice	620	29	4	12	2	75	1690	39	2	26	2 1/2 starch, 3 medium-fat meat, 5 fat
Pepperoni	1 slice	390	16	4	7	1.5	50	1320	39	2	19	2 1/2 starch, 2 medium-fat meat, 1 1/2 fat
Pepperoni & Mushroom	1 slice	360	18	5	7	1.5	40	1090	37	2	18	2 1/2 starch, 2 medium-fat meat, 2 fat
Quartered Ham & Pineapple	1 slice	350	14	4	7	1.5	40	1090	39	2	17	2 1/2 starch, 1 medium-fat meat, 1 fat
Supreme	1 slice	420	21	5	9	1.5	50	1320	39	2	21	2 1/2 starch, 2 medium-fat meat, 2 fat

✔ = Healthiest Bets

(*Continued*)

14" LARGE STUFFED CRUST PIZZA (*Continued*)	Amount	Cal.	Fat (g)	% Cal. Fat	Sat. Fat (g)	Trans Fat (g)	Chol. (mg)	Sod. (mg)	Carb. (g)	Fiber (g)	Pro. (g)	Choices/Exchanges
Veggie Lovers	1 slice	340	14	4	7	1.5	35	1030	38	2	16	2 1/2 starch, 1 medium-fat meat, 1 fat
14" LARGE THIN N' CRISPY PIZZA												
Cheese Only	1 slice	280	12	4	6	0	35	810	30	1	14	2 starch, 1 medium-fat meat, 1 fat
Italian Sausage & Red Onion	1 slice	320	15	4	7	0	40	870	32	2	14	2 starch, 1 medium-fat meat, 2 fat
Meat Lovers	1 slice	430	25	5	10	0.5	65	1430	31	2	21	2 starch, 2 medium-fat meat, 3 fat
Pepperoni	1 slice	300	14	4	6	0	40	920	29	1	14	2 starch, 1 medium-fat meat, 1 1/2 fat
Pepperoni & Mushroom	1 slice	270	12	4	5	0	30	800	30	1	13	2 starch, 1 medium-fat meat, 1 fat

Quartered Ham & Pineapple	1 slice	260	9	3	4.5	0	30	810	32	1	12	2 starch, 1 medium-fat meat, 1 fat
Supreme	1 slice	330	16	4	7	0.5	40	1040	31	2	16	2 starch, 1 medium-fat meat, 2 fat
Veggie Lovers	1 slice	260	10	3	4.5	0	25	770	31	2	12	2 starch, 1 medium-fat meat, 1 fat
6" PERSONAL PAN PIZZA												
Cheese Only	Whole Pizza	620	26	4	11	0.5	60	1370	69	3	28	4 1/2 starch, 2 medium-fat meat, 2 fat
Italian Sausage & Red Onion	Whole Pizza	690	33	4	12	0.5	70	1530	71	4	29	4 1/2 starch, 2 medium-fat meat, 4 fat
Meat Lovers	Whole Pizza	890	49	5	18	1	115	2460	70	4	41	4 1/2 starch, 4 medium-fat meat, 5 fat
Pepperoni	Whole Pizza	640	29	4	11	0.5	65	1530	67	3	28	4 1/2 starch, 2 medium-fat meat, 3 fat

✔ = Healthiest Bets

(*Continued*)

6" PERSONAL PAN PIZZA (*Continued*)	Amount	Cal.	Fat (g)	% Cal. Fat	Sat. Fat (g)	Trans Fat (g)	Chol. (mg)	Sod. (mg)	Carb. (g)	Fiber (g)	Pro. (g)	Choices/Exchanges
Pepperoni & Mushroom	Whole Pizza	600	25	4	10	0.5	55	1350	68	3	26	4 1/2 starch, 2 medium-fat meat, 2 1/2 fat
Quartered Ham & Pineapple	Whole Pizza	570	21	3	8	0	50	1380	70	3	25	4 1/2 starch, 2 medium-fat meat, 2 fat
Supreme	Whole Pizza	710	34	4	13	1	70	1800	70	4	32	4 1/2 starch, 3 medium-fat meat, 3 fat
Veggie Lovers	Whole Pizza	560	22	4	8	0	40	1250	70	4	24	4 1/2 starch, 1 medium-fat meat, 2 fat
APPETIZERS												
✔Breadsticks	1	150	6	4	1	0	0	230	20	1	4	1 1/2 starch, 1 fat
Cheese Breadsticks	1	200	10	5	3	0	15	370	21	1	7	1 1/2 starch, 2 fat
Hot Wings	2 pcs	120	7	5	2	0	65	500	1	0	11	2 lean meat, 1/2 fat
Mild Wings	2 pcs	110	7	6	2	0	65	390	2	0	11	2 lean meat, 1/2 fat

DESSERTS												
Apple Dessert Pizza	1 slice	260	5	2	1	0.5	0	290	52	1	4	3 1/2 carb, 1/2 fat
Cherry Dessert Pizza	1 slice	260	4.5	2	1	0.5	0	280	47	1	4	3 carb, 1 fat
✔Cinnamon Sticks	2 pcs	170	5	3	1	0	0	180	27	1	4	2 carb, 1 fat
White Icing Dipping Cup	2 oz.	190	0	0	0	0	0	0	47	0	0	3 carb
DIPPING SAUCES												
✔Breadstick	3 oz.	40	0	0	0	0	0	270	8	0	1	1/2 carb
Wing Blue Cheese	1.5 oz.	220	23	9	4	0	15	400	3	0	1	4 1/2 fat
Wing Ranch	1.5 oz.	220	23	9	4	0	25	400	3	0	1	4 1/2 fat
DRESSINGS												
French	2 Tbsp.	150	13	8	2	0	0	180	9	0	0	1/2 carb, 2 1/2 fat
Italian	2 Tbsp.	140	15	10	2.5	0	0	360	2	0	0	3 fat

✔ = Healthiest Bets

(*Continued*)

DRESSINGS (*Continued*)	Amount	Cal.	Fat (g)	% Cal. Fat	Sat. Fat (g)	Trans Fat (g)	Chol. (mg)	Sod. (mg)	Carb. (g)	Fiber (g)	Pro. (g)	Choices/Exchanges
✔Lite Italian	2 Tbsp.	70	5	6	1	0	0	510	5	0	0	1/2 carb, 1 fat
✔Lite Ranch	2 Tbsp.	60	6	9	1	0	15	260	1	0	0	1 fat
✔Ranch	2 Tbsp.	100	10	9	1.5	0	5	220	2	0	1	2 fat
Thousand Island	2 Tbsp.	120	11	8	1.5	0	10	220	5	0	0	1/2 carb, 2 fat
XL FULL HOUSE PIZZA												
Cheese Only	1 slice	260	12	4	5	0	30	690	30	2	12	2 starch, 1 medium-fat meat, 1 fat
Italian Sausage & Red Onion	1 slice	300	14	4	5	0	30	720	32	2	12	2 starch, 1 medium-fat meat, 2 fat
Meat Lovers	1 slice	370	20	5	8	0	45	1090	31	2	17	2 starch, 2 medium-fat meat, 2 fat
Pepperoni	1 slice	280	13	4	5	0	30	750	30	2	12	2 starch, 1 medium-fat meat, 1 1/2 fat

Pepperoni & Mushroom	1 slice	270	11	4	1.5	0	25	670	30	2	11	2 starch, 1 medium-fat meat, 1 1/2 fat
Quartered Ham & Pineapple	1 slice	260	10	3	4	0	20	680	32	2	11	2 starch, 1 medium-fat meat, 1 fat
Supreme	1 slice	310	14	4	6	0	30	830	31	2	13	2 starch, 1 medium-fat meat, 2 fat
Veggie Lovers	1 slice	260	10	3	4	0	20	650	31	2	10	2 starch, 1 medium-fat meat, 1 1/2 fat

✔ = Healthiest Bets

Exclusive Web Content

Be sure to visit the following restaurants online at http://www.diabetes.org/healthyrestaurant

Carvel	**Godfather's**	**Whataburger**
Del Taco	**Jersey Mike's**	**Wienerschnitzel**
El Pollo Loco	**Jimmy John's**	**Zaxby's**
Frëshens	**Tim Hortons**	

Tacos, Burritos, and All Else Mexican

RESTAURANTS

Chipotle
Moe's Southwest Grill
Taco Bell
Taco John's

EXCLUSIVE WEB CONTENT

Del Taco (**http://www.diabetes.org/healthyrestaurant**)

NUTRITION PROS

- Beans used in Mexican cooking, such as pinto beans and black beans, contain soluble fiber. This kind of fiber may allow your blood glucose to rise more slowly and not go as high. Beans are also a terrific source of vitamins and minerals.
- In most of the fast-food Mexican restaurants, ordering is à la carte. This helps you order less and eat less.
- In the Mexican made-to-your-specifications restaurants, such as Chipotle and Moe's Southwest Grill, you can pick and choose what you want on or left out of your order.
- High-fat items, such as guacamole, cheese, and sour cream, are added onto and not mixed into some dishes. That's a plus because you can ask the kitchen to hold or serve them on the side.
- Choose guacamole over sour cream, as it contains healthier monounsaturated fat. Calorie for calorie, it's better for you.

- Hot and spicy sauces—red sauce, green sauce, salsa, and pico de gallo—add zest without adding fat and calories.
- Garlic, cilantro, chilies, and onions add flavor with few calories.
- Mexican cuisine is naturally low in protein. You don't get 8-oz hunks of meat. You find a small amount of protein mixed into dishes.
- Most fast-food Mexican restaurants now fry in 100% vegetable oil. That's better than lard because it contains no cholesterol and less saturated fat. However, it may contain a few grams of trans fat. But remember, teaspoon for teaspoon, the calories are the same.
- In the walk-up-and-order Mexican restaurants, the bet-you-can't-eat-just-one tortilla chips don't greet you at the table.

NUTRITION CONS

- Fried items seem almost unavoidable—tortilla chips, taco shells, tortilla shells (in which a salad might be served), and chimichangas are just a few items to cross off your list.
- Your carbohydrate count can escalate quickly with tortillas, beans, rice, and those hard-to-resist tortilla chips.
- Cheese—shredded, melted, or sauced—is a mainstay ingredient.
- Vegetables are few and far between—a few shreds of lettuce or pieces of tomato.
- Fruit is unavailable.

- High-fiber beans are often served refried. Some restaurants still use lard to make them.
- The bet-you-can't-eat-just-one tortilla chips are waiting at your table in most sit-down Mexican or Tex-Mex restaurants.

Get It Your Way

★ Hold the guacamole, cheese, and sour cream or ask for them on the side.
★ If a menu item is served with melted cheese, request a light helping.
★ Substitute black beans for refried beans (if available).
★ Ask for extra tomatoes and lettuce.
★ Request extra salsa or other zesty, low-calorie topper.

Exclusive Web Content

Be sure to visit the following restaurants online at http://www.diabetes.org/healthyrestaurant

Carvel	**Godfather's**	**Whataburger**
Del Taco	**Jersey Mike's**	**Wienerschnitzel**
El Pollo Loco	**Jimmy John's**	**Zaxby's**
Frëshens	**Tim Hortons**	

Healthy Tips

- ★ If the fried tortilla chips greet you when you sit down, keep your hands off. Send them back or to the opposite side of the table.
- ★ Use extra salsa and other hot sauces to add flavor with very few calories.
- ★ Use salsa or another hot sauce as a salad dressing.
- ★ Don't feel like you have to order an entree. Choose from appetizers and side dishes to control your portions.
- ★ Take advantage of ordering à la carte. Mix and match a healthy meal.
- ★ As a starter, try a cup of black bean soup or chili to fill you up and not out.
- ★ Make a bowl of black bean soup or chili the main course, with a salad on the side.
- ★ Look for menu items that use soft tortillas rather than crispy fried ones. For example, choose a burrito or an enchilada rather than a taco or a chimichanga.
- ★ Fajitas are great to split. There's always enough for two.
- ★ Split a side dish—Mexican rice, refried beans, or black beans—to get more carbohydrates and fiber.
- ★ Take advantage of light or nonfat sour cream, if it's served.

Chipotle

(www.chipotle.com)

Light 'n Lean Choice

6" Soft Tortillas (3)
Chicken *(1 order, 4 oz)*
Black Beans *(1 order, 4 oz)*
Red Tomatillo Sauce *(4 Tbsp)*

Calories	613	Cholesterol (mg)	110
Fat (g)	17	Sodium (mg)	1,826
% calories from fat	25	Carbohydrate (g)	66
Saturated fat (g)	4.5	Fiber (g)	15
Trans fat (g)	na	Protein (g)	49

Exchanges: 4 starch, 1 veg, 4 lean meat, 1 1/2 fat

Healthy 'n Hearty Choice

6" Soft Tortillas (3)
Fajita Vegetables *(1 order, 3 oz)*
Pinto Beans *(1 order, 4 oz)*
Corn Salsa *(4 Tbsp)*
Guacamole *(1 order, 4 oz)*

Calories	733	Cholesterol (mg)	0
Fat (g)	28	Sodium (mg)	2,579
% calories from fat	34	Carbohydrate (g)	99
Saturated fat (g)	5.5	Fiber (g)	26
Trans fat (g)	na	Protein (g)	21

Exchanges: 5 starch, 2 veg, 1/2 lean meat, 5 fat

(Continued)

Chipotle

	Amount	Cal.	Fat (g)	% Cal. Fat	Sat. Fat (g)	Trans Fat (g)	Chol. (mg)	Sod. (mg)	Carb. (g)	Fiber (g)	Pro. (g)	Choices/Exchanges
DRESSINGS												
Vinaigrette	2 oz.	330	31	8	4	na	0	960	12	0	0	1 starch, 6 fat
SALSAS												
✔Corn Salsa	4 oz.	100	1	1	0	na	0	540	22	3	3	1/2 starch, 1 veg
✔Green Tomatillo	2 oz.	15	0	0	0	na	0	227	3	1	1	Free
✔Red Tomatillo	2 oz.	28	1	3	0	na	0	493	4	1	1	1 veg
✔Tomato Salsa	4 oz.	20	0	0	0	na	0	490	3	0	2	1 veg
SIDES												
Chips	4 oz.	570	27	4	3.5	na	0	500	73	8	8	5 starch, 5 fat
✔Guacamole	4 oz.	140	10	6	1.5	na	0	240	10	10	2	1/2 starch, 2 fat

✔Sour Cream	2 oz.	120	10	8	7	na	40	30	2	0	2	2 1/2 fat
TACO SHELLS												
✔Crispy Taco Shells	3	180	7	4	1.5	na	0	30	26	1.5	3	1 1/2 starch, 1 1/2 fat
TOPPINGS												
✔Barbacoa	4 oz.	170	7	4	2	na	55	490	2	0	24	3 lean meat
✔Black Beans	4 oz.	130	1	1	0	na	0	318	22	12	9	1 1/2 starch, 1 lean meat
Carnitas	4 oz.	210	11	5	3	na	60	690	2	0	26	4 lean meat
Cheese	1 oz.	110	9	7	6	na	30	180	0	0	7	1 medium-fat meat, 1 fat
✔Chicken	4 oz.	200	7	3	1.5	na	110	430	2	0	33	4 lean meat
✔Fajita Vegetables	3 oz.	100	8	7	1	na	0	640	6	1	1	1 veg, 1 1/2 fat
✔Lettuce	1 oz.	5	0	0	0	na	0	0	0	0	0	Free
Pinto Beans	4 oz.	138	1	1	0	na	0	374	23	10	9	1 1/2 starch, 1 lean meat
Rice	3.5 oz.	160	4	2	0	na	0	330	30	0	3	2 starch, 1 fat

✔ = Healthiest Bets; na = not available

(*Continued*)

TOPPINGS (Continued)	Amount	Cal.	Fat (g)	% Cal. Fat	Sat. Fat (g)	Trans Fat (g)	Chol. (mg)	Sod. (mg)	Carb. (g)	Fiber (g)	Pro. (g)	Choices/Exchanges
✔Steak	4 oz.	190	7	3	2	na	65	420	2	0	29	4 lean meat
TORTILLAS												
✔Burrito Size Flour Tortilla	1	290	9	3	2	na	0	670	44	2	7	3 starch, 2 fat
✔Taco Size Flour Tortilla	3	255	8	3	3	na	0	585	38	2	6	2 1/2 starch, 1 1/2 fat

✔ = Healthiest Bets; na = not available

Exclusive Web Content

Be sure to visit the following restaurants online at http://www.diabetes.org/healthyrestaurant

Carvel
Del Taco
El Pollo Loco
Frëshens
Godfather's
Jersey Mike's
Jimmy John's
Tim Hortons
Whataburger
Wienerschnitzel
Zaxby's

Moe's Southwest Grill

(www.moes.com)

Light 'n Lean Choice

Funk Meister Tacos with soft tortilla, ground beef, black beans, cheese, and pico de gallo *(2)*

Calories	586	Cholesterol (mg)	82
Fat (g)	24	Sodium (mg)	1,616
% calories from fat	37	Carbohydrate (g)	52
Saturated fat (g)	10	Fiber (g)	18
Trans fat (g)	0	Protein (g)	34

Exchanges: 3 1/2 starch, 1 veg, 3 1/2 lean meat, 1 1/2 fat

Healthy 'n Hearty Choice

Instant Friend Quesadilla with tortilla, black beans, rice, and cheese *(1)*

Calories	655	Cholesterol (mg)	60
Fat (g)	25	Sodium (mg)	1,670
% calories from fat	34	Carbohydrate (g)	73
Saturated fat (g)	12	Fiber (g)	20
Trans fat (g)	0	Protein (g)	27

Exchanges: 5 starch, 1 veg, 2 lean meat, 4 fat

(*Continued*)

Moe's

	Amount	Cal.	Fat (g)	% Cal. Fat	Sat. Fat (g)	Trans Fat (g)	Chol. (mg)	Sod. (mg)	Carb. (g)	Fiber (g)	Pro. (g)	Choices/Exchanges
BURRITOS												
Art Vandalay w/ tortilla, black beans, rice, cheese & pico de gallo	1	635	19	3	8	0	30	1750	87	18	23	6 starch, 1 lean meat, 3 fat
Homewrecker w/ black beans, rice & pico de gallo	1	500	9	2	3	0	0	1520	84	16	16	5 1/2 starch, 2 fat
Homewrecker w/ steak, rice, pico de gallo & no tortilla	1	235	6	2	1.5	0	60	1498	20	0	23	1 1/2 starch, 2 medium-fat meat
Homewrecker w/ tortilla, chicken, rice, sour cream cheese, guacamole, pico de gallo & chipotle ranch dressing	1	1060	63	5	18.5	0	128	2895	80	4	42	5 1/2 starch, 4 lean meat, 10 fat

Homewrecker w/ tortilla, fish, black beans, rice & pico de gallo	1	635	14	2	3	0	45	1655	84	16	37	5 1/2 starch, 3 lean meat, 1 fat
Joey Bag of Donuts w/ tortilla, black beans, rice & pico de gallo	1	525	10	2	3	0	0	1570	87	18	16	6 starch, 2 fat
Joey Bag of Donuts w/ tortilla, steak, rice & pico de gallo	1	660	15	2	4.5	0	60	2170	90	18	37	6 starch, 3 medium-fat meat, 1/2 fat
Triple Lindy w/ ground beef, black beans, rice & pico de gallo	1	675	20	3	6.5	0	53	2045	88	16	30	6 starch, 2 medium-fat meat, 2 fat
Triple Lindy w/ tortilla, tofu, black beans, rice & pico de gallo	1	588	14	2	3	0	0	1808	87	19	24	6 starch, 1 lean meat, 2 fat

✔ = Healthiest Bets

(*Continued*)

	Amount	Cal.	Fat (g)	% Cal. Fat	Sat. Fat (g)	Trans Fat (g)	Chol. (mg)	Sod. (mg)	Carb. (g)	Fiber (g)	Pro. (g)	Choices/Exchanges
FAJITAS												
Alfredo Garcia w/ tortilla, chicken, sour cream, cheese, guacamole, pico de gallo	1	1433	52	3	21.3	0	210	3975	145	38	82	9 1/2 starch, 8 lean meat, 6 fat
Fat Sam w/ ground beef, lettuce, pico de gallo, veggies & no tortilla	1	460	24	5	7	0	105	1390	23	6	28	1 1/2 starch, 3 medium-fat meat, 2 fat
NACHOS												
Billy Barou - black bean	1	1340	81	5	28.5	0	120	2573	114	23	34	7 1/2 starch, 2 lean meat, 14 fat
Billy Barou - chicken	1	1350	84	6	30	0	180	2593	97	7	49	6 1/2 starch, 4 lean meat, 14 fat
Billy Barou - ground beef	1	1410	91	6	32	0	173	2858	100	8	42	6 1/2 starch, 3 medium-fat meat, 15 fat

Ruprict - vegetarian	1	1340	81	5	28.5	0	120	2573	114	23	34	7 1/2 starch, 2 medium-fat meat, 14 1/2 fat
QUESADILLAS												
Instant Friend w/ tortilla, black beans, rice & cheese	1	655	26	4	12	0	60	1670	73	20	27	5 starch, 2 lean meat, 4 fat
John Coctosan w/ tortilla, chicken, pico de gallo & veggies	1	380	13	3	3.5	0	60	1270	40	3	26	2 1/2 starch, 3 lean meat, 1 fat
Super Kingpin w/ tortilla, cheese, pico de gallo & no meat	1	420	24	5	12	0	60	1070	33	1	19	2 starch, 2 medium-fat meat, 3 fat
SALADS												
Close Talker w/ crispy salad bowl, chicken, pico de gallo & southwest vinaigrette	1	845	50	5	8	0	60	1765	66	19	32	3 1/2 starch, 3 veg, 2 lean meat, 9 fat

✓ = Healthiest Bets

(*Continued*)

SALADS *(Continued)*	Amount	Cal.	Fat (g)	% Cal. Fat	Sat. Fat (g)	Trans Fat (g)	Chol. (mg)	Sod. (mg)	Carb. (g)	Fiber (g)	Pro. (g)	Choices/Exchanges
✔Personal Trainer w/ black beans, guacamole, lettuce, chipotle ranch dressing & no crispy salad bowl	1	425	30	6	4	0	8	845	32	19	8	1 starch, 3 veg, 6 fat
TACOS												
✔Overachiever w/ soft shell, chicken, black beans, & pico de gallo	1	225	6	2	2	0	30	710	26	9	17	1 1/2 starch, 2 lean meat
The Funk Meister w/ crispy corn shell, black beans, guacamole, sour cream, & cheese	1	489	30	6	15	0	111	1191	25	10	25	1 1/2 starch, 3 lean meat, 4 1/2 fat
✔The Funk Meister w/ ground beef, rice, pico de gallo & no shell	1	143	6	4	2	0	26	513	12	1	8	1 starch, 1 medium-fat meat, 1/2 fat

✔The Funk Meister w/ soft shell, ground beef, black beans, cheese, & pico de gallo	1	293	12	4	5	0	41	808	26	9	17	1 1/2 starch, 2 medium-fat meat, 1/2 fat
✔Unanimous Decision w/ crispy shell, black beans, cheese, & veggies	1	188	9	4	3	0	15	330	20	10	8	1 1/2 starch, 1 lean meat, 1 1/2 fat

✔ = Healthiest Bets

Exclusive Web Content

Be sure to visit the following restaurants online at http://www.diabetes.org/healthyrestaurant

Carvel **Frëshens** **Jimmy John's** **Wienerschnitzel**
Del Taco **Godfather's** **Tim Hortons** **Zaxby's**
El Pollo Loco **Jersey Mike's** **Whataburger**

Taco Bell

(www.tacobell.com)

Light 'n Lean Choice

Freso Menu: Beef Soft Taco *(1)*
Bean Burrito *(1)*
Salsa, side *(1.5 oz, 3 Tbsp)*

Calories	545	Cholesterol (mg)	25
Fat (g)	16	Sodium (mg)	2,000
% calories from fat	26	Carbohydrate (g)	78
Saturated fat (g)	6.5	Fiber (g)	11
Trans fat (g)	0.5	Protein (g)	21

Exchanges: 5 starch, 1/2 lean meat, 2 fat

Healthy 'n Hearty Choice

Gordita Supreme Steak *(1)*
Spicy Chicken Soft Taco *(1)*
Pintos 'n' Cheese *(1 serving)*

Calories	620	Cholesterol (mg)	80
Fat (g)	25	Sodium (mg)	1,780
% calories from fat	36	Carbohydrate (g)	67
Saturated fat (g)	10	Fiber (g)	11
Trans fat (g)	0.5	Protein (g)	34

Exchanges: 4 1/2 starch, 3 medium-fat meat, 2 fat

Taco Bell

	Amount	Cal.	Fat (g)	Cal. Fat	Sat. Fat (g)	Trans Fat (g)	Chol. (mg)	Sod. (mg)	Carb. (g)	Fiber (g)	Pro. (g)	Choices/Exchanges
BURRITOS												
1/2 lb Beef & Potato Burrito	1	530	23	4	7	1	30	1720	66	6	15	4 1/2 starch, 4 fat
1/2 lb Beef Combo Burrito	1	440	18	4	7	1	45	1630	51	8	21	3 1/2 starch, 2 medium-fat meat, 1 1/2 fat
7-Layer Burrito	1	490	18	3	7	1	25	1350	65	9	17	4 1/2 starch, 1 medium-fat meat, 2 1/2 fat
Burrito Supreme - Beef	1	420	17	4	8	1	40	1340	51	7	17	3 1/2 starch, 1 medium-fat meat, 2 fat
Burrito Supreme - Chicken	1	400	13	3	6	0.5	45	1360	49	6	20	3 1/2 starch, 1 lean meat, 1 1/2 fat

✓ = Healthiest Bets

(*Continued*)

BURRITOS *(Continued)*	**Amount**	**Cal.**	**Fat (g)**	**% Cal. Fat**	**Sat. Fat (g)**	**Trans Fat (g)**	**Chol. (mg)**	**Sod. (mg)**	**Carb. (g)**	**Fiber (g)**	**Pro. (g)**	**Choices/Exchanges**
Burrito Supreme - Steak	1	390	14	3	6	1	40	1250	49	6	18	3 1/2 starch, 1 medium-fat meat, 1 fat
Fiesta Burrito - Beef	1	370	13	3	5	0	25	1200	49	4	14	3 1/2 starch, 1 medium-fat meat, 2 fat
Fiesta Burrito - Chicken	1	350	10	3	3.5	0	30	1220	47	3	18	3 starch, 1 lean meat, 1 fat
Fiesta Burrito - Steak	1	340	11	3	4	0	25	1110	47	3	15	3 starch, 1 medium-fat meat, 1 fat
Grilled Stuft Burrito - Beef	1	680	30	4	10	1	55	2120	76	9	27	5 starch, 2 medium-fat meat, 4 fat
Grilled Stuft Burrito - Chicken	1	640	23	3	7	0.5	65	2160	73	7	34	5 starch, 3 lean meat, 3 fat
Grilled Stuft Burrito - Steak	1	630	25	4	8	1	55	1930	72	7	30	5 starch, 2 medium-fat meat, 2 fat

Spicy Chicken Burrito	1	400	17	4	4	0	30	1190	48	3	14	3 starch, 1 lean meat, 3 fat
CHALUPAS												
Chalupa Baja - Beef	1	410	27	6	6	0	35	780	30	4	13	2 starch, 1 medium-fat meat, 4 fat
Chalupa Baja - Chicken	1	390	23	5	4	0	40	800	29	3	17	2 starch, 2 lean meat, 3 1/2 fat
Chalupa Baja - Steak	1	390	24	6	4.5	0	35	690	28	3	15	2 starch, 1 medium-fat meat, 3 1/2 fat
Chalupa Nacho Cheese - Beef	1	370	22	5	4	0	20	770	32	3	12	2 starch, 1 medium-fat meat, 3 fat
✔Chalupa Nacho Cheese - Chicken	1	350	18	5	2	0	25	790	30	2	16	2 starch, 1 lean meat, 2 1/2 fat
✔Chalupa Nacho Cheese - Steak	1	340	19	5	2.5	0	20	670	30	2	14	2 starch, 1 medium-fat meat, 2 fat

✔ = Healthiest Bets

(Continued)

CHALUPAS *(Continued)*	Amount	Cal.	Fat (g)	% Cal. Fat	Sat. Fat (g)	Trans Fat (g)	Chol. (mg)	Sod. (mg)	Carb. (g)	Fiber (g)	Pro. (g)	Choices/Exchanges
✔Chalupa Supreme - Beef	1	380	23	5	7	0.5	40	620	30	3	14	2 starch, 1 medium-fat meat, 3 fat
✔Chalupa Supreme - Chicken	1	360	20	5	5	0	45	650	29	2	17	2 starch, 2 lean meat, 3 fat
Chalupa Supreme - Steak	1	360	21	5	6	0	40	530	28	2	15	2 starch, 1 medium-fat meat, 3 fat
FRESCO MENU												
Bean Burrito	1	330	7	2	2.5	0.5	0	1200	54	9	12	3 1/2 starch, 1 1/2 fat
Burrito Supreme - Chicken	1	330	8	2	2.5	0	25	1360	49	7	18	3 1/2 starch, 1 medium-fat meat, 1/2 fat
Burrito Supreme - Steak	1	330	8	2	3	0.5	20	1250	48	7	16	3 starch, 1 medium-fat meat, 1/2 fat
✔Crunchy Taco	1	150	8	5	2.5	0	20	370	13	3	7	1 starch, 1 medium-fat meat, 1 fat

Fiesta Burrito - Chicken	1	330	8	2	2.5	0	25	1240	48	3	16	3 starch, 1 lean meat, 1 fat
✔Grilled Steak Soft Taco	1	160	5	3	1.5	0	20	550	20	2	10	1 1/2 starch, 1 medium-fat meat
✔Ranchero Chicken Soft Taco	1	170	4	2	1.5	0	25	730	21	3	12	1 1/2 starch, 1 lean meat
✔Soft Taco - Beef	1	180	7	4	3	0	20	650	21	3	8	1 1/2 starch, 1 medium-fat meat, 1 fat
Zesty Chicken Border Bowl w/o Dressing	1 srvg	350	8	2	1.5	0.5	25	1600	51	10	19	3 1/2 starch, 1 lean meat, 1 fat
GORDITAS												
Gordita Baja - Beef	1	340	19	5	5	0	35	780	29	4	13	2 starch, 1 medium-fat meat, 3 fat
Gordita Baja - Chicken	1	320	16	5	3.5	0	40	800	28	3	17	2 starch, 2 lean meat, 2 fat
Gordita Baja - Steak	1	320	17	5	4	0	35	690	27	3	15	2 starch, 1 medium-fat meat, 2 fat

✔ = Healthiest Bets

(*Continued*)

GORDITAS *(Continued)*	Amount	Cal.	Fat (g)	% Cal. Fat	Sat. Fat (g)	Trans Fat (g)	Chol. (mg)	Sod. (mg)	Carb. (g)	Fiber (g)	Pro. (g)	Choices/Exchanges
Gordita Nacho Cheese - Beef	1	300	14	4	3.5	0	20	770	31	3	12	2 starch, 1 medium-fat meat, 2 fat
✔Gordita Nacho Cheese - Chicken	1	280	11	4	2	0	25	790	29	2	16	2 starch, 1 lean meat, 1 1/2 fat
✔Gordita Nacho Cheese - Steak	1	270	12	4	2	0	20	680	29	2	14	2 starch, 1 medium-fat meat, 1 fat
Gordita Supreme - Beef	1	310	16	5	6	0.5	40	620	29	3	14	2 starch, 1 medium-fat meat, 2 fat
✔Gordita Supreme - Chicken	1	290	12	4	5	0	45	650	28	2	17	2 starch, 2 lean meat, 1 1/2 fat
Gordita Supreme - Steak	1	290	13	4	5	0	40	530	28	2	15	2 starch, 1 medium-fat meat, 1 1/2 fat
NACHOS												
Nachos	1 srvg	330	21	6	2	0	0	520	31	2	4	2 starch, 4 fat

Nachos BellGrande	1 srvg	770	44	5	8	1	30	1270	77	12	19	5 starch, 1 medium-fat meat, 8 fat
Nachos Supreme	1 srvg	440	26	5	6	1	30	790	40	7	12	2 1/2 starch, 1 medium-fat meat, 4 fat
REGIONAL MENU ITEMS												
Cheese Quesadilla	1	470	26	5	12	0.5	50	1100	39	2	19	2 1/2 starch, 2 medium-fat meat, 3 1/2 fat
Chili Cheese Burrito	1	370	16	4	8	0.5	40	1060	40	3	16	2 1/2 starch, 1 medium-fat meat, 2 fat
✔Tostada	1 srvg	240	10	4	3.5	0.5	15	730	27	7	11	2 starch, 1 medium-fat meat, 1 fat
SIDES												
Cheesy Fiesta Potatoes	1 srvg	290	17	5	3.5	0	15	830	29	2	4	2 starch, 3 1/2 fat
✔Mexican Rice	1 srvg	110	3	2	0	0	0	460	19	1	2	1 1/2 starch, 1/2 fat

✔ = Healthiest Bets

(*Continued*)

SIDES *(Continued)*	Amount	Cal.	Fat (g)	% Cal. Fat	Sat. Fat (g)	Trans Fat (g)	Chol. (mg)	Sod. (mg)	Carb. (g)	Fiber (g)	Pro. (g)	Choices/Exchanges
Pintos n Cheese	1 srvg	160	6	3	3	0.5	15	670	19	7	9	1 1/2 starch, 1 medium-fat meat, 1/2 fat
SPECIALTIES												
Chicken Fiesta Taco Salad	1 srvg	790	38	4	8	1	75	1830	77	13	37	4 starch, 3 veg, 4 lean meat, 5 fat
Chicken Fiesta Taco Salad w/o Shell	1 srvg	430	18	4	6	1	75	1560	38	11	30	1 starch, 3 veg, 4 lean meat, 1 1/2 fat
Chicken Quesadilla	1	520	28	5	12	0.5	75	1420	40	3	28	2 1/2 starch, 3 lean meat, 4 fat
Chicken Taquitos	1 srvg	310	11	3	4.5	0	40	980	37	2	18	2 1/2 starch, 2 lean meat, 1 1/2 fat
Crunchwrap Supreme	1	560	24	4	8	0.5	30	1430	68	5	17	4 1/2 starch, 4 1/2 fat
Enchirito - Beef	1	360	17	4	8	1	50	1420	34	7	18	2 1/2 starch, 2 medium-fat meat, 2 fat

Enchirito - Chicken	1	340	13	3	7	0.5	50	1450	33	6	22	2 starch, 2 lean meat, 1 1/2 fat
Enchirito - Steak	1	330	14	4	7	1	45	1330	33	6	20	2 starch, 2 medium-fat meat, 1 fat
Express Taco Salad	1 srvg	610	32	5	10	1.5	65	1420	56	14	25	2 1/2 starch, 3 veg, 3 lean meat, 5 fat
Fiesta Taco Salad	1 srvg	840	45	5	11	1.5	65	1780	80	15	30	4 starch, 3 veg, 3 lean meat, 7 fat
Fiesta Taco Salad w/o Shell	1 srvg	470	24	5	10	1.5	65	1510	40	13	23	1 1/2 starch, 3 veg, 3 lean meat, 3 fat
✔Guacamole Side	1.5 oz.	70	5	6	1	0	0	180	5	2	1	1/2 starch, 1 fat
Mexican Pizza	1 srvg	530	30	5	8	1	40	1000	46	6	20	3 starch, 2 medium-fat meat, 4 fat
✔MexiMelt	1 srvg	280	14	5	7	0.5	40	860	22	3	15	1 1/2 starch, 2 medium-fat meat, 1 1/2 fat
✔Salsa Side	1.5 oz.	15	0	0	0	0	0	160	3	0	0	Free

✔ = Healthiest Bets

(*Continued*)

SPECIALTIES *(Continued)*	Amount	Cal.	Fat (g)	% Cal. Fat	Sat. Fat (g)	Trans Fat (g)	Chol. (mg)	Sod. (mg)	Carb. (g)	Fiber (g)	Pro. (g)	Choices/Exchanges
Sour Cream Side	1.5 oz.	80	7	8	4.5	0	25	30	3	0	1	1 1/2 fat
Southwest Steak Border Bowl	1 srvg	600	24	4	6	1	55	2120	68	9	28	4 1/2 starch, 2 medium-fat meat, 2 fat
Spicy Chicken Crunchwrap Supreme	1 wrap	540	23	4	7	0	40	1360	67	4	19	4 1/2 starch, 1 lean meat, 3 fat
Steak Quesadilla	1	520	28	5	13	1	70	1300	39	3	26	2 1/2 starch, 3 medium-fat meat, 3 fat
✔Steak Taquitos	1 srvg	310	11	3	5	0	35	870	36	2	16	2 1/2 starch, 1 medium-fat meat, 1 fat
Zesty Chicken Border Bowl	1 srvg	640	35	5	6	1	30	1800	60	10	22	4 starch, 1 lean meat, 6 fat
Zesty Chicken Border Bowl w/o Dressing	1 srvg	440	15	3	2.5	0.5	30	1540	57	10	21	4 starch, 1 lean meat, 2 fat

TACOS

✔Crunchy Taco Supreme	1	210	13	6	6	0.5	40	370	15	3	9	1 starch, 1 medium-fat meat, 1 1/2 fat
Double Decker Taco	1	320	13	4	5	0.5	25	810	38	6	14	2 1/2 starch, 1 medium-fat meat, 1 fat
Double Decker Taco Supreme	1	370	17	4	7	1	40	820	40	7	14	2 1/2 starch, 1 medium-fat meat, 2 fat
Grilled Steak Soft Taco	1	260	15	5	4.5	0	30	640	20	2	12	1 1/2 starch, 1 medium-fat meat, 2 fat
Ranchero Chicken Soft Taco	1	270	14	5	4	0	35	820	21	2	14	1 1/2 starch, 1 lean meat, 2 fat
Soft Taco Supreme - Beef	1	250	13	5	6	0.5	40	650	23	3	11	1 1/2 starch, 1 medium-fat meat, 1 1/2 fat
Spicy Chicken Soft Taco	1	170	6	3	2	0	25	580	20	2	10	1 1/2 starch, 1 lean meat, 1/2 fat

✔ = Healthiest Bets

(*Continued*)

	Amount	Cal.	Fat (g)	% Cal. Fat	Sat. Fat (g)	Trans Fat (g)	Chol. (mg)	Sod. (mg)	Carb. (g)	Fiber (g)	Pro. (g)	Choices/Exchanges
VALUE MENU												
1/2 lb Cheesy Bean & Rice Burrito	1	470	20	4	5	0	10	1390	58	6	13	4 starch, 4 fat
Bean Burrito	1	350	9	2	3.5	0.5	5	1190	54	8	13	3 1/2 starch, 1 fat
Big Taste Taco	1	420	22	5	6	0	35	1030	43	4	14	3 starch, 1 medium-fat meat, 3 fat
Caramel Apple Empanada	1	290	15	5	2.5	0	0	270	38	2	3	2 1/2 carb, 2 fat
✔Cheese Roll-Up	1 srvg	200	10	5	5	0	20	490	19	1	9	1 1/2 starch, 1 medium-fat meat, 1 1/2 fat
Cheesy Double Beef Burrito	1	460	20	4	6	0.5	40	1610	52	5	18	3 1/2 starch, 1 medium-fat meat, 3 fat
✔Cinnamon Twists	1 srvg	170	7	4	0	0	0	200	26	1	1	1 1/2 carb, 1 fat

✔Crunchy Taco	1	170	10	5	3.5	0	25	350	13	3	8	1 starch, 1 medium-fat meat, 1 fat
✔Soft Taco - Beef	1	200	9	4	4	0	25	630	21	3	10	1 1/2 starch, 1 medium-fat meat, 1 fat
Triple Layer Nachos	1 srvg	340	18	5	1.5	0	0	720	38	6	7	2 1/2 starch, 3 fat

✔ = Healthiest Bets

Exclusive Web Content

Be sure to visit the following restaurants online at http://www.diabetes.org/healthyrestaurant

Carvel
Del Taco
El Pollo Loco
Frëshens
Godfather's
Jersey Mike's
Jimmy John's
Tim Hortons
Whataburger
Wienerschnitzel
Zaxby's

Taco John's

(www.tacojohns.com)

Light 'n Lean Choice

Chicken Softshell Taco *(1)*
Bean Burrito *(1)*

Calories	570	Cholesterol (mg)	45
Fat (g)	15	Sodium (mg)	1,530
% calories from fat	24	Carbohydrate (g)	77
Saturated fat (g)	6	Fiber (g)	10
Trans fat (g)	0	Protein (g)	28

Exchanges: 5 starch, 1 1/2 lean meat, 2 fat

Healthy 'n Hearty Choice

Chicken and Rice Burritos *(1)*
Refried Beans *(1/2 serving)*

Calories	630	Cholesterol (mg)	38
Fat (g)	17	Sodium (mg)	1,930
% calories from fat	24	Carbohydrate (g)	91
Saturated fat (g)	6	Fiber (g)	11
Trans fat (g)	1	Protein (g)	28

Exchanges: 6 starch, 2 lean meat, 2 fat

Taco John's

	Amount	Cal.	Fat (g)	% Cal. Fat	Sat. Fat (g)	Trans Fat (g)	Chol. (mg)	Sod. (mg)	Carb. (g)	Fiber (g)	Pro. (g)	Choices/Exchanges
10G OR LESS OF FAT												
Bean Burrito w/o Cheese	1	320	5	1	0	0	0	740	58	9	11	4 starch, 1 fat
✔Chicken Softshell Taco	1	190	6	3	3	0	30	700	19	1	13	1 1/2 starch, 1 lean meat, 1/2 fat
✔Crispy Taco	1	180	10	5	3.5	0	25	270	13	2	9	1 starch, 1 medium-fat meat, 1 fat
Mexican Rice	1 srvg	250	6	2	0	0	0	1080	45	0	5	3 starch, 1/2 fat
Refried Beans w/o Cheese	1 srvg	280	2	1	0.5	0.5	0	980	50	11	15	3 1/2 starch, 1 lean meat
✔Softshell Taco w/o Cheese	1	190	8	4	3	0	20	530	20	2	9	1 1/2 starch, 1 medium-fat meat, 1 fat

✔ = Healthiest Bets

(Continued)

10G OR LESS OF FAT *(Continued)*	Amount	Cal.	Fat (g)	% Cal. Fat	Sat. Fat (g)	Trans Fat (g)	Chol. (mg)	Sod. (mg)	Carb. (g)	Fiber (g)	Pro. (g)	Choices/Exchanges
✔Taco Burger w/o Cheese	1	250	9	3	2.5	0	25	560	28	3	12	2 starch, 1 medium-fat meat, 1 fat
Texas Chili w/o Cheese	1 srvg	160	6	3	2	0	20	1160	17	4	10	1 starch, 1 medium-fat meat, 1/2 fat
BREAKFAST												
Bacon Burrito	1	550	25	4	6	0	250	1370	56	7	21	3 1/2 starch, 1 medium-fat meat, 3 1/2 fat
Bacon Egg Burrito	1	500	24	4	9	0	275	1120	43	5	26	3 starch, 2 medium-fat meat, 2 fat
Bacon Potato Olés Scrambler	sm	630	41	6	10	0.5	260	1860	45	6	20	3 starch, 2 medium-fat meat, 6 fat
Bacon Potato Olés Scrambler	reg	1030	67	6	17	1	395	3060	72	9	32	5 starch, 3 medium-fat meat, 10 fat

Bacon Scrambler Burrito	1	550	25	4	6	0	250	1370	58	7	21	4 starch, 1 medium-fat meat, 3 fat
✔Bacon Taco	1	270	13	4	4	0	125	810	25	2	10	1 1/2 starch, 1 medium-fat meat, 2 fat
✔Egg Burrito	1	420	19	4	8	0	270	730	42	5	21	3 starch, 2 medium-fat meat, 2 fat
Sausage Burrito	1	640	35	5	10	0	275	1300	56	7	23	3 1/2 starch, 2 medium-fat meat, 5 fat
Sausage Egg Burrito	1	590	34	5	13	0	300	1050	44	6	28	3 starch, 3 medium-fat meat, 3 1/2 fat
Sausage Potato Olés Scrambler	sm	720	50	6	14	0.5	280	1780	45	6	22	3 starch, 2 medium-fat meat, 8 fat
Sausage Potato Olés Scrambler	reg	1140	79	6	22	1	425	2890	72	9	34	5 starch, 3 medium-fat meat, 12 fat
Sausage Scrambler Burrito	1	640	32	5	9	0	270	1440	58	7	21	4 starch, 1 medium-fat meat, 5 fat

✔ = Healthiest Bets; n/a = not available

(*Continued*)

BREAKFAST *(Continued)*	Amount	Cal.	Fat (g)	% Cal. Fat	Sat. Fat (g)	Trans Fat (g)	Chol. (mg)	Sod. (mg)	Carb. (g)	Fiber (g)	Pro. (g)	Choices/Exchanges
✔Sausage Taco	1	310	18	5	6	0	135	770	25	2	11	1 1/2 starch, 1 medium-fat meat, 2 1/2 fat
Waffle Stix - Cinnamon Sugar	1 srvg	740	52	6	4	0	0	560	68	8	5	4 1/2 starch, 10 fat
Waffle Stix - Maple Syrup	1 srvg	880	52	5	4	0	0	600	104	1	4	7 starch, 9 fat
BURRITOS												
Bean Burrito	1	380	9	2	3	0	15	830	58	9	15	4 starch, 2 fat
Beef Grilled Burrito	1	600	32	5	13	1	75	1230	52	8	27	3 1/2 starch, 2 medium-fat meat, 3 fat
✔Beefy Burrito	1	440	20	4	7	1	50	860	45	7	22	3 starch, 2 medium-fat meat, 2 fat
Chicken & Potato Burrito	1	470	19	4	4.5	0	30	1220	56	7	17	3 1/2 starch, 1 lean meat, 3 fat

Chicken & Rice Burrito	1	470	14	3	4	0	30	1420	67	5	19	4 1/2 starch, 1 lean meat, 2 fat
Chicken Grilled Burrito	1	590	29	4	11	0.5	90	1510	50	6	32	3 1/2 starch, 3 lean meat, 3 1/2 fat
✔Combination Burrito	1	400	14	3	5	0.5	35	830	50	8	18	3 1/2 starch, 1 medium-fat meat, 1 fat
Crunchy Chicken & Potato Burrito	1	600	28	4	6	0	35	1320	65	7	20	4 1/2 starch, 1 lean meat, 5 fat
Meat & Potato Burrito	1	500	23	4	6	0.5	30	1100	58	8	15	4 starch, 4 1/2 fat
Steak & Potato Burrito	1	480	22	4	6	0	30	1240	56	10	17	3 1/2 starch, 1 medium-fat meat, 3 fat
Steak & Rice Burrito	1	450	17	3	5	0	35	1440	57	8	20	4 starch, 1 medium-fat meat, 1 1/2 fat
Steak Grilled Burrito	1	610	34	5	13	0.5	85	1540	49	10	31	3 1/2 starch, 3 medium-fat meat, 3 fat

✔ = Healthiest Bets

(Continued)

BURRITOS *(Continued)*	Amount	Cal.	Fat (g)	% Cal. Fat	Sat. Fat (g)	Trans Fat (g)	Chol. (mg)	Sod. (mg)	Carb. (g)	Fiber (g)	Pro. (g)	Choices/Exchanges
Super Burrito	1	450	18	4	7	0.5	40	920	54	9	19	3 1/2 starch, 1 medium-fat meat, 2 fat
CHALUPAS												
✔Beef Chalupa	1	300	17	5	6	0.5	30	430	28	2	13	2 starch, 1 medium-fat meat, 2 fat
✔Beef Chalupa w/o Cheese & Sour Cream	1	240	12	5	2.5	0	20	340	27	2	10	2 starch, 1 medium-fat meat, 1 fat
✔Chipotle Chicken Chalupa	1	240	10	4	1	0	20	650	26	2	13	1 1/2 starch, 1 lean meat, 1 fat
Cilantro Lime Steak Chalupa	1	310	19	6	3.5	0	25	590	25	4	12	1 1/2 starch, 1 medium-fat meat, 3 fat
CONDIMENTS												
Bacon Ranch Dressing	1.5 oz.	130	10	7	1.5	0	10	370	10	0	1	1/2 starch, 2 fat
Creamy Italian Dressing	1.5 oz.	130	15	10	2	0	0	320	3	0	0	3 fat

Guacamole	2 oz.	90	6	6	2	0	0	115	8	2	0	1/2 starch, 1 fat
✔Hot Sauce	1 oz.	10	0	0	0	0	0	125	1	0	0	Free
House Dressing	1.5 oz.	70	7	9	1	0	0	260	2	0	0	1 1/2 fat
✔Mild Sauce	1 oz.	10	0	0	0	0	0	130	1	0	0	Free
Nacho Cheese	3 oz.	120	9	7	4	0	10	520	5	0	4	1/2 starch, 2 fat
✔Pico de Gallo	1 oz.	10	0	0	0	0	0	90	1	0	0	Free
Ranch Dressing	1.5 oz.	140	16	10	2	0	20	350	3	0	1	3 fat
✔Salsa	2 oz.	20	0	0	0	0	0	220	4	1	1	1 veg
Sour Cream	2 oz.	120	12	9	7	0	25	30	2	0	2	2 1/2 fat
✔Super Hot Sauce	1 oz.	10	0	0	0	0	0	25	1	0	0	Free
DESSERTS												
Apple Grande	1 srvg	270	12	4	3	0	5	420	39	2	5	2 1/2 carb, 2 fat
Choco Taco	1 srvg	390	20	5	15	0	15	160	48	1	5	3 carb, 3 fat

✔ = Healthiest Bets

(*Continued*)

DESSERTS *(Continued)*	Amount	Cal.	Fat (g)	% Cal. Fat	Sat. Fat (g)	Trans Fat (g)	Chol. (mg)	Sod. (mg)	Carb. (g)	Fiber (g)	Pro. (g)	Choices/Exchanges
✔Churro	1 srvg	190	7	3	1.5	0	20	170	15	4	2	1 carb, 2 fat
✔Giant Goldfish Grahams	1 srvg	70	2	3	0.5	0	0	55	11	1	1	1/2 carb, 1/2 fat
LOCAL FAVORITES												
Chili Cheese Potato Olés	1 srvg	590	36	5	8	0.5	25	2130	55	8	13	3 1/2 starch, 7 fat
Chili Enchilada	1 srvg	310	16	5	7	1	50	1000	24	4	18	1 1/2 starch, 2 medium-fat meat, 1 1/2 fat
Chilito	1 srvg	360	15	4	7	0	35	670	40	5	15	2 1/2 starch, 3 fat
✔Mexi Rolls w/o Nacho Cheese	2 pc	160	7	4	2	0	15	190	16	6	8	1 starch, 1 medium-fat meat, 1/2 fat
Mexi Rolls w/o Nacho Cheese	4 pc	310	14	4	4.5	1	30	390	32	12	16	2 starch, 1 medium-fat meat, 1 fat
Mexi Rolls w/o Nacho Cheese	6 pc	470	21	4	7	1	50	580	47	18	24	3 starch, 2 medium-fat meat, 1 1/2 fat

Ranch Burrito - Beef	1	440	22	5	6	0	45	850	45	6	17	3 starch, 1 medium-fat meat, 3 fat
Ranch Burrito - Chicken	1	400	17	4	4.5	0	45	970	44	5	19	3 starch, 1 lean meat, 2 fat
Smothered Burrito	1	510	20	4	8	1	45	1330	60	10	23	4 starch, 2 medium-fat meat, 2 fat
SIDES												
Mexican Rice	1 srvg	250	6	2	0	0	0	1080	45	0	5	3 starch, 1/2 fat
Nachos	1 srvg	380	23	5	6	0	10	750	38	1	6	2 1/2 starch, 4 fat
Potato Olés - Kids Meal/ Breakfast Portion	1 srvg	290	18	6	2.5	0	0	840	31	4	3	2 starch, 3 fat
Potato Olés	sm	430	26	5	3.5	0	0	1220	45	6	4	3 starch, 4 1/2 fat
Potato Olés	med	600	36	5	5	0.5	0	1710	62	8	6	4 starch, 6 fat
Potato Olés	lg	770	46	5	6	1	0	2200	80	11	7	5 1/2 starch, 8 fat
Refried Beans	1 srvg	320	6	2	3.5	1	15	1020	47	11	18	3 starch, 1 medium-fat meat

✓ = Healthiest Bets

(*Continued*)

SIDES *(Continued)*	Amount	Cal.	Fat (g)	% Cal. Fat	Sat. Fat (g)	Trans Fat (g)	Chol. (mg)	Sod. (mg)	Carb. (g)	Fiber (g)	Pro. (g)	Choices/Exchanges
Refried Beans w/o Cheese	1 srvg	260	2	1	0	0.5	0	940	47	11	14	3 starch, 1 lean meat
Texas Chili w/o Crackers	1 srvg	220	11	5	5	0	35	1240	17	4	14	1 starch, 2 medium-fat meat, 1/2 fat
Texas Chili w/o Crackers & Cheese	1 srvg	160	6	3	2	0	20	1160	17	4	10	1 starch, 1 medium-fat meat, 1/2 fat
SPECIALTIES												
Cheese Quesadilla	1	450	23	5	12	0	45	930	43	5	20	3 starch, 2 lean meat, 3 fat
Chicken Quesadilla	1	500	24	4	13	0	65	1240	44	5	29	3 starch, 3 lean meat, 2 1/2 fat
Chicken Taco Salad w/o Dressing	1 srvg	480	27	5	9	0.5	65	1020	35	6	24	1 starch, 3 veg, 3 lean meat, 3 1/2 fat
Crunchy Chicken Taco Salad w/o Dressing	1 srvg	660	40	5	10	0.5	70	1180	47	6	29	2 starch, 3 veg, 3 lean meat, 6 fat

Steak Quesadilla	1	510	27	5	14	0	65	1260	43	8	28	3 starch, 3 medium-fat meat, 2 fat
Steak Taco Salad w/o Dressing	1 srvg	490	30	6	11	0.5	60	1040	34	9	24	1 starch, 3 veg, 3 lean meat, 4 fat
Super Nachos	sm	450	27	5	9	0	35	650	38	3	12	2 1/2 starch, 5 1/2 fat
Super Nachos	reg	810	48	5	16	1	55	1450	74	5	22	5 starch, 9 1/2 fat
Super Potato Olés	sm	620	39	6	11	1	35	1270	53	7	14	3 1/2 starch, 8 fat
Super Potato Olés	reg	1030	65	6	19	1.5	55	2850	87	13	24	6 starch, 13 fat
Taco Salad w/o Dressing	1 srvg	520	33	6	11	1	60	860	37	7	21	1 starch, 3 veg, 3 lean meat, 5 fat

TACOS

✔Chicken Softshell Taco	1	190	6	3	3	0	30	700	19	1	13	1 1/2 starch, 1 lean meat, 1/2 fat
✔Chicken Softshell Taco w/o Cheese	1	160	3.5	2	1.5	0	20	650	19	1	12	1 1/2 starch, 1 lean meat

✔ = Healthiest Bets

(*Continued*)

TACOS *(Continued)*	Amount	Cal.	Fat (g)	% Cal. Fat	Sat. Fat (g)	Trans Fat (g)	Chol. (mg)	Sod. (mg)	Carb. (g)	Fiber (g)	Pro. (g)	Choices/Exchanges
✔Chipotle Chicken Softshell Taco	1	200	7	3	3	0	30	780	20	1	13	1 1/2 starch, 1 lean meat, 1/2 fat
Cilantro Lime Steak Softshell Taco	1	240	14	5	4.5	0	30	760	19	4	13	1 1/2 starch, 1 medium-fat meat, 1 fat
✔Crispy Taco	1	180	10	5	3.5	0	25	270	13	2	9	1 starch, 1 medium-fat meat, 1 fat
✔Softshell Taco	1	220	11	5	4.5	0.5	25	580	21	2	11	1 1/2 starch, 1 medium-fat meat, 1 fat
Taco Bravo	1	340	13	3	4.5	0.5	25	750	40	5	15	2 1/2 starch, 1 medium-fat meat, 1 fat
✔Taco Burger	1	270	12	4	4	0.5	30	600	28	3	14	2 starch, 1 medium-fat meat, 1 fat

✔ = Healthiest Bets

Frozen Sweets and Treats

RESTAURANTS

Baskin Robbins
Cold Stone Creamery
TCBY

EXCLUSIVE WEB CONTENT

Carvel (**http://www.diabetes.org/healthyrestaurant**)
Frëshens Premium Yogurt
(**http://www.diabetes.org/healthyrestaurant**)

The Scoop: Nutrition information is for 4-fluid-ounce servings. Yes, that's small, but it is the industry standard serving size. In many cases the nutrition information is only for vanilla or several other flavors. Flavors that have nuts, fudge, or chocolate pieces will most likely have more calories. Several companies base their nutrition information on an average of all flavors.

No meals are provided for this chapter because these foods are usually eaten as a snack or in addition to a meal.

NUTRITION PROS

- Small portions are an option.
- Some restaurants offer a kiddie or junior size. That's portion control at work, and hopefully it's enough to satisfy your sweet tooth.
- Healthier toppings are easy to spot: fresh fruit, granola, nuts, or raisins.

- Low-fat, fat-free, and/or sugar-free frozen treats abound.
- Desserts are easy to split. Just ask for two forks or spoons.
- You can watch the server's every move. Make sure they do what you want.

NUTRITION CONS

- Overindulgence is easy.
- Unhealthy toppers are plentiful: candy bar pieces, cookies, hot fudge, or butterscotch.
- Sometimes the low-fat, fat-free, and/or sugar-free desserts are not that much lower in calories than the regular varieties. Check it out.
- Often the low-fat or fat-free products are higher in carbohydrate. The fat gets swapped for the carbohydrate.
- Fruit smoothies or shakes are often light on the "real fruit" and heavy on the sugar.

Get It Your Way

- ★ Low-fat or fat-free; frozen yogurt, light ice cream, or sorbet; and kiddie and small—options are aplenty for healthful eating.

Healthy Tips

- ★ Don't think kiddie or junior sizes are just for kids. They're great small sizes for calorie and carbohydrate counters too.
- ★ Order one dessert and two spoons. Just a few bites often quiets your sweet tooth.

Exclusive Web Content

Be sure to visit the following restaurants online at http://www.diabetes.org/healthyrestaurant

Carvel
Del Taco
El Pollo Loco
Frëshens
Godfather's
Jersey Mike's
Jimmy John's
Tim Hortons
Whataburger
Wienerschnitzel
Zaxby's

Baskin Robbins
(www.baskinrobbins.com)

Baskin Robbins

	Amount	Cal.	Fat (g)	% Cal. Fat	Sat. Fat (g)	Trans Fat (g)	Chol. (mg)	Sod. (mg)	Carb. (g)	Fiber (g)	Pro. (g)	Choices/Exchanges
BEVERAGES: CAPPUCCINO BLAST												
Caramel	16 oz.	480	16	3	10	0	60	300	81	0	7	5 1/2 carb, 2 fat
Caramel	24 oz.	720	24	3	15	0.5	90	440	121	0	10	8 carb, 4 fat
Caramel	32 oz.	1000	30	3	19	1	115	650	173	0	13	11 1/2 carb, 5 fat
Low Fat	16 oz.	220	2	1	1.5	0	10	115	45	0	6	3 carb
Mocha	16 oz.	380	12	3	7	0	45	85	64	0	5	4 1/2 carb, 2 fat
Mocha	24 oz.	540	18	3	12	0	70	140	87	0	8	6 carb, 3 fat
Mocha	32 oz.	750	23	3	15	0	90	170	128	0	11	8 1/2 carb, 4 fat
Mocha w/ Whipped Cream	16 oz.	370	13	3	8	0	50	100	58	0	6	4 carb, 2 fat
Mocha w/ Whipped Cream	24 oz.	620	21	3	13	0	80	160	100	0	9	6 1/2 carb, 3 fat

✓ = Healthiest Bets

(*Continued*)

BEVERAGES: CAPPUCCINO BLAST *(Continued)*	Amount	Cal.	Fat (g)	% Cal. Fat	Sat. Fat (g)	Trans Fat (g)	Chol. (mg)	Sod. (mg)	Carb. (g)	Fiber (g)	Pro. (g)	Choices/Exchanges
Mocha w/ Whipped Cream	32 oz.	790	25	3	16	0	100	190	136	0	11	9 carb, 4 fat
Nonfat	16 oz.	210	0	0	0	0	5	120	45	0	7	3 carb
Nonfat	24 oz.	340	0	0	0	0	5	190	78	0	11	5 carb
Nonfat	32 oz.	440	0.5	0	0	0	5	240	102	1	14	7 carb
Original	16 oz.	300	12	4	7	0	45	95	43	0	6	3 carb, 2 fat
Original	24 oz.	460	19	4	12	0	75	150	66	0	9	4 1/2 carb, 3 fat
Original	32 oz.	620	24	3	15	0	95	200	94	0	12	6 1/2 carb, 4 fat
w/ Whipped Cream	16 oz.	330	14	4	9	0	55	110	48	0	6	3 carb, 2 fat
w/ Whipped Cream	24 oz.	480	21	4	13	0	80	160	67	0	9	4 1/2 carb, 3 fat
w/ Whipped Cream	32 oz.	660	28	4	17	0	105	220	97	0	12	6 1/2 carb, 4 fat
BEVERAGES: FREEZES												
w/ Orange Sherbet	16 oz.	370	4	1	2.5	0	15	120	82	0	3	5 1/2 carb, 1/2 fat

w/ Orange Sherbet	23 oz.	510	5	1	3.5	0	20	160	112	1	3	7 1/2 carb, 1/2 fat
w/ Orange Sherbet	33 oz.	740	8	1	5	0	30	240	164	1	5	11 carb, 1 fat
BEVERAGES: FRUIT BLAST												
Berry Pomegranate	16 oz.	370	0	0	0	0	0	15	93	1	0	6 carb
Berry Pomegranate	24 oz.	510	0	0	0	0	0	20	128	1	1	8 1/2 carb
Berry Pomegranate	32 oz.	740	0	0	0	0	0	30	186	1	1	12 1/2 carb
Peach Passion	16 oz.	270	0	0	0	0	0	10	68	2	1	4 1/2 carb
Peach Passion	24 oz.	370	0.5	0	0	0	0	10	94	3	2	6 1/2 carb
Peach Passion	32 oz.	50	1	2	0	0	0	15	136	4	3	9 carb
Strawberry Citrus	16 oz.	350	1	0	0	0	0	10	89	3	1	6 carb
Strawberry Citrus	24 oz.	480	1	0	0	0	0	15	122	4	2	8 carb
Strawberry Citrus	32 oz.	700	1.5	0	0	0	0	20	178	6	3	12 carb
Wild Mango	16 oz.	340	1	0	0	0	0	10	84	2	1	5 1/2 carb

✓ = Healthiest Bets

(*Continued*)

BEVERAGES: FRUIT BLAST *(Continued)*	Amount	Cal.	Fat (g)	% Cal. Fat	Sat. Fat (g)	Trans Fat (g)	Chol. (mg)	Sod. (mg)	Carb. (g)	Fiber (g)	Pro. (g)	Choices/Exchanges
Wild Mango	24 oz.	470	1.5	0	0	0	0	15	116	2	1	7 1/2 carb
Wild Mango	32 oz.	690	2	0	0	0	0	20	169	3	1	11 1/2 carb
BEVERAGES: FRUIT BLAST SMOOTHIE												
Berry Pomegranate Banana	16 oz.	510	0.5	0	0	0	0	80	125	2	5	8 1/2 carb
Berry Pomegranate Banana	24 oz.	710	1	0	0	0	5	125	172	3	7	11 1/2 carb
Berry Pomegranate Banana	32 oz.	1020	1.5	0	0.5	0	5	160	250	5	9	16 1/2 carb
Mango	16 oz.	440	1.5	0	0	0	0	75	104	2	4	7 carb
Mango	24 oz.	620	2	0	0	0	5	120	148	3	7	10 carb
Mango	32 oz.	870	3	0	0	0	5	150	209	4	8	14 carb
Peach Passion	16 oz.	420	1	0	0	0	0	70	102	4	6	7 carb
Peach Passion	24 oz.	540	1	0	0	0	5	110	131	5	8	8 1/2 carb
Peach Passion	32 oz.	830	1.5	0	0.5	0	5	140	204	8	11	13 1/2 carb

Strawberry Banana	16 oz.	490	1.5	0	0	0	0	75	121	5	5	8 carb
Strawberry Banana	24 oz.	730	2	0	0	0	5	120	178	7	9	12 carb
Strawberry Banana	32 oz.	980	2.5	0	0.5	0	5	150	242	9	11	16 carb
BEVERAGES: ICE CREAM FLOATS												
w/ Vanilla Ice Cream & Root Beer	17 oz.	470	20	4	13	0.5	80	130	69	0	6	4 1/2 carb, 3 fat
w/ Vanilla Ice Cream & Root Beer	24 oz.	680	30	4	19	1	120	190	99	0	8	6 1/2 carb, 5 fat
w/ Vanilla Ice Cream & Root Beer	34 oz.	940	40	4	25	1.5	155	260	138	0	11	9 carb, 7 fat
BEVERAGES: ICE CREAM SODAS												
w/ Vanilla Ice Cream	14 oz.	480	20	4	13	0.5	80	130	69	0	6	4 1/2 carb, 3 fat
w/ Vanilla Ice Cream	21 oz.	720	30	4	19	1	120	190	103	0	8	7 carb, 5 fat
w/ Vanilla Ice Cream	29 oz.	960	40	4	25	1.5	155	260	138	0	11	9 carb, 7 fat

✔ = Healthiest Bets

(Continued)

	Amount	Cal.	Fat (g)	% Cal. Fat	Sat. Fat (g)	Trans Fat (g)	Chol. (mg)	Sod. (mg)	Carb. (g)	Fiber (g)	Pro. (g)	Choices/Exchanges
BEVERAGES: PREMIUM SHAKES												
Chocolate Oreo	16 oz.	1040	56	5	26	1.5	85	630	126	5	16	8 1/2 carb, 9 fat
Chocolate Oreo	24 oz.	1490	79	5	36	1.5	110	950	186	7	23	12 1/2 carb, 14 fat
Chocolate Oreo	32 oz.	2600	135	5	59	2.5	185	1770	333	13	38	22 carb, 24 fat
Heath	16 oz.	990	46	4	28	1	130	670	129	1	16	8 1/2 carb, 8 fat
Heath	24 oz.	1420	67	4	40	1.5	180	960	184	1	23	12 1/2 carb, 11 fat
Heath	32 oz.	2310	108	4	64	2.5	295	1560	303	2	35	20 carb, 18 fat
Jamoca Oreo	16 oz.	790	31	4	18	1	90	560	117	1	14	8 carb, 5 fat
Jamoca Oreo	24 oz.	1170	44	3	25	1	120	890	177	2	21	12 carb, 7 fat
Jamoca Oreo	32 oz.	1890	73	3	41	2	205	1380	283	4	32	19 carb, 12 fat
Oreo Cookies n Cream	16 oz.	990	46	4	25	1	110	660	132	2	16	9 carb, 7 fat
Oreo Cookies n Cream	24 oz.	1410	62	4	33	1.5	145	940	195	4	23	13 carb, 11 fat

Oreo Cookies n Cream	32 oz.	2210	100	4	54	2	245	1400	302	5	35	20 carb, 17 fat
Reeses Peanut Butter Cup	16 oz.	1010	62	6	27	1	110	560	93	4	24	6 carb, 12 fat
Reeses Peanut Butter Cup	24 oz.	1430	93	6	36	1	140	830	122	6	36	8 carb, 18 fat
Reeses Peanut Butter Cup	32 oz.	2320	150	6	60	2	235	1320	204	10	56	13 1/2 carb, 27 fat
York Peppermint Pattie	16 oz.	960	44	4	25	1	100	290	132	2	14	9 carb, 7 fat
York Peppermint Pattie	24 oz.	1390	62	4	35	1	135	440	195	3	20	13 carb, 11 fat
York Peppermint Pattie	32 oz.	2210	103	4	57	2	225	680	304	6	31	20 1/2 carb, 17 fat
BEVERAGES: SHAKES												
Chocolate Chip	16 oz.	540	21	4	14	0.5	65	300	77	1	15	5 carb, 3 fat
Chocolate Chip	24 oz.	750	28	3	18	1	85	410	106	2	21	7 carb, 5 fat
Chocolate Chip	32 oz.	1220	48	4	31	1.5	145	680	170	3	34	11 1/2 carb, 8 fat
Chocolate w/ Chocolate Ice Cream	16 oz.	620	30	4	18	1	105	300	81	1	15	5 1/2 carb, 5 fat

✓ = Healthiest Bets

(Continued)

BEVERAGES: SHAKES *(Continued)*	Amount	Cal.	Fat (g)	% Cal. Fat	Sat. Fat (g)	Trans Fat (g)	Chol. (mg)	Sod. (mg)	Carb. (g)	Fiber (g)	Pro. (g)	Choices/Exchanges
Chocolate w/ Chocolate Ice Cream	24 oz.	990	40	4	25	1	135	440	149	1	20	10 carb, 6 fat
Chocolate w/ Chocolate Ice Cream	32 oz.	1290	58	4	36	0	200	630	176	1	28	11 1/2 carb, 10 fat
Chocolate w/ Vanilla Ice Cream	16 oz.	690	33	4	21	0	130	210	85	0	13	5 1/2 carb, 5 fat
Chocolate w/ Vanilla Ice Cream	24 oz.	1000	45	4	28	0	175	290	133	0	19	9 carb, 7 fat
Chocolate w/ Vanilla Ice Cream	32 oz.	1300	66	5	42	0	260	420	152	0	27	10 carb, 11 fat
Mint Chocolate Chip	16 oz.	760	36	4	24	0	115	320	94	1	16	6 1/2 carb, 6 fat
Mint Chocolate Chip	24 oz.	970	47	4	31	0	155	410	116	2	21	7 1/2 carb, 8 fat
Mint Chocolate Chip	32 oz.	1520	72	4	47	0	225	630	189	3	31	12 1/2 carb, 13 fat

Strawberry w/ Very Berry Strawberry Ice Cream	16 oz.	470	14	3	9	0	50	270	75	1	13	5 carb, 2 fat
Strawberry w/ Very Berry Strawberry Ice Cream	24 oz.	650	19	3	12	0.5	70	370	104	1	18	7 carb, 3 fat
Strawberry w/ Very Berry Strawberry Ice Cream	32 oz.	1120	46	4	29	1.5	185	440	154	2	24	10 1/2 carb, 7 fat
Vanilla	16 oz.	680	33	4	21	0	130	380	81	0	13	5 1/2 carb, 6 fat
Vanilla	24 oz.	980	45	4	28	0	175	640	125	0	19	8 1/2 carb, 7 fat
Vanilla	32 oz.	1290	66	5	42	0	260	650	147	0	27	10 carb, 11 fat
CAKES: ROLL ICE CREAM CAKES												
Chocolate Chip Ice Cream/Chocolate	1 slice	290	15	5	6	0	40	340	41	2	4	2 1/2 carb, 2 fat
Mint Chocolate Chip Ice Cream/ Chocolate	1 slice	290	14	4	6	0	45	240	36	2	5	2 1/2 carb, 3 fat
Vanilla Ice Cream/Chocolate	1 slice	270	14	5	4	0	45	340	39	2	4	2 1/2 carb, 2 fat

✔ = Healthiest Bets

(*Continued*)

	Amount	Cal.	Fat (g)	% Cal. Fat	Sat. Fat (g)	Trans Fat (g)	Chol. (mg)	Sod. (mg)	Carb. (g)	Fiber (g)	Pro. (g)	Choices/Exchanges
CAKES: ROUND ICE CREAM CAKES												
Chocolate Chip Cookie Dough Ice Cream/ Devils Food 6"	1 slice	460	23	5	11	0	65	380	59	1	7	4 carb, 4 fat
Chocolate Chip Ice Cream/ Devils Food 9"	1 slice	410	23	5	11	0	70	320	51	2	6	3 1/2 carb, 4 fat
Oreo Cookies n Cream Ice Cream/ Devils Food 6"	1 slice	440	23	5	10	0	65	400	56	1	7	3 1/2 carb, 4 fat
Oreo Cookies n Cream Ice Cream/ Devils Food 9"	1 slice	430	23	5	10	0.5	65	390	55	1	7	3 1/2 carb, 4 fat
Pralines n Cream Ice Cream/ White Sponge 9"	1 slice	430	20	4	8	0	50	380	65	1	6	4 1/2 carb, 3 fat
Vanilla & Chocolate Ice Cream/ Fudge Crunch 9"	1 slice	340	18	5	12	1	45	170	41	1	5	2 1/2 carb, 3 fat

CAKES: SHEET ICE CREAM CAKES

Chocolate Chip Ice Cream/Devils Food	1 slice	330	18	5	8	0	55	240	41	1	5	2 1/2 carb, 3 fat
Mint Chocolate Chip Ice Cream/Devils Food	1 slice	330	18	5	8	0	55	240	41	1	5	2 1/2 carb, 3 fat
Oreo Cookies n Cream Ice Cream/White Sponge	1 slice	350	16	4	7	0	45	270	47	1	5	3 carb, 3 fat
Pralines n Cream Ice Cream/White Sponge	1 slice	360	16	4	6	0	40	280	49	1	5	3 1/2 carb, 3 fat
Vanilla & Chocolate Ice Cream/Fudge Crunch	1 slice	330	18	5	12	1	45	160	40	1	5	2 1/2 carb, 3 fat
Vanilla Ice Cream/Devils Food	1 slice	340	19	5	9	0	60	220	39	1	5	2 1/2 carb, 4 fat
Very Berry Strawberry Ice Cream/White Sponge	1 slice	310	13	4	6	0	40	210	44	1	4	3 carb, 2 fat

✔ = Healthiest Bets

(*Continued*)

	Amount	Cal.	Fat (g)	% Cal. Fat	Sat. Fat (g)	Trans Fat (g)	Chol. (mg)	Sod. (mg)	Carb. (g)	Fiber (g)	Pro. (g)	Choices/Exchanges
CAKES: SPECIALTY ICE CREAM CAKES												
Chocolate Chip Ice Cream/ Devils Food Heart	1 slice	330	18	5	8	0	55	240	40	1	5	2 1/2 carb, 3 fat
Vanilla Ice Cream/ Devils Food Heart	1 slice	340	19	5	9	0	60	220	39	1	5	2 1/2 carb, 3 fat
GRAB-N-GO: FRUIT BLAST BARS												
✔Blue Raspberry	1 bar	50	0	0	0	0	0	0	14	0	0	1 carb
✔Mango	1 bar	50	0	0	0	0	0	0	14	0	0	1 carb
✔Strawberry	1 bar	50	0	0	0	0	0	0	13	0	0	1 carb
GRAB-N-GO: PRE-PACKED ICE CREAM												
✔Chocolate Chip Ice Cream Quart	1/2 cup	170	10	5	6	0	35	55	18	0	3	1 carb, 2 fat

✔Chocolate Cookie Dough Ice Cream Quart	1/2 cup	200	10	5	6	0	30	85	23	0	3	1 1/2 carb, 2 fat
✔Chocolate Ice Cream Quart	1/2 cup	170	9	5	6	0	30	85	21	1	3	1 1/2 carb, 2 fat
✔Chocolate Oreo Ice Cream Quart	1/2 cup	200	11	5	5	0	25	110	24	1	3	1 1/2 carb, 2 fat
✔Gold Medal Ribbon Ice Cream Quart	1/2 cup	170	8	4	5	0	30	105	22	0	3	1 1/2 carb, 1 1/2 fat
✔Heath Ice Cream Quart	1/2 cup	200	10	5	6	0	30	115	25	0	3	1 1/2 carb, 2 fat
✔Jamoca Almond Fudge Ice Cream Quart	1/2 cup	180	10	5	5	0	30	55	21	1	4	1 1/2 carb, 2 fat
✔Love Potion #31 Ice Cream Quart	1/2 cup	180	9	5	6	0	30	55	22	1	3	1 1/2 carb, 2 fat
✔Mint Chocolate Chip Ice Cream Quart	1/2 cup	170	10	5	6	0	35	55	18	0	3	1 carb, 2 fat
Old Fashioned Butter Pecan Ice Cream Quart	1/2 cup	180	12	6	6	0	35	70	16	1	3	1 carb, 2 1/2 fat

✔ = Healthiest Bets

(*Continued*)

GRAB-N-GO: PRE-PACKED ICE CREAM *(Continued)*	Amount	Cal.	Fat (g)	% Cal. Fat	Sat. Fat (g)	Trans Fat (g)	Chol. (mg)	Sod. (mg)	Carb. (g)	Fiber (g)	Pro. (g)	Choices/Exchanges
✔Oreo Cookies n Cream Ice Cream Quart	1/2 cup	180	10	5	6	0	30	100	21	0	3	1 1/2 carb, 2 fat
Peanut Butter n Chocolate Ice Cream Quart	1/2 cup	200	13	6	6	0	30	115	20	1	5	1 1/2 carb, 2 1/2 fat
✔Pralines n Cream Ice Cream Quart	1/2 cup	190	9	4	5	0	30	125	24	0	3	1 1/2 carb, 2 fat
✔Rainbow Sherbet Quart	1/2 cup	120	2	2	1	0	5	30	26	0	1	1 1/2 carb, 1/2 fat
Reeses Peanut Butter Cup Ice Cream Quart	1/2 cup	190	11	5	6	0	30	85	20	0	4	1 1/2 carb, 2 fat
✔Rocky Road Ice Cream Quart	1/2 cup	190	10	5	5	0	30	85	23	1	4	1 1/2 carb, 2 fat
✔Vanilla Ice Cream Quart	1/2 cup	170	10	5	7	0	40	45	17	0	3	1 carb, 2 fat
✔Very Berry Strawberry Ice Cream Quart	1/2 cup	140	7	5	4.5	0	25	45	18	0	2	1 carb, 1 1/2 fat

GRAB-N-GO: SUNDAE CUPS												
Oreo	1 cup	330	15	4	7	0	40	190	45	0	4	3 carb, 2 fat
Pralines n Cream	1 cup	330	16	4	8	0	45	170	43	1	4	3 carb, 3 fat
Reeses Peanut Butter Cup	1 cup	390	24	6	9	0	40	190	36	2	8	2 1/2 carb, 5 fat
ICE CREAM: CLASSIC FLAVORS												
Cherries Jubilee	1 scoop	240	12	5	7	0	45	80	30	1	4	2 carb, 2 1/2 fat
Chocolate	1 scoop	260	14	5	9	0	50	130	33	0	5	2 carb, 2 1/2 fat
Chocolate Chip	1 scoop	270	16	5	10	0	55	95	28	1	5	2 carb, 3 fat
Chocolate Chip Cookie Dough	1 scoop	290	15	5	9	1	55	130	36	1	5	2 1/2 carb, 3 fat
Chocolate Fudge	1 scoop	270	15	5	10	0	50	140	35	0	4	2 carb, 3 fat
French Vanilla	1 scoop	280	18	6	11	0.5	120	85	26	0	4	1 1/2 carb, 3 1/2 fat
Gold Medal Ribbon	1 scoop	260	13	5	8	0	45	150	34	0	5	2 1/2 carb, 2 fat
Heath	1 scoop	300	15	5	9	0	45	180	38	0	5	2 1/2 carb, 2 1/2 fat

✔ = Healthiest Bets

(*Continued*)

ICE CREAM: CLASSIC FLAVORS *(Continued)*	Amount	Cal.	Fat (g)	% Cal. Fat	Sat. Fat (g)	Trans Fat (g)	Chol. (mg)	Sod. (mg)	Carb. (g)	Fiber (g)	Pro. (g)	Choices/Exchanges
Jamoca	1 scoop	240	13	5	9	0	55	90	26	0	5	1 1/2 carb, 2 1/2 fat
Jamoca Almond Fudge	1 scoop	270	15	5	7	0	40	80	31	1	6	2 carb, 2 1/2 fat
Mint Chocolate Chip	1 scoop	270	16	5	10	0	55	95	28	1	5	2 carb, 3 fat
Nutty Coconut	1 scoop	300	20	6	9	0	45	90	28	1	6	2 carb, 4 fat
Old Fashioned Butter Pecan	1 scoop	280	18	6	9	0	50	95	24	1	5	1 1/2 carb, 3 1/2 fat
Peanut Butter n Chocolate	1 scoop	320	20	6	9	0	45	180	31	1	7	2 carb, 4 fat
Pistachio Almond	1 scoop	290	19	6	9	0	50	85	25	1	7	1 1/2 carb, 4 fat
Pralines n Cream	1 scoop	270	14	5	8	0	45	170	34	0	4	2 1/2 carb, 2 1/2 fat
Reeses Peanut Butter Cup	1 scoop	300	18	5	10	0	50	130	31	0	6	2 carb, 3 fat
Rocky Road	1 scoop	290	15	5	8	0	45	120	36	1	5	2 1/2 carb, 2 1/2 fat
Vanilla	1 scoop	260	16	6	10	0.5	65	70	26	0	4	1 1/2 carb, 3 fat

✔Very Berry Strawberry	1 scoop	220	11	5	7	0	40	70	28	0	4	2 carb, 1 1/2 fat
World Class Chocolate	1 scoop	280	16	5	11	0	45	95	31	0	5	2 carb, 3 fat
ICE CREAM: CONES												
✔Cake	1 cone	25	0	0	0	0	0	15	5	0	0	1/2 carb
✔Sugar	1 cone	45	1	2	0	0	0	35	9	0	1	1/2 carb
Waffle	1 cone	160	4	2	1	0	10	5	28	0	2	2 carb, 1 fat
ICE CREAM: FLAVORS OF THE MONTH												
Chocolate Oreo	1 scoop	360	20	5	8	0	35	210	44	2	5	3 carb, 3 fat
Jamoca Oreo	1 scoop	270	12	4	7	0	40	135	36	1	4	2 1/2 carb, 2 1/2 fat
Oreo Cookies n Cream	1 scoop	280	15	5	9	0	50	150	32	1	5	2 carb, 3 fat
ICE CREAM: LIGHTER SIDE												
✔Berries n Banana w/o Sugar	1 scoop	110	2	2	1	n/a	125	125	25	1	5	1 1/2 carb
Caramel Turtle w/o Sugar	1 scoop	160	4	2	3	0	10	170	37	0	5	2 1/2 carb, 1/2 fat

✔ = Healthiest Bets

(*Continued*)

ICE CREAM: LIGHTER SIDE *(Continued)*	Amount	Cal.	Fat (g)	% Cal. Fat	Sat. Fat (g)	Trans Fat (g)	Chol. (mg)	Sod. (mg)	Carb. (g)	Fiber (g)	Pro. (g)	Choices/Exchanges
✔Chocolate Chocolate Chip w/o Sugar	1 scoop	150	5	3	3.5	0	10	140	31	1	6	2 carb, 1/2 fat
✔Espresso n Cream	1 scoop	180	4	2	1.5	0	10	120	32	1	5	2 carb, 1 fat
✔Lemon Sorbet	1 scoop	130	0	0	0	0	0	15	33	0	0	2 carb
✔Lime Daiquiri Ice	1 scoop	130	0	0	0	0	0	15	33	0	0	2 carb
Maui Brownie Madness Frozen Yogurt	1 scoop	210	4	2	1.5	n/a	10	135	40	2	6	2 1/2 carb, 1/2 fat
Orange Sherbet	1 scoop	160	2	1	1.5	0	10	40	34	0	1	2 1/2 carb, 1/2 fat
✔Pineapple Coconut Low Fat w/o Sugar	1 scoop	120	2	2	1.5	0	10	140	27	0	5	2 carb
Rainbow Sherbet	1 scoop	160	2	1	1.5	0	10	40	34	0	1	2 1/2 carb
Raspberry Cheese Louise Frozen Yogurt	1 scoop	190	3.5	2	2.5	0	10	150	35	1	5	2 1/2 carb, 1/2 fat

Red Raspberry Sherbet	1 scoop	160	2	1	1	0	10	40	35	1	2	2 1/2 carb
Rock n Pop Swirl Sherbet	1 scoop	190	4	2	3	0	10	45	37	0	1	2 1/2 carb, 1/2 fat
✔Splish Splash Sherbet/ Ice Swirl	1 scoop	140	1	1	0.5	0	5	25	33	0	1	2 carb
✔Strawberry Sorbet	1 scoop	130	0	0	0	0	0	10	34	0	0	2 carb
✔Tin Roof Sundae w/o Sugar	1 scoop	150	4	2	2	0	10	160	33	1	5	2 carb
Tropical Ice	1 scoop	140	0	0	0	0	0	15	35	0	0	2 1/2 carb
✔Vanilla Nonfat Frozen Yogurt	1 scoop	150	0	0	0	0	5	105	32	0	6	2 carb
Wild n Reckless Sherbet	1 scoop	160	2	1	1.5	0	10	40	33	0	1	2 carb
ICE CREAM: REGIONAL FLAVORS												
Banana Nut	1 scoop	250	15	5	7	0	45	75	25	1	5	1 1/2 carb, 3 fat
Bananas n Strawberries	1 scoop	230	11	4	7	0	45	85	31	0	4	2 carb, 1 1/2 fat
Black Walnut	1 scoop	280	19	6	9	0	50	90	25	1	6	1 1/2 carb, 3 1/2 fat

✔ = Healthiest Bets

(*Continued*)

ICE CREAM: REGIONAL FLAVORS *(Continued)*	Amount	Cal.	Fat (g)	% Cal. Fat	Sat. Fat (g)	Trans Fat (g)	Chol. (mg)	Sod. (mg)	Carb. (g)	Fiber (g)	Pro. (g)	Choices/Exchanges
Chocolate Almond	1 scoop	300	18	5	9	0	45	120	32	1	7	2 carb, 3 fat
Chocolate Mousse Royale	1 scoop	310	18	5	13	0	40	140	35	1	5	2 1/2 carb, 3 fat
✔Creole Cream Cheese	1 scoop	190	7	3	4.5	0	25	130	28	0	28	2 carb, 1 1/2 fat
Fudge Brownie	1 scoop	310	18	5	11	0	45	140	35	2	5	2 1/2 carb, 3 fat
Lemon Custard	1 scoop	260	13	5	8	0	75	105	30	0	5	2 carb, 2 1/2 fat
Makin Cookies	1 scoop	310	13	4	9	0	45	180	40	0	4	2 1/2 carb, 2 fat
Mississippi Mud	1 scoop	270	13	4	8	0	45	150	38	1	4	2 1/2 carb, 2 1/2 fat
Oregon Blackberry	1 scoop	250	12	4	8	0	50	85	28	1	4	2 carb, 2 1/2 fat
Rum Raisin	1 scoop	250	11	4	7	0	45	80	34	0	4	2 1/2 carb, 1 1/2 fat
Tiramisu	1 scoop	210	8	3	5	0	35	150	32	0	5	2 carb, 1 fat
ICE CREAM: SEASONAL FLAVORS												
Americas Birthday Cake	1 scoop	280	15	5	10	0	50	105	33	0	4	2 carb, 3 fat

Baseball Nut	1 scoop	280	14	5	8	0	45	160	34	0	5	2 1/2 carb, 3 fat
Cotton Candy	1 scoop	260	12	4	7	0	45	210	32	0	4	2 carb, 2 1/2 fat
Egg Nog	1 scoop	250	13	5	8	0	70	85	31	0	5	2 carb, 2 fat
Everyone's Favorite Candy Bar	1 scoop	250	10	4	5	0	25	190	36	0	5	2 1/2 carb, 2 fat
German Chocolate Cake	1 scoop	300	16	5	9	0	45	150	37	1	5	2 1/2 carb, 2 1/2 fat
Icing on the Cake	1 scoop	290	15	5	10	0.5	45	90	35	0	5	2 1/2 carb, 2 1/2 fat
Love Potion #31	1 scoop	270	14	5	9	0	45	85	32	1	4	2 carb, 2 1/2 fat
✔Peppermint	1 scoop	210	8	3	6	0	25	125	30	0	5	2 carb, 1 fat
Pink Bubblegum	1 scoop	260	12	4	8	0	50	80	36	0	4	2 1/2 carb, 2 fat
✔Pumpkin Pie	1 scoop	180	6	3	4	0	25	125	29	0	4	2 carb, 1/2 fat
Quarterback Crunch	1 scoop	250	12	4	9	0	25	180	33	0	5	2 carb, 2 fat
Strawberry Cheesecake	1 scoop	270	14	5	9	0.5	55	115	32	0	5	2 carb, 3 fat
Tax Crunch	1 scoop	280	15	5	8	0	20	150	32	1	5	2 carb, 2 1/2 fat

✔ = Healthiest Bets

(*Continued*)

ICE CREAM: SEASONAL FLAVORS *(Continued)*	Amount	Cal.	Fat (g)	% Cal. Fat	Sat. Fat (g)	Trans Fat (g)	Chol. (mg)	Sod. (mg)	Carb. (g)	Fiber (g)	Pro. (g)	Choices/Exchanges
✔Winter White Chocolate	1 scoop	220	9	4	7	0	20	120	30	1	4	2 carb, 2 fat
York Peppermint Pattie	1 scoop	310	18	5	10	0	45	75	37	1	4	2 1/2 carb, 3 fat
SOFT SERVE: 31 BELOW												
Chocolate Oreo	sm (12 oz.)	910	39	4	21	0.5	65	750	131	2	15	8 1/2 carb, 6 fat
Chocolate Oreo	med (16 oz.)	1280	55	4	29	1	85	1060	185	3	21	12 1/2 carb, 9 fat
Chocolate Oreo	lg (24 oz.)	1740	75	4	40	1.5	120	1430	251	4	29	16 1/2 carb, 10 fat
Fudge Brownie	sm (12 oz.)	970	43	4	19	1	125	650	136	1	16	9 carb, 7 fat
Fudge Brownie	med (16 oz.)	1390	62	4	26	1	175	930	194	1	22	13 carb, 10 fat

Fudge Brownie	lg (24 oz.)	1900	85	4	36	1.5	245	1270	265	2	31	17 1/2 carb, 15 fat
Heath	sm (12 oz.)	850	39	4	23	1	85	630	113	1	14	7 1/2 carb, 7 fat
Heath	med (16 oz.)	1150	54	4	31	1	115	840	149	1	19	10 carb, 9 fat
Heath	lg (24 oz.)	1660	77	4	44	1.5	165	1220	219	2	27	14 1/2 carb, 14 fat
Oreo	sm (12 oz.)	710	29	4	15	0.5	65	650	101	2	15	6 1/2 carb, 5 fat
Oreo	med (16 oz.)	980	41	4	21	1	85	900	141	3	20	9 1/2 carb, 7 fat
Oreo	lg (24 oz.)	1350	56	4	29	1.5	120	1230	192	4	28	13 carb, 9 fat
Reese's Peanut Butter Cup	sm (12 oz.)	950	53	5	21	0.5	65	630	97	4	24	6 1/2 carb, 10 fat

✓ = Healthiest Bets

(*Continued*)

SOFT SERVE: 31 BELOW *(Continued)*	Amount	Cal.	Fat (g)	% Cal. Fat	Sat. Fat (g)	Trans Fat (g)	Chol. (mg)	Sod. (mg)	Carb. (g)	Fiber (g)	Pro. (g)	Choices/Exchanges
Reese's Peanut Butter Cup	med (16 oz.)	1230	67	5	27	1	90	820	132	5	31	9 carb, 13 fat
Reese's Peanut Butter Cup	lg (24 oz.)	1800	101	5	39	1	125	1190	184	8	45	12 1/2 carb, 19 fat
Strawberry Banana	sm (12 oz.)	530	17	3	11	0.5	65	310	84	3	13	5 1/2 carb, 3 fat
Strawberry Banana	med (16 oz.)	690	23	3	15	0.5	85	420	110	3	18	7 1/2 carb, 3 1/2 fat
Strawberry Banana	lg (24 oz.)	1010	33	3	21	1	120	590	161	5	26	10 1/2 carb, 6 fat
SOFT SERVE: 31 BELOW PIES												
Heath	1 slice	310	14	4	7	0	20	290	43	1	5	3 carb, 2 fat
Oreo	1 slice	290	13	4	6	0	20	290	40	1	5	2 1/2 carb, 2 fat

Reeses Peanut Butter Cup	1 slice	340	18	5	8	0	20	160	38	1	7	2 1/2 carb, 3 fat
SOFT SERVE: CUPS & CONES												
Chocolate Dipped Vanilla	kids (3 oz.)	230	14	5	11	0	20	110	24	1	4	1 1/2 carb, 3 fat
Chocolate Dipped Vanilla Vanilla	reg (6 oz.)	520	33	6	27	0	45	220	51	2	9	3 1/2 carb, 6 fat
Chocolate Dipped Vanilla	lg (9 oz.)	760	47	6	38	0.5	65	330	75	2	13	5 carb, 8 fat
✔Vanilla	kids (3 oz.)	140	6	4	3.5	0	20	100	19	0	4	1 1/2 carb, 1 fat
Vanilla	reg (6 oz.)	280	11	4	7	0	40	200	37	0	8	2 1/2 carb, 2 fat
Vanilla	lg (9 oz.)	420	17	4	11	0.5	35	300	56	0	12	3 1/2 carb, 3 fat

✔ = Healthiest Bets

(*Continued*)

	Amount	Cal.	Fat (g)	% Cal. Fat	Sat. Fat (g)	Trans Fat (g)	Chol. (mg)	Sod. (mg)	Carb. (g)	Fiber (g)	Pro. (g)	Choices/Exchanges
SOFT SERVE: FRUIT CREAM												
Berry Pomegranate	sm (12 oz.)	530	15	3	10	0	55	290	89	1	12	6 carb, 2 fat
Berry Pomegranate	med (16 oz.)	670	19	3	12	0.5	70	860	112	1	15	7 1/2 carb, 3 fat
Berry Pomegranate	lg (24 oz.)	920	25	2	16	1	90	470	160	1	19	10 1/2 carb, 4 fat
Mango	sm (12 oz.)	510	14	2	9	0	50	250	89	1	10	6 carb, 2 fat
Mango	med (16 oz.)	640	18	3	11	0.5	65	320	110	1	13	7 1/2 carb, 3 fat
Mango	lg (24 oz.)	890	24	2	15	0.5	85	430	155	2	18	10 1/2 carb, 4 fat

Strawberry Fruit Cream	sm (12 oz.)	530	15	3	10	0	55	290	90	2	12	6 carb, 2 fat
Strawberry Fruit Cream	med (16 oz.)	660	19	3	12	0.5	70	360	112	2	15	7 1/2 carb, 3 fat
Strawberry Fruit Cream	lg (24 oz.)	920	25	2	16	1	90	470	160	3	19	10 1/2 carb, 4 fat

SOFT SERVE: SUNDAES

Caramel	reg (10 oz.)	580	21	3	13	0.5	70	470	89	1	13	6 carb, 3 fat
Caramel	lg (16 oz.)	850	29	3	18	1	100	700	132	1	20	9 carb, 5 fat
Hot Fudge	reg (10 oz.)	620	28	4	17	0	65	400	85	1	13	5 1/2 carb, 5 fat
Hot Fudge	lg (16 oz.)	910	40	4	24	0.5	90	590	126	1	19	8 1/2 carb, 7 fat

✓ = Healthiest Bets

(Continued)

SOFT SERVE: SUNDAES *(Continued)*	Amount	Cal.	Fat (g)	% Cal. Fat	Sat. Fat (g)	Trans Fat (g)	Chol. (mg)	Sod. (mg)	Carb. (g)	Fiber (g)	Pro. (g)	Choices/Exchanges
Strawberry	reg (10 oz.)	450	18	4	11	0	65	310	59	1	12	4 carb, 3 fat
Strawberry	lg (16 oz.)	650	26	4	16	0.5	90	460	87	1	18	6 carb, 4 fat
SUNDAES: CLASSIC SUNDAES												
Banana Royale	1 srvg	630	31	4	18	0.5	85	180	87	3	8	6 carb, 5 fat
Brownie	1 srvg	890	42	4	17	1	150	370	123	1	10	8 carb, 7 fat
Classic Banana Split	1 srvg	980	31	3	18	0.5	100	260	172	8	12	11 1/2 carb, 5 fat
SUNDAES: PREMIUM SUNDAES												
Candy Rush	1 srvg	850	40	4	25	2.5	85	210	115	2	8	7 1/2 carb, 7 fat
Chocolate Oreo	1 srvg	1100	55	5	24	0.5	75	760	151	5	12	10 carb, 10 fat
Heath	1 srvg	1050	50	4	32	1	110	680	142	2	12	9 1/2 carb, 8 fat

Jamoca Oreo	1 srvg	830	32	3	17	1	85	540	130	2	10	8 1/2 carb, 5 fat
Oreo	1 srvg	1330	61	4	31	1	100	950	189	4	14	12 1/2 carb, 10 fat
Reese's Peanut Butter Cup	1 srvg	1250	81	6	32	1	100	680	108	6	27	7 carb, 15 fat
York Peppermint Pattie Brownie	1 srvg	1610	80	4	32	1	195	740	222	3	16	15 carb, 14 fat

✔ = Healthiest Bets

Exclusive Web Content

Be sure to visit the following restaurants online at http://www.diabetes.org/healthyrestaurant

Carvel
Del Taco
El Pollo Loco
Frëshens
Godfather's
Jersey Mike's
Jimmy John's
Tim Hortons
Whataburger
Wienerschnitzel
Zaxby's

Cold Stone Creamery

(www.coldstonecreamery.com)

Cold Stone Creamery

	Amount	Cal.	Fat (g)	% Cal. Fat	Sat. Fat (g)	Trans Fat (g)	Chol. (mg)	Sod. (mg)	Carb. (g)	Fiber (g)	Pro. (g)	Choices/Exchanges
ICE CREAM												
Amaretto	5 oz.	330	20	5	12	0.5	80	80	33	0	5	2 carb, 4 fat
Amaretto	8 oz.	530	31	5	20	1	125	130	53	0	8	3 1/2 carb, 6 fat
Amaretto	12 oz.	790	47	5	30	1.5	185	190	80	0	12	5 1/2 carb, 9 fat
Banana	5 oz.	310	18	5	12	0.5	70	70	33	0	5	2 carb, 3 fat
Banana	8 oz.	500	29	5	18	1	115	115	53	0	8	3 1/2 carb, 5 fat
Banana	12 oz.	750	44	5	28	1	175	170	80	0	11	5 1/2 carb, 8 fat
Black Cherry	5 oz.	330	19	5	12	0.5	75	75	36	0	5	2 1/2 carb, 3 1/2 fat
Black Cherry	8 oz.	530	30	5	19	1	120	120	58	0	8	4 carb, 5 fat
Black Cherry	12 oz.	790	44	5	28	1	175	180	86	0	11	5 1/2 carb, 8 fat

✔ = Healthiest Bets

(*Continued*)

ICE CREAM *(Continued)*	Amount	Cal.	Fat (g)	% Cal. Fat	Sat. Fat (g)	Trans Fat (g)	Chol. (mg)	Sod. (mg)	Carb. (g)	Fiber (g)	Pro. (g)	Choices/Exchanges
Blueberry Muffin	5 oz.	330	19	5	12	0.5	70	120	38	0	5	2 1/2 carb, 3 fat
Blueberry Muffin	8 oz.	530	30	5	20	1	115	190	61	0	9	4 carb, 5 fat
Blueberry Muffin	12 oz.	800	45	5	30	1	170	280	91	0	13	6 carb, 7 fat
Butter Pecan	5 oz.	320	19	5	12	0.5	75	105	32	0	5	2 carb, 3 1/2 fat
Butter Pecan	8 oz.	520	31	5	20	1	125	170	53	0	8	3 1/2 carb, 5 fat
Butter Pecan	12 oz.	780	47	5	30	1.5	185	260	79	0	12	5 1/2 carb, 8 fat
Cake Batter	5 oz.	340	19	5	12	0.5	70	180	41	0	5	2 1/2 carb, 3 fat
Cake Batter	8 oz.	550	30	5	19	1	115	280	66	0	8	4 1/2 carb, 5 fat
Cake Batter	12 oz.	830	45	5	28	1.5	170	420	99	0	12	6 1/2 carb, 8 fat
Candy Cane	5 oz.	350	20	5	12	1	75	75	40	0	5	2 1/2 carb, 3 fat
Candy Cane	8 oz.	560	32	5	19	2	115	120	64	0	7	4 1/2 carb, 6 fat
Candy Cane	12 oz.	850	47	5	28	3	175	180	95	0	11	6 1/2 carb, 8 1/2 fat

Cheesecake	5 oz.	330	18	5	11	0.5	70	75	37	0	5	2 1/2 carb, 3 1/2 fat
Cheesecake	8 oz.	520	29	5	18	1	115	120	59	0	8	4 carb, 6 fat
Cheesecake	12 oz.	790	43	5	27	1	170	180	89	0	11	6 carb, 7 1/2 fat
Chocolate	5 oz.	320	20	6	13	0.5	75	95	33	1	6	2 carb, 4 fat
Chocolate	8 oz.	520	32	6	20	1	125	160	53	2	9	3 1/2 carb, 6 fat
Chocolate	12 oz.	780	48	6	30	1	185	230	79	3	13	5 1/2 carb, 8 fat
Chocolate Cake Batter	5 oz.	340	19	5	11	0.5	70	210	42	1	5	3 carb, 3 fat
Chocolate Cake Batter	8 oz.	550	30	5	18	1	110	340	68	2	9	4 1/2 carb, 5 fat
Chocolate Cake Batter	12 oz.	820	45	5	27	1.5	160	510	101	3	13	6 1/2 carb, 8 fat
Cinnamon	5 oz.	330	20	5	12	0.5	80	80	34	0	5	2 1/2 carb, 4 fat
Cinnamon	8 oz.	530	32	5	20	1	125	125	55	1	8	3 1/2 carb, 6 fat
Cinnamon	12 oz.	790	47	5	30	1.5	185	190	82	2	12	5 1/2 carb, 8 fat
Cinnamon Bun	5 oz.	370	21	5	12	0.5	70	100	43	0	4	3 carb, 3 fat

✔ = Healthiest Bets

(*Continued*)

ICE CREAM *(Continued)*	Amount	Cal.	Fat (g)	% Cal. Fat	Sat. Fat (g)	Trans Fat (g)	Chol. (mg)	Sod. (mg)	Carb. (g)	Fiber (g)	Pro. (g)	Choices/Exchanges
Cinnamon Bun	8 oz.	600	33	5	19	1	115	160	68	0	7	4 1/2 carb, 6 fat
Cinnamon Bun	12 oz.	890	50	5	29	1.5	170	240	102	0	11	7 carb, 8 fat
Coconut	5 oz.	330	20	5	12	0.5	75	80	33	0	5	2 carb, 4 fat
Coconut	8 oz.	520	31	5	20	1	125	125	52	0	8	3 1/2 carb, 5 fat
Coconut	12 oz.	780	47	5	30	1.5	185	190	79	0	12	5 1/2 carb, 8 fat
Coffee	5 oz.	330	20	5	12	0.5	80	80	34	0	5	2 1/2 carb, 4 fat
Coffee	8 oz.	530	31	5	20	1	125	125	54	0	8	3 1/2 carb, 6 fat
Coffee	12 oz.	790	47	5	30	1.5	185	190	81	0	12	5 1/2 carb, 8 fat
Cookie Batter	5 oz.	380	20	5	11	0	65	240	44	0	5	3 carb, 4 fat
Cookie Batter	8 oz.	600	32	5	17	1	105	380	71	0	7	4 1/2 carb, 6 fat
Cookie Batter	12 oz.	900	49	5	26	1	155	570	107	0	11	7 carb, 8 fat
Cotton Candy	5 oz.	330	19	5	12	0.5	75	75	34	0	5	2 1/2 carb, 4 fat

Cotton Candy	8 oz.	530	31	5	20	1	125	120	55	0	8	3 1/2 carb, 6 fat
Cotton Candy	12 oz.	790	47	5	29	1.5	185	180	82	0	12	5 1/2 carb, 8 1/2 fat
Dark Chocolate	5 oz.	340	20	5	12	0.5	75	95	32	3	7	2 carb, 4 fat
Dark Chocolate	8 oz.	540	32	5	20	1	115	150	51	5	11	3 1/2 carb, 6 fat
Dark Chocolate	12 oz.	800	47	5	30	1	175	230	77	7	16	5 carb, 9 fat
Dark Chocolate Peppermint	5 oz.	340	20	5	12	0.5	75	95	32	3	7	2 carb, 4 fat
Dark Chocolate Peppermint	8 oz.	540	32	5	20	1	115	150	54	5	11	3 1/2 carb, 6 fat
Dark Chocolate Peppermint	12 oz.	810	47	5	29	1	175	230	80	7	16	5 1/2 carb, 9 fat
French Toast	5 oz.	330	19	5	12	0.5	75	150	35	0	5	2 1/2 carb, 4 fat
French Toast	8 oz.	530	31	5	19	1	120	250	56	0	8	3 1/2 carb, 6 fat
French Toast	12 oz.	790	46	5	29	1.5	180	370	84	0	12	5 1/2 carb, 8 fat
French Vanilla	5 oz.	340	19	5	14	0.5	100	80	37	0	5	2 1/2 carb, 4 fat
French Vanilla	8 oz.	540	30	5	22	1	60	125	60	0	8	4 carb, 5 fat

✔ = Healthiest Bets

(Continued)

ICE CREAM *(Continued)*	Amount	Cal.	Fat (g)	% Cal. Fat	Sat. Fat (g)	Trans Fat (g)	Chol. (mg)	Sod. (mg)	Carb. (g)	Fiber (g)	Pro. (g)	Choices/Exchanges
French Vanilla	12 oz.	810	46	5	33	1.5	240	190	89	0	12	6 carb, 8 fat
Ghirardelli Chocolate	5 oz.	330	20	5	12	0.5	75	75	37	4	7	2 1/2 carb, 4 fat
Ghirardelli Chocolate	8 oz.	520	31	5	20	1	115	125	59	6	11	4 carb, 5 fat
Ghirardelli Chocolate	12 oz.	780	47	5	30	1	175	180	88	8	16	6 carb, 8 fat
Irish Cream	5 oz.	330	20	5	13	0.5	80	80	33	0	5	2 carb, 4 fat
Irish Cream	8 oz.	530	32	5	20	1	125	125	54	0	8	3 1/2 carb, 6 fat
Irish Cream	12 oz.	790	47	5	30	1.5	190	190	80	0	12	5 1/2 carb, 9 fat
Macadamia Nut	5 oz.	330	20	5	12	0.5	80	75	34	0	5	2 1/2 carb, 4 fat
Macadamia Nut	8 oz.	530	31	5	20	1	125	125	54	0	8	3 1/2 carb, 6 fat
Macadamia Nut	12 oz.	790	47	5	30	1.5	185	190	81	0	12	5 1/2 carb, 9 fat
Mango	5 oz.	310	18	5	12	0.5	70	70	33	0	5	2 carb, 3 fat
Mango	8 oz.	490	29	5	18	1	115	115	53	0	7	3 1/2 carb, 5 fat

Mango	12 oz.	740	44	5	28	1	175	170	80	0	11	5 1/2 carb, 8 fat
Mint	5 oz.	330	19	5	12	0.5	75	75	36	0	5	2 1/2 carb, 4 fat
Mint	8 oz.	530	30	5	19	1	120	120	57	0	8	4 carb, 5 fat
Mint	12 oz.	790	45	5	29	1.5	180	180	86	0	12	5 1/2 carb, 8 fat
Mocha	5 oz.	320	20	6	12	0.5	75	95	33	1	6	2 carb, 4 fat
Mocha	8 oz.	520	31	5	20	1	120	150	53	2	9	3 1/2 carb, 5 fat
Mocha	12 oz.	780	47	5	30	1.5	180	230	80	3	14	5 1/2 carb, 8 fat
Oatmeal Cookie Batter	5 oz.	340	19	5	12	0.5	75	110	36	0	5	2 1/2 carb, 4 fat
Oatmeal Cookie Batter	8 oz.	540	31	5	19	1	120	170	58	0	9	4 carb, 5 1/2 fat
Oatmeal Cookie Batter	12 oz.	810	46	5	29	1.5	180	260	87	0	13	6 carb, 8 fat
Orange Dreamsicle	5 oz.	320	19	5	12	0.5	75	75	35	0	5	2 1/2 carb, 4 fat
Orange Dreamsicle	8 oz.	510	30	5	19	1	120	120	55	0	8	3 1/2 carb, 5 fat
Orange Dreamsicle	12 oz.	760	45	5	28	1.5	180	180	83	0	11	5 1/2 carb, 8 fat

✔ = Healthiest Bets

(*Continued*)

ICE CREAM *(Continued)*	Amount	Cal.	Fat (g)	% Cal. Fat	Sat. Fat (g)	Trans Fat (g)	Chol. (mg)	Sod. (mg)	Carb. (g)	Fiber (g)	Pro. (g)	Choices/Exchanges
Peach	5 oz.	310	17	5	11	0	65	70	36	0	4	2 1/2 carb, 3 fat
Peach	8 oz.	500	27	5	17	1	105	110	58	0	7	4 carb, 5 fat
Peach	12 oz.	740	41	5	26	1	160	160	86	0	11	5 1/2 carb, 7 fat
Peanut Butter	5 oz.	370	24	6	13	0.5	75	130	33	0	7	2 carb, 5 fat
Peanut Butter	8 oz.	590	39	6	20	1	115	210	53	1	12	3 1/2 carb, 8 fat
Peanut Butter	12 oz.	890	58	6	30	1	175	310	79	2	18	5 1/2 carb, 11 fat
Pecan Praline	5 oz.	330	19	5	12	0.5	75	90	37	0	5	2 1/2 carb, 4 fat
Pecan Praline	8 oz.	530	30	5	19	1	115	150	58	0	8	4 carb, 5 fat
Pecan Praline	12 oz.	800	45	5	28	1	175	220	88	0	11	6 carb, 8 fat
Pistachio	5 oz.	330	20	5	12	0.5	80	85	34	0	5	2 1/2 carb, 4 fat
Pistachio	8 oz.	520	31	5	20	1	125	135	54	0	8	3 1/2 carb, 5 1/2 fat
Pistachio	12 oz.	780	47	5	30	1.5	185	200	80	0	12	5 1/2 carb, 8 fat

Pumpkin	5 oz.	290	15	5	10	0	60	105	33	1	4	2 carb, 3 fat
Pumpkin	8 oz.	460	24	5	15	0.5	95	170	53	2	7	3 1/2 carb, 5 fat
Pumpkin	12 oz.	680	37	5	23	1	145	260	80	3	10	5 1/2 carb, 6 1/2 fat
Raspberry	5 oz.	330	19	5	12	0.5	75	75	36	0	5	2 1/2 carb, 4 fat
Raspberry	8 oz.	520	30	5	19	1	120	125	57	0	8	4 carb, 5 fat
Raspberry	12 oz.	780	44	5	28	1	175	180	85	0	12	5 1/2 carb, 7 1/2 fat
Sinless Sans Fat Sweet Cream	5 oz.	140	0	0	0	0	<5	110	34	0	6	2 carb
Sinless Sans Fat Sweet Cream	8 oz.	220	0	0	0	0	5	180	55	1	10	3 1/2 carb
Sinless Sans Fat Sweet Cream	12 oz.	330	0	0	0	0	10	270	83	2	15	5 1/2 carb
Strawberry	5 oz.	320	18	5	12	0.5	75	75	35	0	5	2 1/2 carb, 3 1/2 fat
Strawberry	8 oz.	510	30	5	19	1	115	120	55	0	8	3 1/2 carb, 5 fat
Strawberry	12 oz.	770	44	5	28	1	175	180	83	0	11	5 1/2 carb, 8 fat

✓ = Healthiest Bets

(Continued)

ICE CREAM *(Continued)*	Amount	Cal.	Fat (g)	% Cal. Fat	Sat. Fat (g)	Trans Fat (g)	Chol. (mg)	Sod. (mg)	Carb. (g)	Fiber (g)	Pro. (g)	Choices/Exchanges
Sweet Cream	5 oz.	330	20	5	13	0.5	80	80	33	0	5	2 carb, 4 fat
Sweet Cream	8 oz.	530	32	5	20	1	125	125	53	0	8	3 1/2 carb, 6 fat
Sweet Cream	12 oz.	790	48	5	30	1.5	190	190	80	0	12	5 1/2 carb, 9 fat
Vanilla Bean	5 oz.	330	19	5	12	0.5	75	75	32	0	5	2 carb, 4 fat
Vanilla Bean	8 oz.	530	31	5	19	1	120	120	52	0	8	3 1/2 carb, 6 fat
Vanilla Bean	12 oz.	790	46	5	29	1.5	180	180	77	0	12	5 carb, 9 fat
White Chocolate	5 oz.	320	19	5	12	0.5	75	75	33	0	5	2 carb, 4 fat
White Chocolate	8 oz.	520	31	5	20	1	125	125	53	0	8	3 1/2 carb, 6 fat
White Chocolate	12 oz.	780	47	5	29	1.5	185	180	79	0	12	5 1/2 carb, 9 fat
SORBET & YOGURT												
Green Apple Gummy Bear	5 oz.	160	0	0	0	0	0	15	41	0	0	2 1/2 carb
Green Apple Gummy Bear	8 oz.	250	0	0	0	0	0	25	65	1	0	4 1/2 carb

Green Apple Gummy Bear	12 oz.	380	0	0	0	0	0	35	97	2	0	6 1/2 carb
Lemon Sorbet	5 oz.	150	0	0	0	0	0	15	40	0	0	2 1/2 carb
Lemon Sorbet	8 oz.	250	0	0	0	0	0	25	64	0	0	4 carb
Lemon Sorbet	12 oz.	370	0	0	0	0	0	35	96	0	0	6 1/2 carb
✔Nrgize Yogurt	5 oz.	140	0	0	0	0	0	70	33	0	3	2 carb
Nrgize Yogurt	8 oz.	230	0	0	0	0	0	115	53	0	5	3 1/2 carb
Nrgize Yogurt	12 oz.	340	0	0	0	0	0	170	79	0	8	5 carb
Raspberry Sorbet	5 oz.	160	0	0	0	0	0	15	42	0	0	3 carb
Raspberry Sorbet	8 oz.	260	0	0	0	0	0	30	67	0	0	4 1/2 carb
Raspberry Sorbet	12 oz.	390	0	0	0	0	0	40	101	0	0	6 1/2 carb
Watermelon Sorbet	5 oz.	160	0	0	0	0	0	15	41	0	0	3 carb
Watermelon Sorbet	8 oz.	260	0	0	0	0	0	25	66	0	0	4 1/2 carb
Watermelon Sorbet	12 oz.	380	0	0	0	0	0	40	99	0	0	6 1/2 carb

✔ = Healthiest Bets

TCBY
(www.tcby.com)

TCBY

	Amount	Cal.	Fat (g)	% Cal. Fat	Sat. Fat (g)	Trans Fat (g)	Chol. (mg)	Sod. (mg)	Carb. (g)	Fiber (g)	Pro. (g)	Choices/Exchanges
SOFT SERVE FROZEN YOGURT												
✔Cake Batter	1/2 cup	110	2	2	1.5	0	5	90	23	3	4	1 1/2 carb, 1/2 fat
✔Chocolate	1/2 cup	110	2	2	1	0	5	95	23	3	4	1 1/2 carb, 1/2 fat
✔Fat Free Dutch Chocolate	1/2 cup	110	0	0	0	0	0	100	24	3	4	1 1/2 carb
✔Golden Vanilla	1/2 cup	120	2	2	1	0	5	85	23	3	4	1 1/2 carb, 1/2 fat
✔Mango Sorbet	1/2 cup	110	0	0	0	0	0	15	26	0	0	1 1/2 carb
✔NSA Fat Free Mountain Blackberry	1/2 cup	90	0	0	0	0	0	90	24	4	4	1 1/2 carb
✔NSA Fat Free Peach	1/2 cup	90	0	0	0	0	0	90	24	4	4	1 1/2 carb
✔NSA Fat Free Vanilla	1/2 cup	90	0	0	0	0	0	85	24	4	4	1 1/2 carb

✔ = Healthiest Bets; NSA = no sugar added

(*Continued*)

SOFT SERVE FROZEN YOGURT *(Continued)*	Amount	Cal.	Fat (g)	% Cal. Fat	Sat. Fat (g)	Trans Fat (g)	Chol. (mg)	Sod. (mg)	Carb. (g)	Fiber (g)	Pro. (g)	Choices/Exchanges
✔NSA White Chocolate Macadamia	1/2 cup	90	0	0	0	0	5	85	24	4	4	1 1/2 carb
✔Old Fashioned Vanilla	1/2 cup	110	0	0	0	0	0	90	24	3	4	1 1/2 carb
✔Orange Sorbet	1/2 cup	100	0	0	0	0	0	30	24	0	0	1 1/2 carb
✔Raspberry Sorbet	1/2 cup	100	0	0	0	0	0	10	25	0	0	1 1/2 carb
✔Strawberry	1/2 cup	110	2	2	1.5	0	5	90	23	3	4	1 1/2 carb, 1/2 fat
✔Strawberry Kiwi Sorbet	1/2 cup	100	0	0	0	0	0	20	24	0	0	1 1/2 carb
✔White Chocolate Mousse	1/2 cup	110	2	1	1.5	0	5	85	23	3	4	1 1/2 carb, 1/2 fat

✔ = Healthiest Bets; NSA = no sugar added